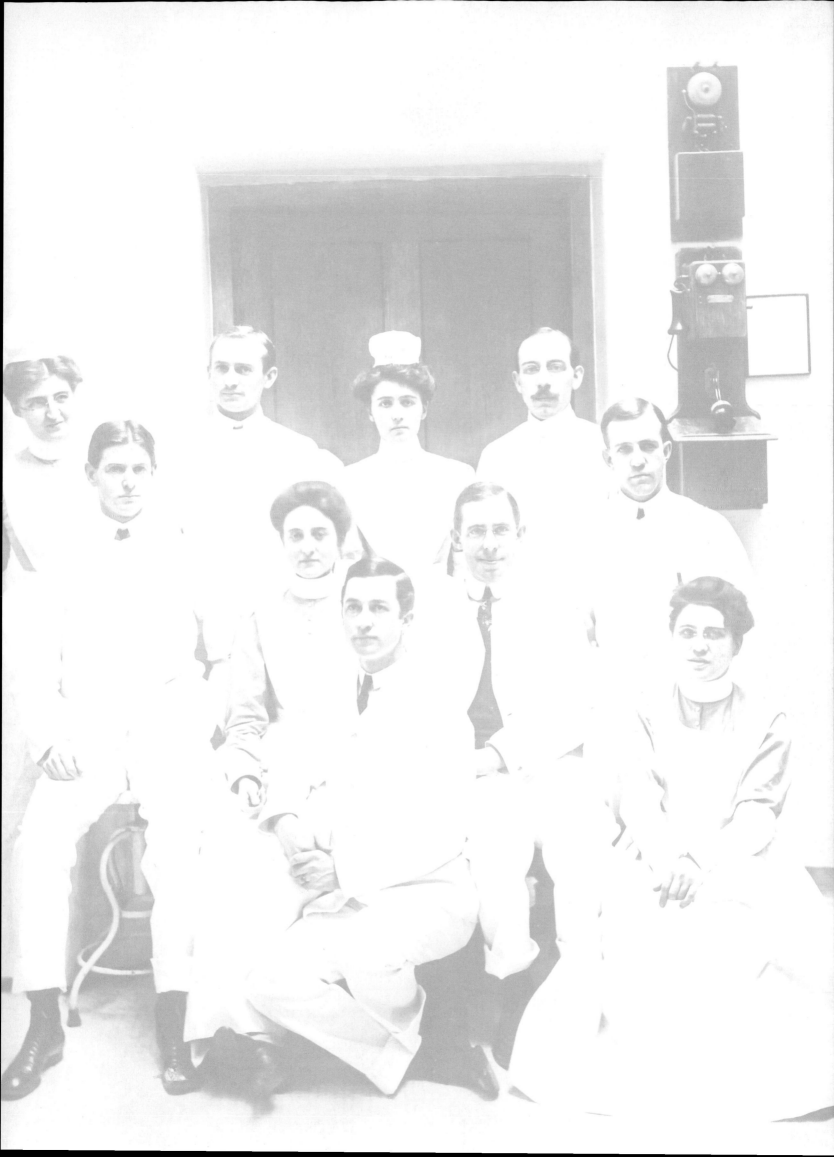

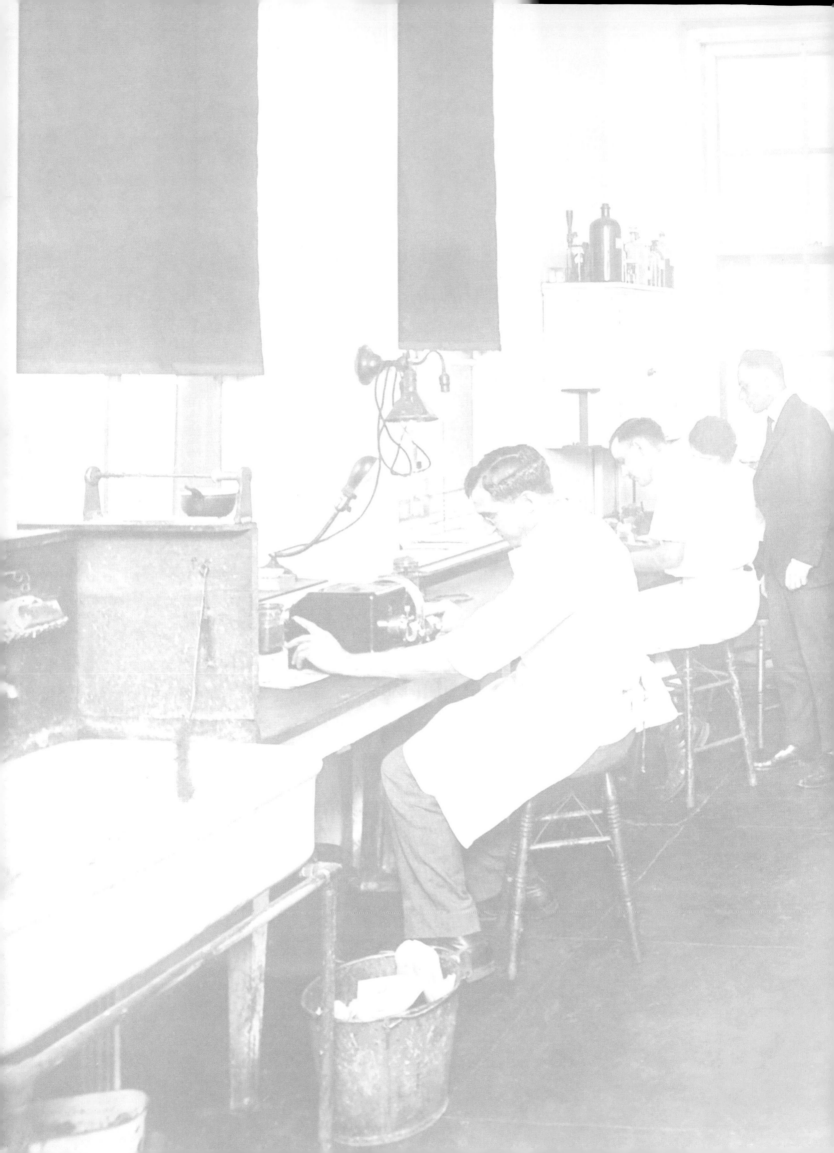

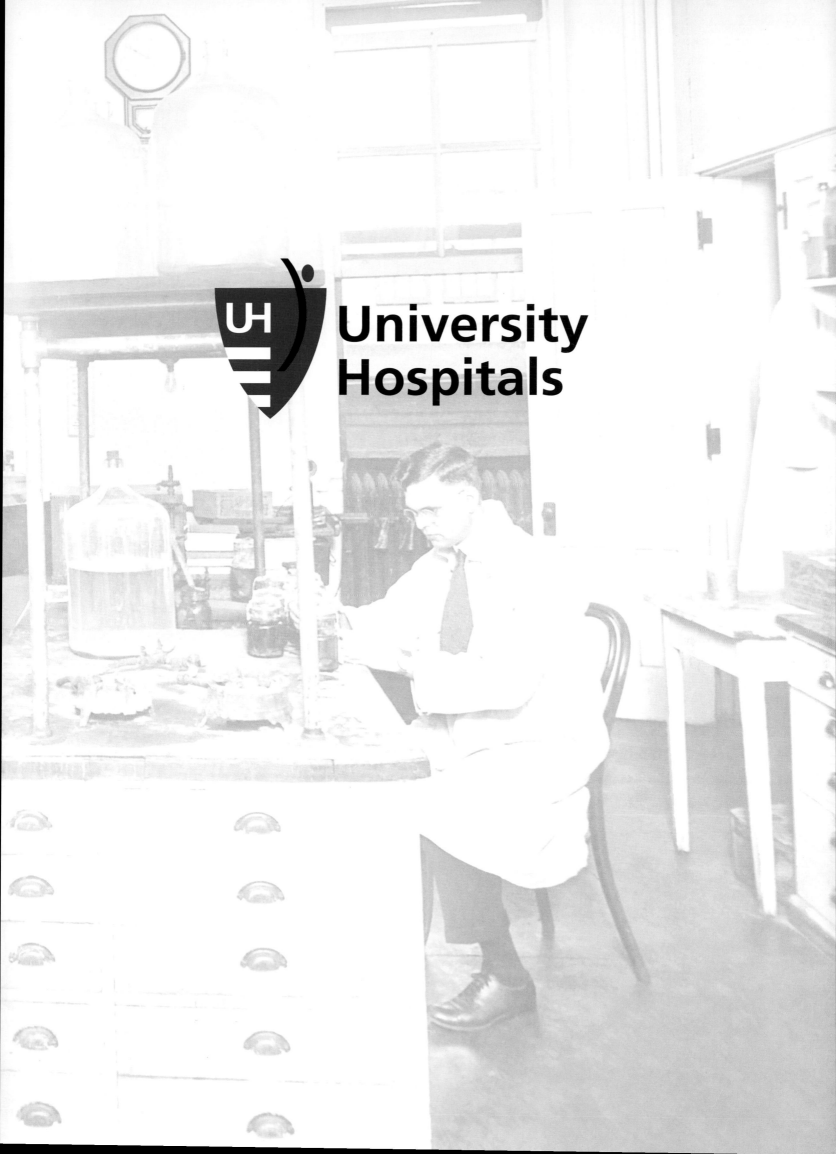

University
Hospitals

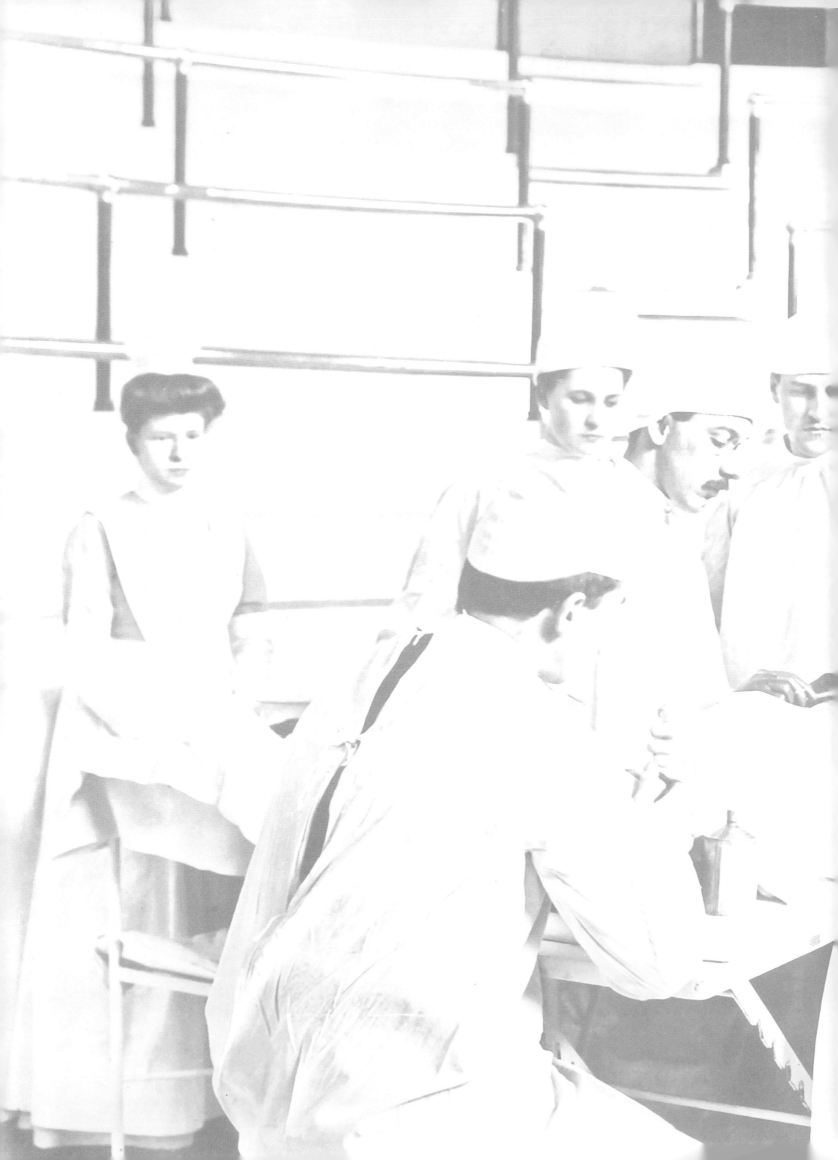

150 YEARS

Advancing the Science of Health and the Art of Compassion

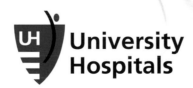
University Hospitals

Laura Taxel

ORANGE *frazer* PRESS
Wilmington, Ohio

ISBN 978-1939710-802
Copyright©2019 University Hospitals

No part of this publication may be reproduced in any material
form (including photocopying or storing in any medium by
electronic means and whether or not transiently or incidentally
to some other use of this publication) without the written
permission of the copyright holder except in accordance with
the provisions of the Copyright, Designs and Patents Act 1988.

Published for University Hospitals:
Orange Frazer Press
P.O. Box 214
Wilmington, OH 45177
Telephone: 937.382.3196 for price and shipping information.
Website: www.orangefrazer.com

Book design: Alyson Rua and Orange Frazer Press
Cover design: Justin Brabander

Page 16: *Nationally ranked University Hospitals Rainbow
Babies & Children's Hospital's main entrance is made more
welcoming through the colorful statue, "Where Dreams
Come True," designed by Hector Vega and generously
donated by Iris and the late Mort November in celebration of
the life of Debra Ann November.*

All content contained in University Hospitals' *150 Years:
Advancing the Science of Health and the Art of Compassion*
is accurate as of July 1, 2018.

Library of Congress Control Number: 2018964859

Printed in China

First Printing

Acknowledgments

The story of how University Hospitals came into existence, endured, and grew is a long and complicated narrative that encompasses more than 150 years. There are many key players, critical turning points, and significant accomplishments. A comprehensive account would require multiple volumes. We have a different aim. Our goal is to celebrate this medical institution and the consistency of its commitment to serve the people of this community as well as show the impact it has had on the city, the region, the nation, and the world. So rather than organize the book chronologically, I chose a thematic structure that spotlights the big ideas that have defined and driven this organization. Each chapter concentrates on a core principle or subject that represents the bedrock of the UH mission and its relationships with patients and their families, the health care providers in its employ, and all who come to study here.

Delving deep into a history that begins in 1866, getting a grasp on all that is going on today, and articulating the vision for the future and the work being done to make that future vision a reality, required a team effort. This was an undertaking with many moving parts, and there would be no book without project manager Lisa Linden. Her expertise, dedication, and guidance kept us on track and moving forward. As an editor, she helped me be a better writer, and her creative sensibilities influenced every page.

Christopher Dawson, a trained historian and senior researcher with the UH Department of Institutional Relations & Development, gave generously of his time and extensive knowledge of Cleveland's development, the hospital, and the families that built them both. At the beginning of the process, he was an invaluable mentor, pointing me in all the right directions. As the work progressed, he made important contributions of fact and detail. His close reading of the manuscript at every stage and insightful commentary made this book more accurate and more interesting.

The development of the book involved several years of research and interviews, during which time a number of personnel changes, retirements, and untimely passings affected the project. We worked with two outstanding archivists at the Stanley A. Ferguson Archives of University Hospitals.

Dianne O'Malia introduced us to the wealth of materials in her charge and helped us understand what was important. Margaret Burzynski-Bays took us over the finish line after her predecessor's retirement, fact-checking material, and serving as a member of our editorial review board. Stephanie Liscio, PhD, was of great assistance in finding, organizing, dating, and scanning photographs and relevant documents. She also did additional research, finding answers to the many questions that arose, and conducted numerous interviews. Additionally, a special thanks to a number of senior leaders at UH, who took the time out of their busy schedules to review various chapters and drafts and provide guidance on a number of issues.

I took advantage of the collection at Cleveland's Dittrick Medical History Center, and chief curator James Edmonson educated me about a number of relevant topics. I also drew on the assets of the Western Reserve Historical Society; the Archives of Case Western Reserve University; The Cleveland Memory Project, a searchable collection of digitized photographs, documents, and other materials focused on local and regional history created by the Michael Schwartz Library at the Cleveland State University; and The Photograph Collection and *Plain Dealer* historical digital database, both at the Cleveland Public Library.

But my deepest and profound thanks goes to all the people who talked with me, taking time to tell me about their work, their illnesses, their memories, and their experiences.

It is through hundreds of these personal stories that I truly came to understand what University Hospitals is, what it does, and what it means.

—Laura Taxel, *author*

Contents

Foreword by John J. Grabowski, PhD pg. xi

Introduction by Thomas F. Zenty III pg. xv

1 Coming Together pg. 3

2 Beds and Buildings pg. 21

3 Purpose and Promise pg. 47

4 Breakthroughs pg. 73

5 Caring pg. 107

6 Giving pg. 129

7 Reach pg. 159

8 The Work Continues pg. 177

Endnotes pg. 193

Photograph Credits pg. 197

Index pg. 199

Foreword by John J. Grabowski, PhD

Today, there are but a handful of organizations in Northeast Ohio that can claim a century and a half of continuous existence devoted to a single mission. As we commemorate the 150th anniversary of University Hospitals, we should praise the foresight of those who created this organization and the generations who have nurtured it up to the present. This achievement is remarkable and certainly against the odds.

Yet, as we celebrate a milestone such as this and look back at the 150 years that separate then from now, we need to be careful not to see the past as divorced from the present. Within the health care industry, complexity, rapidity of change, and indeed, degrees of uncertainty seem to be the challenges of our 21st century world and we might assume that earlier times were less difficult for the hospital's founders. Perhaps, the past, as some wish to believe, was a simpler place and one, from our position in the present, that we also feel we can come to fully understand.

Neither assumption is correct. Those who founded what has become University Hospitals did so in a world of swirling change not unlike that which we are experiencing today. And, it is hard to truly know their world. We do know, however, that success was not foreordained, begging the question of why the organization not only survived but also grew in both size and stature.

The key to the longevity of University Hospitals is its ability to adapt to changing times and unexpected challenges without losing sight of its core mission in the process. Throughout all of the changes UH has experienced over the years—in location, size, operating models, staffing, shifting patterns of disease and illness—one aspect has remained a constant: its focus on the patient and a concern for the broader needs and welfare of its community.

This focus was the concern of a small group of women from Cleveland's First Presbyterian Church who created a "Home for the Friendless" to assist refugees during the Civil War. They were acting on their faith and, particularly, on the concept of stewardship, asking each citizen to take responsibility for his or her community. As documented in this historical account, the efforts of these women were the seeds of what would become the Cleveland Hospital Society in 1866, the progenitor of University Hospitals.

The earliest years of the hospital were set in an era of sadness and persistent national division. Those who founded the Cleveland City Hospital Association had to contend with a city and a nation economically and socially transformed by the Civil War. Cleveland's population had increased by 50 percent between 1860 and 1866 and its demographic composition was becoming increasingly diverse—over a third of the population was of foreign birth. What had been somewhat a model of a New England mercantile town in the mid-1830s was now an industrial center. Indeed, by the 1870s, refining petroleum was the primary economic driver and, by the following decade, the manufacturing and fabrication of iron and steel would move into primary position. This was the beginning of the post-war "Gilded Age"—a period of enormous economic change, class conflict, and uncertainty. It was a time when typhoid and cholera persisted and tuberculosis outbreaks challenged heavily populated cities such as Cleveland. It was also a time when injuries from industrial accidents would increase the burdens on the fledgling health care organization that began in a small residence on Wilson Street (today's Davenport Street). These competing stressors made for a fragile beginning.

As ably detailed by Laura Taxel in this book, the hospital was able to adapt to these circumstances by moving into ever-larger structures and rapidly recognizing and adopting a wealth of new procedures, inventions, and advancements in medical science that came about at a remarkable pace in the late nineteenth and early twentieth centuries. Within 54 years of its founding, the hospital was firmly established. The city it served had become the fifth largest in the nation and far more complex in terms of demography and economics than it was even only three decades earlier. Known for its turn-of-the century Progressive approach to government and social problems, the city of Cleveland found able partners in Lakeside, Babies and Childrens, and

Maternity hospitals as well as Rainbow Cottage. To say that all who served the institution were absent the prejudices of their times would be incorrect, but a look at the record at this time and beyond shows a clear engagement with and compassion for an ever-changing community. For example, Babies' Dispensary and Hospital reached out to mothers and infants from an increasing number of foreign-born residents and African-Americans who came to the community in search of jobs and equality in the early years of the 20th century, working with settlement houses and similar agencies to curb infant mortality.

Although many people paid for their care and helped keep the hospital functioning, this revenue source has never been enough to cover all of the operating expenses. The endurance of the organization and its ability to grow relied on charitable support from the families of its founders and increasingly from newer wealth in Cleveland. For example, Samuel Mather, a man with unquestionable New England roots and a long connection to the city and the hospital, supported the organization until his death and also promoted its move to University Circle. It was fortunate, and still is, that the community saw and continues to see growth as positive and necessary, particularly because this kind of philanthropic support advances the core mission of the hospital.

The hospital's move to University Circle did not come at the most propitious time. The Depression and World War II occurred in quick succession after the hospital's relocation and the decades following the war had complexities of their own. Accelerating changes in medicine, rising costs for care, the near collapse of the city's industrial economy and the diminution of its population, as well as an increasingly diverse population in Northeast Ohio, posed challenges to both the community and its health care system. Yet, after the war, University Hospitals began a period of growth and expansion that continues to today.

Many remember this period of expansion and indeed, it is the one that has reshaped the contemporary organization. University Hospitals has responded to suburbanization by creating and absorbing branch medical centers; responded to urban decline and poverty by maintaining a progressive outreach to the community; and rapidly responded to technological change through investments not only in equipment but also in hiring expert physicians, many of whom have backgrounds that reflect the globalization of modern medicine. It is this global perspective that is the best symbol of the organization's ability to adapt to a diverse and changing world.

Today, University Hospitals is considered a key economic driver of what some characterize as a post-industrial city. This recognition, perhaps, would astound the founders, considering UH originated as a humanitarian endeavor rather than as a growth agent in the then industrializing community. Certainly, it is valid to position this 150-year-old organization in the cultural future of the community and to see it as a critical asset in the revitalization of Greater Cleveland. However, to view UH and predicate its future only in that guise obscures its core. That core is embodied in the word "hospital," which has as its root the Latin word "hospes"—a stranger or guest. So, while it remains a place once known as the "Home for the Friendless"—or, more appropriately, a place for those facing a personal or family health crisis—it is also an organization that has evolved to more clearly define its mission: To Heal. To Teach. To Discover. This proof of continuity, coupled with an ability to adapt to change, would please not only the founders but also all of those who have worked at and contributed to University Hospitals for the past 150 years.

John J. Grabowski, PhD
Historian
Case Western Reserve University and
Western Reserve Historical Society

Introduction by Thomas F. Zenty III

Dear Friend,

A great civic institution is a living expression of its community. It embodies a spirit of common purpose and generosity and a shared heritage and commitment among neighbors that spans past, present, and future. A great civic institution also evolves in step with its community's needs.

This book celebrates the community relationship behind University Hospitals. Many of Cleveland's pillars of business, religion, and medicine came together on May 14, 1866, and resolved to build a great charity hospital for their booming city. This hospital, they declared, would be focused on an important founding principle of "the most needy being considered the most worthy." Our founders knew they were doing something special. Could they have imagined, though, that 150 years later, we would still be celebrating their foresight? Could they have predicted that their grandchildren, great-grandchildren, and generations to follow would continue to benefit from their creation and keep nurturing it to become ever larger, stronger, and more responsive to the needs of our community?

The hospital they established in an old house has grown into a biomedical powerhouse.

UH today provides over 1 million patients each year with the highest-quality care, the most personalized experiences, and the most meaningful innovations. We've delivered babies, nurtured our community, saved countless lives, and tended to the most fragile. Physicians and clinicians from all over the globe come to make a difference in our patients' lives. By providing excellent bedside care, innovating new treatment protocols, or mentoring and training others, these medical practitioners espouse a passion to touch and save lives near and far. Our innovators have transformed standards of care all over the world.

Although many of our patients, alumni, and supporters are scattered across continents, our system is focused around a vision of helping every patient live life to the fullest with optimal health while bringing world-class care as close to home as possible. That's why UH is pioneering new ways to address the health of our entire community. Our population health initiatives align thousands of care providers and support services to catalyze distinct and measurable health improvements. We're joining with other community leaders to address root causes of health disparities. We're forming new partnerships and using our civic and economic influence to create jobs and stimulate investment because prosperity and health are closely correlated.

Indeed, UH's 150th anniversary reminds us that while our past is filled with milestones, our future depends on undaunted innovation. Our momentum is growing and our future is bright, impressively aided by our community's generous philanthropy. Nearly 90,000 individuals and organizations are powering UH forward with funding that now approaches $150 million annually.

Inspired by this support and by a growing demand for UH's uniquely personal compassion and care excellence, we are preparing for a dynamic future. Through strategic investments, UH is improving access to our services, expanding our geographic reach, and deepening our roster of world-renowned experts. We're empowering consumers to be more engaged in their care through new technology that puts health care data, diagnostic capabilities, scheduling flexibility, and cost-saving opportunities at their fingertips.

It is my hope that as you read this book, you'll feel proud to be part of the community that supports UH and proud to be a part of the community that University Hospitals supports in return. It is through you, and for you, that we renew, at our 150-year anniversary, our mission: To Heal. To Teach. To Discover.

Thomas F. Zenty III
Chief Executive Officer

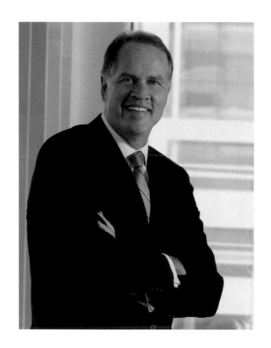

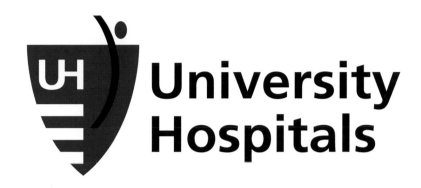

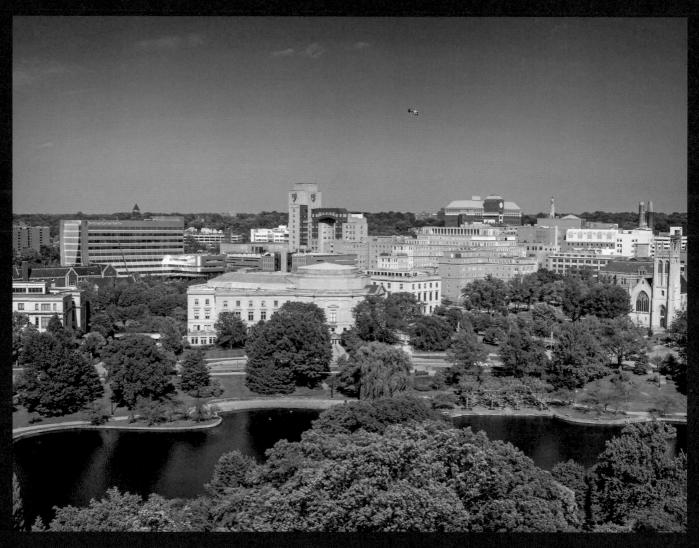

University Circle has experienced tremendous growth over the past 100 years. The continuous expansion of University Hospitals' flagship academic medical center and its proximity to Case Western Reserve University, along with the establishment of numerous cultural institutions, has earned University Circle a national reputation as a learning and cultural center in Cleveland.

Coming Together

"I believe the realization of the complete plan for the university group of hospitals will greatly advance Cleveland in the field of public health… [and] place Cleveland in a very select group of cities at the very peak of medical progress and teaching."

– William R. Hopkins, City Manager and chair of the citizens committee for the Medical Center campaign, *The Plain Dealer,* April 10, 1927

Cartez Scott graduated from high school in May 2015. What makes this rite of passage extra special is that he had a stroke before his second birthday and was not expected to live. Cartez was diagnosed with sickle cell disease at 3 months. It is a serious and painful blood disorder with no known cure that affects 100,000 people in this country and is particularly prevalent among African-Americans. Cartez has been a University Hospitals Rainbow Babies & Children's Hospital patient since he was a year-and-a-half old. "We'd been going to another hospital," says his mother, Letha Richards. "We switched when I heard about the sickle cell program for children at University Hospitals. He's had to deal with a lot of adversity, a lot of operations and crises, but his doctors and nurses have helped him through." After moving to Summit County, Letha and Cartez continued to make the 45-minute trip to UH for monthly tests, numerous medical emergencies, and various procedures. "We wouldn't consider going anywhere else. This is our hospital. We trust his caregivers, and they are a second family for him," she continues. A transition clinic supports Cartez as he makes the switch from pediatrics to the Adult Sickle Cell Disease Center. "UH means everything to me," Cartez says. "It's the reason I'm here today."

The story of UH, and the four founding institutions that came together to create it, is a long one with more than one beginning. But no matter where the story starts, it always ends with people like Cartez Scott and his mom—people who are sick or hurt and in need of expert, attentive care. Being there for patients has been UH's main purpose for 150 years.

Today, University Hospitals is an integrated health system of 18 hospitals, more than 50 health centers and outpatient facilities, and physician offices at more than 200 locations across 15 Northeast Ohio counties. The system's flagship academic medical center, University Hospitals Cleveland Medical Center, is located in University Circle. The UH organization has a large and many-branched "family tree" that grew out of a sense of civic and social responsibility. It has a formative and enduring relationship with a medical school that dates back over a century and a history of collaborations, partnerships, and affiliations that continue to evolve. Joining forces to better serve the people of this region is what drives the work forward.

The First Four

Lakeside Hospital

The Home for Friendless Strangers, organized by the Ladies' Aid Society of Cleveland's First Presbyterian Church in 1863, assisted men and women displaced and left destitute by the American Civil War. In 1866, a year after the hostilities ended, a number of board members from the Home for Friendless Strangers and other leading citizens met and incorporated as the Cleveland City Hospital Association with the goal of establishing a public facility to care for the sick and disabled. Explaining their vision, Rev. J.H. Rylance said, "The hospital should be free to all—so that no cases of suffering should go unrelieved—none to be excluded on account of poverty, nativity, color, or religion. The doors should be open to all alike—the most needy being considered the most worthy."[1] The small wood-frame house on Wilson Street, purchased by the group in 1868, was the forerunner of today's University Hospitals.

Top left: To provide aid and supplies for sick and wounded soldiers, women organized the Soldiers Aid Society, the first Cleveland division of the U.S. Sanitary Commission, in 1861 at the start of the Civil War. Many of these same women would later found the Home for Friendless Strangers in 1863. *Top right:* Civil War soldiers, ca. 1863.

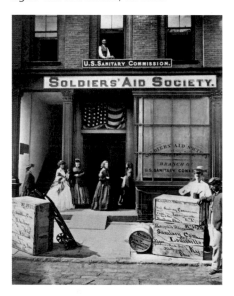

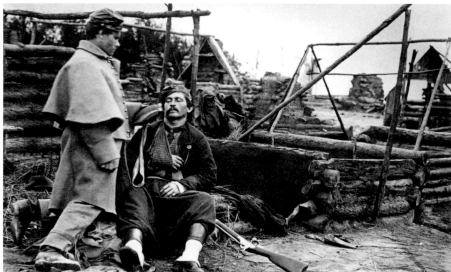

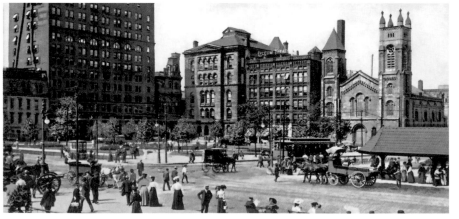

Commonly known as The Old Stone Church, the First Presbyterian Church was located on Public Square in downtown Cleveland, ca. early 1900s.

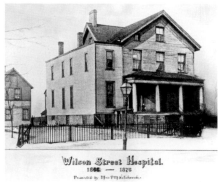

Wilson Street Hospital was located between East 16th and East 18th streets in downtown Cleveland, close to Lake Erie, on what is now Davenport Avenue.

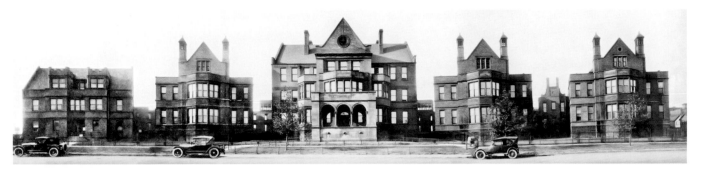

Thirty years after Wilson Street opened, a new home for the hospital was built north of what is now Lakeside Avenue, between East 12th and East 14th streets.

During its first few years, Wilson Street Hospital turned to the community for donations of cash, household goods, and food. In 1868, items requested included washstands, rocking chairs, crockery, and 10 pounds of sirloin roast along with linens, pillows, and blankets. Then, as now, the generosity of Clevelanders kept the doors open and medical services available to all. In the first three months of 1871, 59 people were treated at no charge and an additional 43 paid for services. "Each entry [in the record book] represents days, often weeks and sometimes months of homelike comfort, of skillful surgical and medical attendance, of faithful nursing and patient watching day and night. Five thousand and thirty-eight days of care…are summed up in the pages where these 102 names are entered."[2]

Cleveland was industrializing at a rapid rate—with iron and steel production leading the way—and the population was growing, thanks to an abundance of jobs and a steady influx of immigrants to fill them. Overcrowding in the hospital soon became a problem, with beds in the attic, lining the corridors, and even usurping the matron's room. Marine Hospital, owned by the federal government, was nearby and

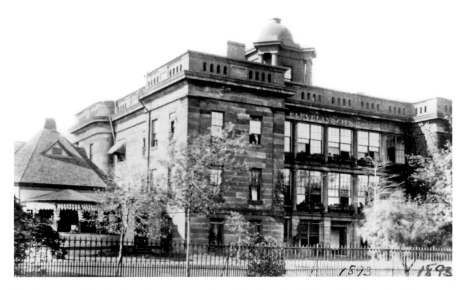

The three-story Marine Hospital was located one block west of Wilson Street on what is now Lakeside Avenue, 1893.

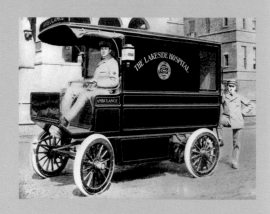

Behind the Scenes

An electric ambulance was put into service in February 1903 for emergency and maternity cases. Although the vehicle had trouble driving up steep grades, it responded to 750 calls and covered 4,000 miles its first year. Around 1910, Samuel Mather donated one of his Packard limousines so Lakeside Hospital's nursing students would not have to ride the streetcar when making house calls during their obstetrical training. The nurses nicknamed his car Maude.

underutilized. The trustees leased it for 20 years and moved the hospital there in 1875. In exchange for an annual rent of $1, they agreed to provide medical care for military men at reduced rates and pay for the extensive repairs and renovations the structure required. Among the benefactors who made this possible were members of prestigious and wealthy Cleveland families who would play a critical and continuing role in the development of both the hospital and the city for generations to come. The 1881 donor list includes names such as the Mather, Severance, Blossom, Wade, Payne, Bingham, Chisholm, and Stone families.

The building was renamed Cleveland City Hospital. In 1889, concerned that their private, philanthropic institution would be confused with the new publicly funded City Hospital, the predecessor of what is now the MetroHealth System, the trustees changed the name again to Lakeside Hospital. With the termination of the lease approaching and demand reaching capacity, the trustees began planning for a larger, more modern facility. Five acres of land next to the Marine Hospital grounds were purchased for $66,833.99 in 1890. When Lakeside's new 250-bed hospital opened on January 12, 1898, it was said that the campus was so impressive that it could easily be mistaken for a great university. The comparison was apt considering that the hospital had established a formal affiliation with the medical department of Western Reserve University. It was a transformative move in every way, setting the hospital on a path of expansion, modernization, and improvement that continues to this day.

Samuel Mather joined the board of Lakeside in its early days and served for the next 46 years, most of them as president. He amassed great wealth through Pickands Mather & Co., a firm he established in 1882 that operated coal and iron ore mines, shipped raw materials, and manufactured pig iron. However, Mather is best known for his philanthropic spirit. It is estimated that over the course of his lifetime he

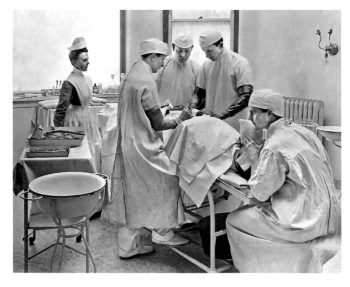

Early operating room, Lakeside Hospital, ca. 1910s.

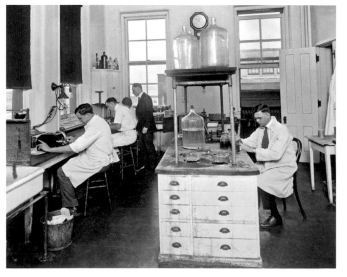

Pathology laboratory, Lakeside Hospital, ca. 1920s.

gave $8 million—the equivalent of more than $110 million today—to civic and community projects. Lakeside and Western Reserve University were major philanthropic beneficiaries. Mather was the driving force in bringing the two together and setting them on a path to become a nationally-recognized academic medical institution.

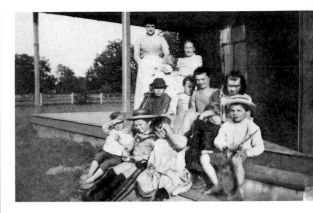

The original Rainbow Cottage building in 1891. The lakefront retreat provided an opportunity for children to convalesce outside of the crowded city during the summer months.

Rainbow Hospital

On Thanksgiving in 1887, nine teenage friends from prominent Cleveland families joined together to form a local branch of the King's Daughters, a national service organization with a mission to alleviate suffering and perform charitable works. The young women dubbed themselves the Rainbow Circle and agreed to focus their efforts on aiding the city's sick and underprivileged children.

Initially, they arranged short stays out in the country during the warm weather months for a few needy youngsters. By 1891, they rented a small lakeside home on 14 bucolic acres at the end of what is now East 105th Street, far from the city's dirty, congested, germ-infested neighborhoods. They called it Rainbow Cottage. Thirty-two children suffering from injury, malnutrition, and disease received medical attention, healthy food, and nurturing care for two weeks during the summer.

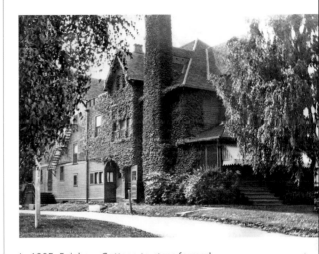

In 1905, Rainbow Cottage trustees formed an association with the Kinderheim Circle, a committee of the Cleveland Day Nursery and Free Kindergarten Association. Together the two leased and then bought Novak Villa.

To prepare Rainbow Cottage for the first occupants, the young women of the Rainbow Circle donated everything from flannel shirts and bibs to cases of oatmeal, baskets of fruit, vegetables, and cash. Drawing on their own and their families' financial resources, they solicited donations and organized events to support their charitable endeavor.

The group formally incorporated in 1896. Edith Harkness, a charter member of the board, and her husband, William, donated $25,000 in 1899 to purchase land in South Euclid and build a permanent facility. However, the new, three-story brick bungalow was destroyed by a fire five years later. Because the cost to rebuild was prohibitive, the following spring Rainbow Cottage relocated to Novak Villa, a nearby private estate that had been converted into a resort and then abandoned.

Children were soon admitted for care year-round, most ranging in age from 2 to 12 and suffering from tuberculosis, bone and joint disease, polio, rickets, pneumonia, and cardiac conditions. Lakeside Hospital physicians served as advisors and, along with doctors from other area hospitals, referred patients to Rainbow Cottage.

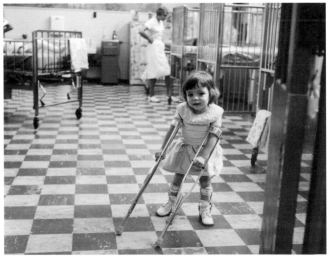

A young girl receives treatment at Rainbow Hospital, ca. 1950s. The checkered floor tiles were a distinctive feature of the 1928 building.

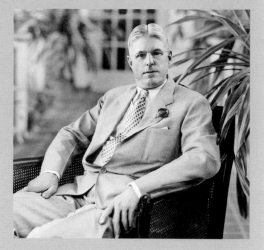

Arthur Bill, MD, ca. 1930.

Pioneer

In the early 1900s, Arthur Bill, MD, ran an independent service out of his home, delivering babies for charity patients at his own expense. His mother played a vital role, answering the telephone calls that came in day and night, sterilizing instruments, and packing the large bag he lugged from house to house all over the city. Dr. Bill brought the benefit of his internships at Lakeside Hospital, Johns Hopkins Hospital, Vassar Hospital, and New York Lying-In Hospital as well as his studies of the latest European obstetrical methods in Berlin, Vienna, and Paris to Cleveland's poorest women. He continued this work even after he became associated with Maternity Hospital in 1906. Under his leadership, the hospital operated neighborhood prenatal dispensaries and the District Delivery Service, which supervised home births until 1951.

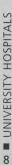

By 1908, with a more formal arrangement in place, Lakeside provided all of the medical and surgical staff. Six years later, with more and more emphasis on medical treatment and long-term support, especially for orthopedically disabled children, the organization adopted the name Rainbow Hospital for Crippled and Convalescent Children and erected a 50-bed hospital on the property. That capacity was soon increased to 75 plus a "summer unit" that could accommodate an additional 25 children.

A November 1921 newspaper story about the hospital's need for support was filled with heart-wrenching stories of children. A patient named Joe, "the tiniest baby at Rainbow Hospital," was only 15 months old with a tubercular spine and "never felt like laughing or gurgling." Joe's parents had neither the knowledge nor the means to care for him.[3] Another child was 12-year-old Carmella who was "crippled during babyhood with infantile paralysis" and rescued by Rainbow Hospital staff from a "hovel" with a floor of clay.[4] Finally, there was the hopeful story of Harry who "is going to walk" and become a "self-supporting citizen some day, as strong as anybody" thanks to multiple operations performed at the hospital."[5]

Maternity Hospital

The Maternity Home Association was an independent, nonsectarian organization established in 1891 by a group of women whose husbands were physicians affiliated with Huron Road Hospital in downtown Cleveland. Maternity Home provided a safe and sanitary setting for labor and delivery, staffed by skilled practitioners. Obstetrics was still an emerging field, and birth typically took place in the home, a practice that would continue through the first half of the 1900s. However, for medically complicated situations and for those living in poverty, home births were not advisable. "In one week," according to an 1897 news story, "12 married women, all wives of men out of employment or deserted by their husbands, were cared for" at the Maternity Home. "It makes ones' heart ache to hear of the emergency causes of women found suffering and helpless on the street or in homes where both mother and child would have perished without the timely aid."[6]

Lack of money necessitated a move from Maternity Home's original quarters on Huron Road to a smaller building on East Prospect Avenue (now Carnegie Avenue) in 1898. This was the same year the group petitioned to change its name to Maternity Hospital. Martha A. Canfield, MD, who was on the surgical staff, explained why. "The word 'home' conveys the idea of a permanent abode, and has imbued the public with the false impression that this institution is a reformatory, a refuge for fallen women. It is truly and simply a lying-in hospital."[7]

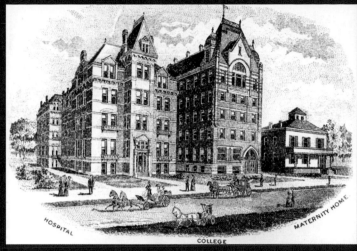

The original Maternity Hospital was located in the small house (far right) from 1891 to 1898, adjacent to Huron Road Hospital and the Cleveland Homeopathic Hospital College.

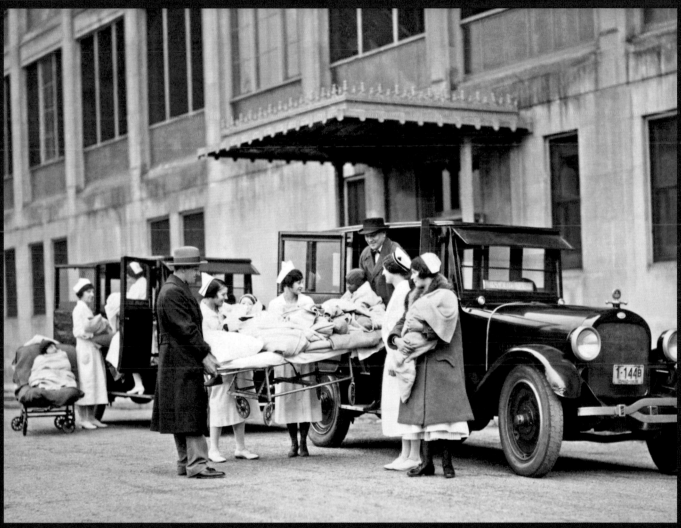

When Maternity Hospital moved into its new building in University Circle in 1925, the easiest way to transport the smallest patients was by stacking them on a stretcher.

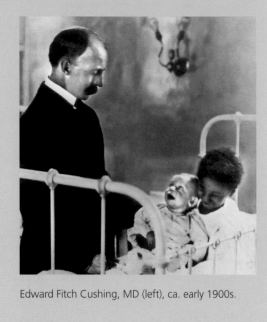
Edward Fitch Cushing, MD (left), ca. early 1900s.

Pioneers

Edward Fitch Cushing, MD, was an obstetrician and one of Cleveland's first pediatric specialists. He was in charge of the children's ward when Lakeside Hospital opened in 1898. His dream was to establish a hospital devoted exclusively to the treatment of children.

Another trailblazer, John Lowman, MD, founder of the Anti-Tuberculosis League of Cleveland, was a nationally-recognized expert on pulmonary disease. He practiced at Lakeside and was on the faculty of the Western Reserve University School of Medicine for four decades. His wife Isabel, a nurse, helped him start the Infants' Clinic, the precursor to Babies' Dispensary and Hospital, and she played an influential role in nursing education at the Lakeside Training School.

Women of means were encouraged to take advantage of Maternity's ideal conditions for child birth. The same services were free to mothers who could not pay and at reduced rates for those with limited means. Arthur Bill, MD, Cleveland's first specialist in obstetrics, was head of the medical staff. He was also chairman of the department at Western Reserve University's medical college and facilitated an important and lasting training relationship between the school and Maternity that was formalized in 1917. After several moves, the hospital relocated to a former hotel and sanitarium on Cedar Avenue, and although the new building was an improvement, it was still inadequate. By the early 1920s, Maternity was added to the plans for a new medical center complex in University Circle.

Babies and Childrens Hospital

By some estimates, as many as one out of every three American infants born to families living in poverty in the early 1900s did not survive their first year of life. Those who did survive often succumbed later to preventable childhood diseases or were left with permanent impairment and deformity. Poor hygiene, lack of medical care and information, and serious infections such as tuberculosis were deemed largely responsible. Two Lakeside Hospital physicians with a keen interest in public health and children's welfare were Edward Fitch Cushing, MD, and John Lowman, MD. Together, they urged two local organizations to cooperate in addressing these issues and provide the city's youngest and most disadvantaged inhabitants an opportunity for better lives.

The Milk Fund Association and the Visiting Nurse Association established the Infants' Clinic in the summer of 1906. The dispensary operated out of three rooms at Central Friendly Inn, a settlement house

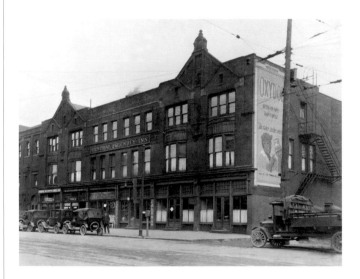
The original Babies' Dispensary and Hospital began in the Central Friendly Inn social settlement in 1906.

in downtown Cleveland's Haymarket district, one of the city's poorest and roughest neighborhoods populated by immigrants of 40 different countries. This account sets the scene: "Outside the big brick building heavy drays thundered. Crates of noisy fowls and barrels of potatoes blocked the way. Piles of cabbages wilting in the July sun scented the air….[I]nside, in a cool, clean room, two doctors were bending over the tiny, weazened [sic] face of a four-month-old baby, the latest patient of the infant clinic at Central Friendly Inn. 'Weighs two pounds less than at birth,' said the nurse, lifting the morsel of a hand gently. 'Inanition. Too weak to hold its head up, you see, but we have another baby who was just as badly off and now is gaining, so we have given the mother hope.'"[8]

The following year the staff moved into a former residence on East 35th Street. A sign was installed over the front door with the organization's new name: Babies' Dispensary and Hospital. There was a laboratory for preparing modified milk, fortified according to doctors' orders for individual cases, and for testing, sterilizing, and bottling milk that was distributed on site and at various stations around the city. It was described in 1910 as "saving children every day," "taking them in half dead of starvation, disease, or lack of care and turning them out strong and healthy, fat and laughing, fairly started on their way to growth… doing it all in an old house, a building whose floors are sagging, whose walls are weak, and which is neither big enough nor properly equipped to half the work which comes to hand."[9] Cleveland's Bureau of Child Hygiene eventually took over the logistics of milk distribution.

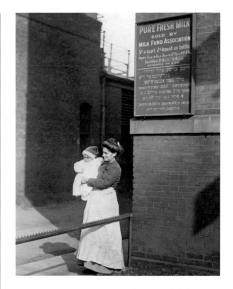

A woman and baby wait for a milk delivery, ca. early 1900s. The milk fund helped impoverished children and families, including recent immigrants.

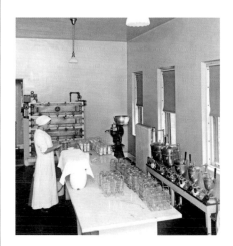

Babies' Dispensary and Hospital milk laboratory, 1911.

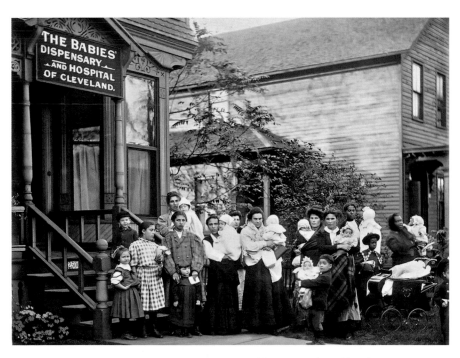

Over the past 150 years, University Hospitals has cared for the needy and less fortunate—adhering to its long-standing mission: To Heal. To Teach. To Discover. Babies' Dispensary and Hospital operated numerous clinics throughout the Cleveland area. This 1907 photo shows women waiting for medical care at one of these dispensary sites.

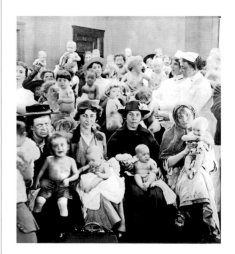

Babies' Dispensary and Hospital waiting room, ca. 1910.

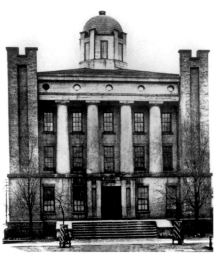

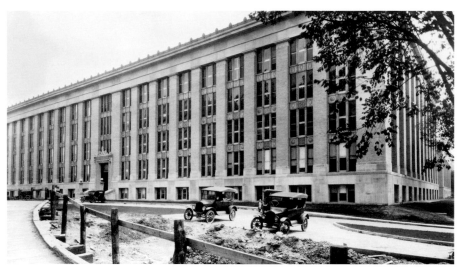

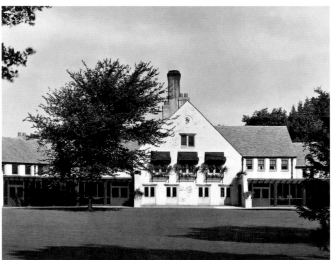

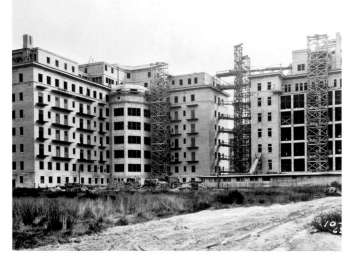

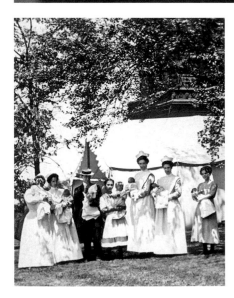

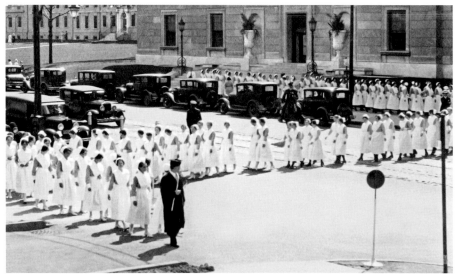

Top left: The original medical school building was located downtown from 1843 to 1885. It was replaced by a newer building in the same location. *Top right:* The new medical school on the campus of Western Reserve University was dedicated in 1924. *Middle left:* Rainbow Hospital moved into this newly built, modern facility in South Euclid in 1928. *Middle right:* Maternity and Babies and Childrens hospitals under construction on the new medical center campus in University Circle. *Bottom left:* In Babies' Dispensary and Hospital's early years, sick children requiring extended care could only be accommodated during the summer, in tents set up outside on the lawn of the Andrews estate nearby. *Bottom right:* Lakeside Hospital dedication ceremony held at Severance Hall in 1931.

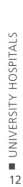

The situation improved with the construction of a larger building on the same site that was completed in 1911. Construction costs were covered by Jeptha H. Wade II and his wife in honor of his mother, Anna. Samuel Mather donated funds for outfitting the laboratory. Physicians attached to Lakeside, Rainbow Cottage, and Western Reserve University served as advisors and staff. Many would become well-known pediatricians and leaders in the fight against infant mortality. One of them was Henry Gerstenberger, MD, a Cushing protégé. He was appointed medical director of Babies' Dispensary and a faculty member in the newly established department of pediatrics at the medical school. Another was Chauncey Wyckoff, MD, the first resident pediatrician at the new Babies' Dispensary and its associate director.

The need in the community for the services provided by Babies' Dispensary prompted multiple moves and expansions, but the organization still lacked an inpatient hospital building in 1914 when it formed an alliance with Western Reserve University to provide training to medical students. Samuel Mather championed the idea of creating a medical campus that would be the new home of Western Reserve University's medical school, and it was decided to locate the children's hospital there, too. However, it would take another decade to make these plans a reality.

A Medical and Educational Center in University Circle

Mather was a longtime board member of both Western Reserve University and Lakeside Hospital, fostering cooperation between the two. He wanted to establish an academic medical center in Cleveland similar to Johns Hopkins University in Baltimore, Maryland, where the school and hospital shared a campus and the task of instructing the next generation of physicians.

At the end of 1913, the Joint Committee on Hospital and Medical School Buildings was inaugurated. The idea of moving the medical school from its location on East 9th Street to Lakeside was abandoned as the downtown site near the railroad tracks was dirty and noisy. University

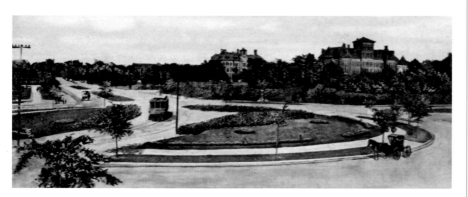

The University Circle neighborhood, late 19th century.

Family Ties

"My whole life," states Henri Pell Junod Jr., "is literally tied up with University Hospitals. My mother was on Rainbow's board. I was born at the hospital in 1944, a preemie with a heart valve defect and not expected to live, but after three months in an incubator, I went home. Chauncey Wyckoff, MD, was my pediatrician when I had a very serious case of pneumonia as a child. He saved me. As an adult I've been treated at UH for diabetes and had triple bypass surgery."

Junod's ties to the hospital go beyond the medical care he has received. His father, Henri Sr., was Executive VP and Vice Chairman of the Board of Pickands Mather & Co., Samuel Mather's iron ore mining and shipping firm, and gave money to furnish and equip a room at the new Rainbow and Babies Childrens Hospital. His uncle and godfather, Robert Livingston Ireland Jr., and his cousin, George M. Humphrey II, were on UH's board. Junod has established two endowed fellowships, one in orthopedics and the other in cardiology, and serves on the Leadership Councils for those specialties.

I Remember

Chauncey Wyckoff, MD, met Florence Wales in 1910. He was a resident in medicine at old Lakeside Hospital, and she was a nurse in training there. Recalling that time in a 1969 interview, he described what happened when matron Lettie Darling caught them together. "Matron was very strict. There was a rule that stipulated no interns, residents, and externs (house staff) were to be found walking with any of the student nurses, who, at that time, were also the hospital's nursing staff." To punish Wales, who had just gotten off night duty, Darling assigned her six more months of the late shift. Undaunted, Dr. Wyckoff and Miss Wales continued to see each other and married three years later. At their 50th anniversary, he told a reporter, "I earned $25 a month and worked seven days and nights a week....My last $75 was spent on our honeymoon to Atlantic City."

Circle, four miles east, where Western Reserve University's other academic programs had been located since 1883, was a better choice.

Years of discussions, negotiations, and planning to secure the necessary parcels of land followed. In 1922, with a site selected and drawings for the new medical school ready, Mather was informed that funds were lacking to move forward. An often-repeated story is that he replied, "Build the building and charge it to me." Even if he did not utter these exact words, the overture made national news.

The new medical school was dedicated on September 9, 1924. An article in *The Plain Dealer* that appeared the next day reported that Mather gave a brief speech but failed to mention his contribution. "[I]t remained for the president [Dr. Robert Vinson, Western Reserve University] to remind the audience that every brick in the building and every pound of steel was his [Mather's] gift." It would not be Mather's last or his largest donation to the ambitious and forward-thinking enterprise of creating an academic medical center.

Babies and Childrens Hospital and Maternity Hospital opened in University Circle in 1925. A May 26 article in *The Plain Dealer* proclaimed that in combination with the new college of medicine, this was "the greatest group of buildings devoted to the physical welfare of mankind anywhere in the country," and positioned the city as a leader in medical education. The public, which had donated generously to help make this possible, turned out in droves to tour the hospitals. Although Rainbow Hospital joined University Hospitals in 1926, it remained in South Euclid, five miles east of University Circle. A new hospital was erected on the property and was ready for patients in 1928.

Construction of the new Lakeside building in University Circle was the next step in fashioning a "modern coalition against disease."[10] Ground was broken in early October 1929, but, within a few weeks, the stock market crashed, sparking the Great Depression. Finances were uncertain, and money that had been pledged was not forthcoming. This slowed but did not stop progress on the building's construction. Lakeside, a grand limestone structure that remains at the heart of the medical center, was dedicated on June 17, 1931. Thanking Mather, Rev. James Delong Williamson said, "May your years be brightened by the knowledge that your work has assured life to thousands who will follow you and us."

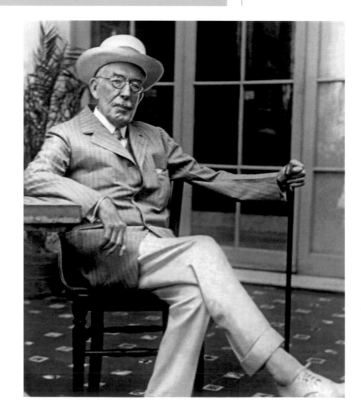

Cleveland industrialist and philanthropist Samuel L. Mather was pivotal to the hospital's survival and growth in its early years, ca. 1930.

Each of the four separate founding institutions went through various name changes in the past 150 years, and so has University Hospitals itself.

Lakeside Hospital

1866   Cleveland City Hospital Association formed

1868   Wilson Street Hospital established

1876   Cleveland City Hospital, located in the former Marine Hospital, replaces Wilson Street Hospital

1889   Lakeside Hospital
(It was informally referred to as "old Lakeside" after the construction of a new hospital building in 1931, which was unofficially known as "new Lakeside.")

Maternity Hospital

1891   Maternity Home Association

1892   Maternity Hospital

1936   MacDonald House

1984   MacDonald Hospital for Women

1990   University Hospitals MacDonald Women's Hospital

Rainbow Hospital

1891   Rainbow Cottage

1914   Rainbow Hospital for Crippled and Convalescent Children

1971   Rainbow Babies and Children's Hospital

1997   University Hospitals Rainbow Babies & Childrens Hospital

Babies and Childrens Hospital

1906   Infants' Clinic

1907   Babies' Dispensary and Hospital

1924   Babies and Childrens Hospital
(Typographical errors in the 1924 incorporation papers eliminated the apostrophe in the name. It appeared as Babies and Childrens Hospital until a rebranding in 1997.)

1971   Rainbow Babies and Childrens Hospital

1997   University Hospitals Rainbow Babies & Children's Hospital

University Hospitals Cleveland Medical Center

1925   The University Hospitals of Cleveland (Lakeside, Maternity, and Babies and Childrens hospitals came together; Rainbow Hospital joined in 1926.)

1940   University Hospitals of Cleveland (Operations were consolidated across the founding hospitals.)

2006   University Hospitals Case Medical Center (used for the main campus of UH's academic medical center in University Circle until 2017).

2017   University Hospitals Cleveland Medical Center (came into public use based on a name change formalized in 2010).

In 1987, University Hospitals Health System, Inc. was formed as UH grew beyond its main campus.

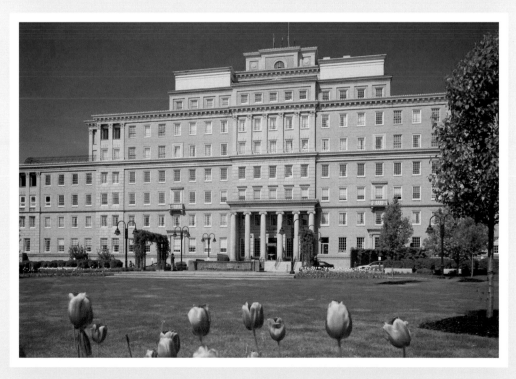

Lakeside Hospital outgrew three different locations before finding its permanent home in University Circle in 1931.

Mather died just four months later, but he had succeeded in what he set out to do. The relationships he fostered and the buildings he funded were the foundation of today's University Hospitals Cleveland Medical Center, the heart and soul of a system of facilities, caregivers, programs, services, and initiatives that reach far beyond University Circle and the city of Cleveland. It stands today as a testament not only to his foresight, vision, and zeal but also to the dedication of all those physicians, nurses, educators, and social activists of the past who were devoted to providing the finest medical care for all.

Going Off Campus

The last member of the UH founding family of institutions moved to University Circle in 1971. Rainbow Hospital consolidated its services with Babies and Childrens Hospital in 1974, formalizing the change in name to Rainbow Babies and Childrens Hospital, which occurred in 1971.

The South Euclid property on Green Road, formerly occupied by Rainbow, became University Suburban Health Center. It was a private group practice made up mostly of physicians affiliated with University Hospitals and the medical school that brought many specialties and services together under one roof. Conveniently located for families that had moved east and out of Cleveland's urban core, it represented a first step in bringing health care services to people where they lived. This idea has also been a guiding principle for UH's more recent expansion into a regional health care delivery system over the past two decades.

UH was the first multi-hospital consortium of its kind in the region. The model foreshadowed

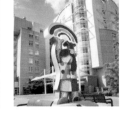

University Hospitals consists of a nationally recognized academic medical center and integrated health system.

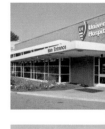
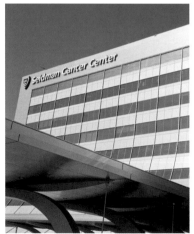
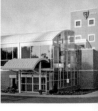
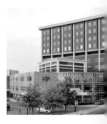
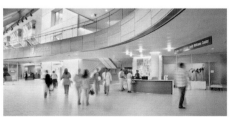
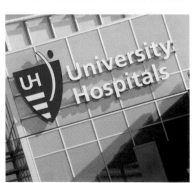
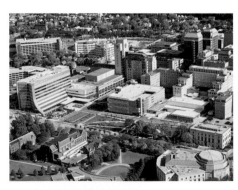
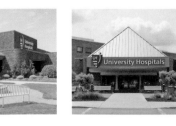
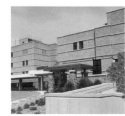
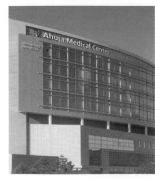
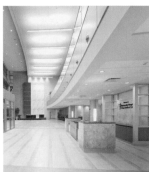
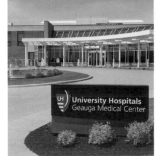
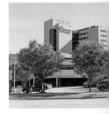
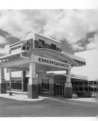

These University Hospitals medical centers each began as a community hospital with its own origin and story.

UH Bedford Medical Center—
The Community Hospital of Bedford traces its start to four beds on the second floor of a private home in 1908. When University Hospitals purchased the hospital in 1993, it had grown to 110 beds. Since then, a state-of-the-art outpatient surgery center, a branch of University Hospitals Harrington Heart & Vascular Institute, a Wound Center, and an MRI suite have been added.

UH Conneaut Medical Center—
Brown Memorial Hospital began operating in a donated mansion. A one-day "Help the Hospital" drive on November 25, 1919, raised enough money to convert it into a hospital. It affiliated with UH in 1997 and now is home to the Ohio Bone & Joint Institute, an intensive care unit, and expanded surgical suite, and is a designated critical access facility.

UH Elyria Medical Center—
After two street cars collided in 1907, killing nine and seriously injuring many more, the Elyria community resolved to build a hospital, and Elyria Memorial Hospital opened in 1908 with 36 beds. One of the early founders, E.H. Allen, who lost a child in the accident, was the founder of the Easter Seals Society. As the hospital grew and expanded its reach into the surrounding area, its name changed to EMH Healthcare, which became part of UH in 2013.

UH Geauga Medical Center—
Geauga Community Hospital opened in 1959 with 56 beds. After joining UH in 1995, the facility added a behavioral health unit, outpatient surgery center, Center for Women's Health, and the county's first UH Harrington Heart & Vascular Institute catheterization laboratory. It also offers comprehensive University Hospitals Seidman Cancer Center services.

UH Geneva Medical Center—
Before a six-bed emergency hospital was established in 1906, the town marshal cared for patients in the local jail until they could be transferred. New facilities were built in 1918, 1951, and 1990. The 25-bed community hospital joined UH in 1997.

UH Parma Medical Center—
Parma Community General Hospital opened in 1961, the result of a joint effort by six municipalities. In 2012, it was ranked among the top hospitals in the state and the best hospital in Ohio for coronary interventions. Parma has been nationally recognized for its orthopedic and cardiovascular programs and ICU. Parma integrated with UH in 2013.

UH Portage Medical Center—
Robinson Memorial Hospital in Ravenna began in 1894 under the auspices of a single surgeon who saw a need for a facility to treat accident victims. Called White Hospital, it was purchased by the county in 1917 and renamed in 1932 to acknowledge a major donation from the Robinson brothers in honor of their parents. After years of expansion and acquisition, it became Robinson Health System and joined UH in June 2015.

UH Richmond Medical Center—
Richmond Heights General Hospital was started by an osteopathic physician in 1961. It joined UH in 2000 and, with 125 beds, offers more than 30 specialties from over 400 physicians.

UH St. John Medical Center—
The Sisters of Charity of St. Augustine have run this nonprofit hospital on Cleveland's Westside since 1916. In 1981, it merged with Bay View Osteopathic General Hospital to form the medical center, serving residents of western Cuyahoga and eastern Lorain counties. The Sisters of Charity Health System entered into a joint venture arrangement in 1999 with UH, which became sole owner of the 240-bed acute care facility in 2015.

UH Samaritan Medical Center—
Philanthropists J.L. Clark and his wife, Mary, gave Ashland a hospital in 1912 with the understanding that "no sick person would ever be refused care." Located between Ohio's two largest cities, Cleveland and Columbus, it grew into the Samaritan Regional Health System, which integrated with UH in 2015.

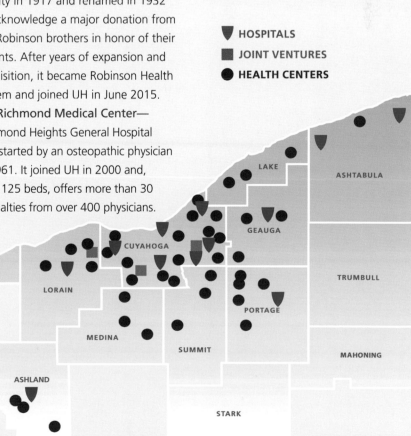

▼ HOSPITALS
■ JOINT VENTURES
● HEALTH CENTERS

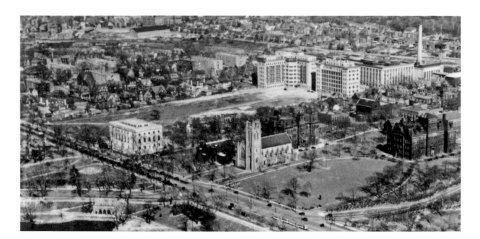

Left: University Hospitals Cleveland Medical Center campus has changed dramatically over the past 90 years. In 1926, the only completed buildings were Maternity Hospital and Babies and Childrens Hospital – open space was plentiful. *Right:* Today, it is the site of a bustling, internationally renowned medical campus.

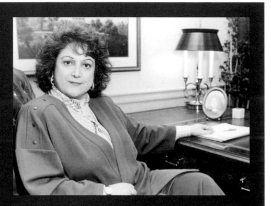

Farah Walters, 1991.

Turning Point

Farah Walters became the first female CEO of University Hospitals in 1992 and led the organization during the transition from a stand-alone academic medical center to an integrated health care delivery system. Reflecting on her tenure, she states, "The 1980s and '90s were turbulent times in health care. Declining reimbursements, Medicaid cuts, and the emergence of managed care as a way to contain costs caused many hospitals to close." UH responded by merging with local community hospitals to expand its patient base. This expansion continued for the next two decades. "We couldn't have survived with our limited geographic reach," continues Walters. "Yet, in spite of the changes we had to make to protect ourselves, we always maintained our commitment to our mission and to preserving our culture."

the realignment and consolidation of medical institutions in response to unprecedented financial pressures that would become a nationwide trend in the 1990s. Small, single-site hospitals could not afford the latest sophisticated and expensive technologies. Some refer to this period as "the hospital wars" in reference to the fight to survive in an increasingly competitive and contracting field.

Against the odds, UH not only survived but thrived. Between 1993 and 2013, it acquired 10 community hospitals and built a brand new one, University Hospitals Ahuja Medical Center in Beachwood. The main Cleveland campus remains the hub of the wheel and the epicenter of clinical research, innovation, and teaching. The health system is an integrated network of 18 hospitals, including a joint venture with Southwest General Health Center, and more than 50 health centers and outpatient facilities located in 15 counties throughout Northeast Ohio. Together, they form University Hospitals, a mission-driven, nonprofit organization motivated by the same set of values that inspired the founders of Lakeside, Rainbow Cottage, Babies and Childrens Hospital, and Maternity Hospital so long ago and united them in a single, shared undertaking.

"We went from a small group of separate hospitals and doctors to this large, multifaceted organization," states Lifetime Trustee Bob Gries. "Who we are is much more than the separate pieces and parts. It's about what we stand for."

The cooperative, connected approach that shaped so much of UH's growth and progress is also redefining relationships with the city and the neighborhood. When Thomas F. Zenty III became Chief Executive Officer of UH in 2003, he reaffirmed the hospital's longstanding commitment to actively engage with different community constituencies to promote the overall health of Northeast Ohio in economic, environmental, and social ways. One such relationship involves UH's participation in the Greater University Circle Initiative (GUCI), a collaborative redevelopment effort

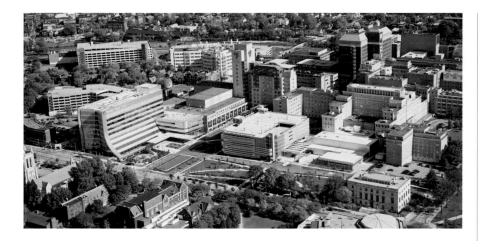

convened by the Cleveland Foundation in 2005. The nation's first charity devoted to local, place-based giving, the Cleveland Foundation was established in 1914, the same year Babies and Childrens Hospital formalized its relationship with Western Reserve University's medical school and agreed to build in University Circle. A 2013 assessment of the program noted that GUCI has made significant inroads in addressing economic inclusion, improving transportation access, and catalyzing business growth in the University Circle area.

Former Cleveland Foundation Executive Vice President Robert Eckardt says the Greater University Circle Initiative is a national model and notes UH's vital role in helping to create vibrant neighborhoods and a better future for Cleveland.

In 2006, UH launched Vision 2010, a five-year strategic plan for a $1.2 billion capital expansion effort. It was another opportunity to affect positive, enduring change in the region. Much of the funds raised by the initiative was allocated to local construction companies and vendors owned by minorities and women. A case study conducted by scholars from MIT and the University of Maryland called it "a path-breaking strategy" that successfully met its goals.

Describing the thinking behind this strategy in a 2008 speech, Zenty said that hospitals should go beyond their traditional and fairly narrow role of being places to help the sick and injured. "Communities and health care leaders are discovering that hospitals can help to heal entire cities."

"Tom Zenty and Steve Standley [UH Chief Administrative Officer] told me they wanted to use Vision 2010 to benefit the community by going beyond basic equal opportunity requirements," says Cleveland Mayor Frank G. Jackson. "It has resulted in hundreds of millions of dollars being invested and has provided opportunities for minority and female business owners to get a foot in the door. Many talk about what they're going to do. University Hospitals actually did it. University Hospitals is a valuable partner for the City of Cleveland and its contributions are immeasurable." ▼

I Work Here

The benefits of working at University Hospitals extend beyond the workplace. Thomas Sanders works in the UH Information Technology & Services department. He took advantage of the Greater Circle Living program, offered through University Hospitals' partnership with the Greater University Circle Initiative to purchase a home in 2013. "It works as a forgivable zero-interest loan," says Sanders. "The condition is you have to stay in the property for five years and work for an organization in University Circle. Sometimes it's tough to be able to purchase. A lot of folks aren't going to have 20 or more percent to put down. This program gives you one of the best opportunities to buy a home."

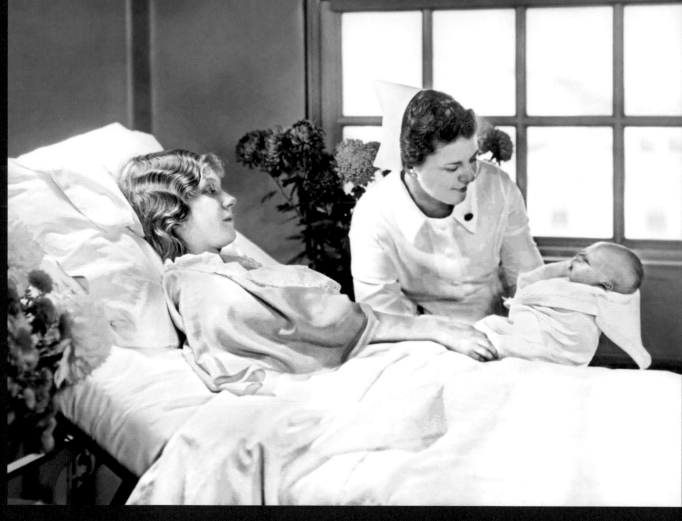

Bedside care at Maternity Hospital, ca. late 1920s. Chronicling the history of University Hospitals' buildings is one way of telling the story of how UH has responded to the community's health care needs for over 150 years, always striving to be the best place, in the right place. University Hospitals is preparing for the coming decades with the same intention and thought.

Beds and Buildings

"In the construction and administration of every hospital the first thought should be for the immediate comfort and well-being of the patients. At the same time it must not be forgotten that the work of such an institution is not for today only and that due regard should be paid to its possibilities from a scientific and medical standpoint."

– Hunter Robb, MD, Professor of Gynecology, Western Reserve University, "A Brief Description of the New Lakeside Hospital," *Cleveland Medical Gazette*, May 1896

John Flemming walked into a police station in downtown Cleveland on the morning of January 23, 1898, with blood streaming from a gash above his left eye and a wound on the back of his head. The victim of a vicious assault, he was lucky. An ambulance took him to the magnificent new Lakeside Hospital on what is now Lakeside Avenue, which had only been admitting patients for a week.[1]

It was "thoroughly equipped" and "fitted with all the modern improvements" for care of the sick.[2] The 1,500 visitors taking pre-opening tours of the hospital on January 13 were surprised and impressed, according to news reports. Thirty-three years later, considered outdated and unusable, it sat empty and abandoned. But this was a sign of progress, not failure—a response to advances in medicine, an improved understanding of health care, and new ideas in hospital architecture. This was the third time the hospital outgrew its location, its grounds continuously transforming, until a permanent home was found in University Circle in 1931.

The last 65 patients were moved on Sunday morning, February 1, 1931, to Lakeside's next home, a nine-story structure in University Circle designed to provide "the latest science could devise."[3] It cost $4.3 million—a sum equivalent to more than $100 million today. But at a time when a quarter bought a dozen eggs and the average hourly wage for a factory worker was 43 cents, it represented a significant outlay.

Lakeside joined the newly-constructed Babies and Childrens Hospital and Maternity Hospital on the burgeoning academic medical center campus. Built to replace the inadequate and makeshift quarters these two institutions had occupied for decades, the new facilities were also acclaimed for "embodying every mechanical device that contributes to the comfort and welfare of the patient."[4] Speaking at the dedication of the two new hospitals on October 28, 1925, Abraham Flexner, an education reformer who had a profound influence on how doctors were trained in America, said, "Here are magnificent buildings, not surpassed in beauty, convenience, or completeness by any in this country or in Europe…They represent civic ambition, civic

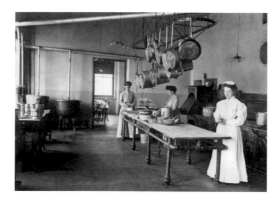

Old Lakeside Hospital's main kitchen, 1905. The American Dietetic Association, predecessor of today's Academy of Nutrition and Dietetics, was co-founded in 1917 by Lulu Graves, head dietitian at Lakeside. The group's inaugural meeting was held in Cleveland, and she served as the organization's first President.

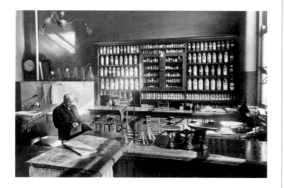

Medicines were made in old Lakeside Hospital's compounding pharmacy, 1905.

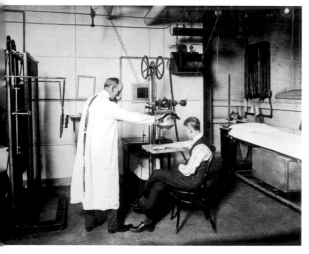

Old Lakeside Hospital's X-ray equipment, ca. 1920s. With radiology playing an increasingly important role at that time, University Hospitals started an on-the-job X-ray technician training program to address the shortage of qualified applicants.

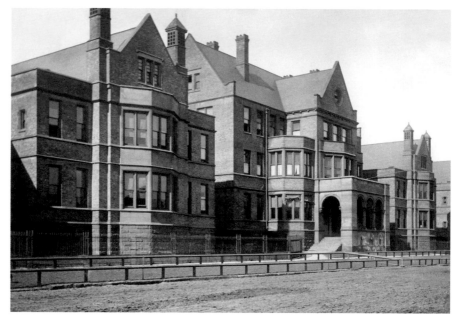

Old Lakeside Hospital, 1898.

effort, civic service. They are to be forever consecrated today to noble uses." His words continued to ring true, year after year, as University Hospitals expanded its footprint and responded to the evolving ideas and forward leaps of medical and surgical practices with new construction, renovation of old buildings, and demolition of those that became obsolete. Because in health care, innovation is a constant, and change a necessity.

Hospital Tour: "Old" Lakeside Hospital, 1898

After 30 years of making do at the Wilson Street and Marine hospitals and a two-year hiatus while it was being built, Lakeside Hospital finally received facilities worthy of its mission and aspirations in 1898. A building committee of hospital board members, led by Samuel Mather, toured hospitals in Europe and nine U.S. cities before choosing the pavilion plan used by Johns Hopkins in Baltimore, deemed one of the country's best and most progressive hospitals. "The new building just completed, furnishes Lakeside Hospital with its third home...The hospital at the present time is one of the most complete in the country in its provision for caring for patients in an advanced and thoroughly scientific manner."[5] Situated on what is now Lakeside Avenue between East 12th and 14th streets, next to Lakeside Hospitals' previous home in Marine Hospital, the five acre site was on open and mostly undeveloped land. It was ideally suited for the sprawling complex of 11 buildings.

There were 10 wards, including one for children and two for emergency patients, a surgical suite, and a drug room for filling

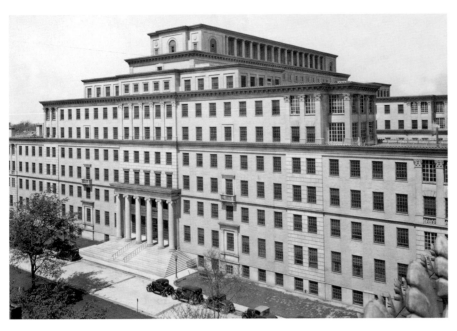

New Lakeside Hospital, ca. 1930s.

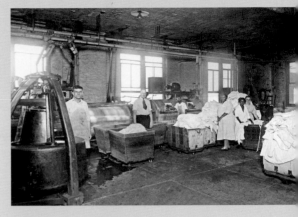

Old Lakeside Hospital laundry, ca. late 1910s.

prescriptions. In a departure from policies of the past, special accommodations and an operating room were devoted to paying patients. But most of the hospital's 250 beds were dedicated to those who paid little or nothing. An outpatient dispensary for non-hospital cases could accommodate 300 people a day. Patients were charged 10 cents per visit, but records show that most of these fees went uncollected. Scientific inquiry was becoming increasingly important during Lakeside's early years. Post-mortems were conducted in a well-equipped pathology building. It contained a morgue room and laboratories for research and the examination of anatomical specimens.

The understanding that germs caused many diseases and infections emerged in Europe in the 1860s and began to be adopted in the United States by the 1880s, prompting Lakeside planners to install a water filtering system and adopt a method of heating and ventilation that ensured the flow of pure, dry air. To discourage the accumulation of dust and dirt and make cleaning easier, angled corners of floors and ceilings were replaced by curved surfaces, and moldings around doors and windows were eliminated. Operating rooms were arranged to encourage germ-free aseptic conditions. Dudley Peter Allen, MD, a Lakeside surgeon and medical college professor, championed the use of sterile procedures in Cleveland after studying them in Europe. But the ideas were not widely or fully understood and were slow to take hold. Howard Dittrick, MD, an obstetrician who was a junior member of Lakeside's house staff in the early 1900s, recalled an attending physician in another hospital who pulled scissors from his pocket and offered them as a replacement for a pair that had fallen on the floor during an operation.[6]

Behind the Scenes

It was reported in 1900 that the laundresses at old Lakeside Hospital washed 18,000 – 20,000 pieces of linen every week, more than any public laundry in the city at that time. "The enormous wash is the result of the fact that no piece of linen is used but once before being washed. A physician wipes his hands on a towel, having just washed them in an anti-septic solution. The towel is sent to the laundry without again being used for any purpose."[7] In contrast, today University Hospitals outsources more than 5 million pounds of washing for University Hospitals Cleveland Medical Center annually.

I Remember

Charles Pimlott started as a hospital bookkeeper in 1931 and was Assistant Treasurer and Secretary of the University Hospitals Board of Trustees when he retired 40 years later. He had experienced Depression-era cutbacks, the staff shortages of WWII, and the medical center building boom of the 1950s and '60s. Recounting the organization's history to a group of longtime employees in 1962, Pimlott described the day the last patients and staff moved out of old Lakeside Hospital: "[F]or the first time in its 32 years of service, the hospital on the lake was left deserted and in darkness, and a new epoch began in the history of University Hospitals of Cleveland."[8]

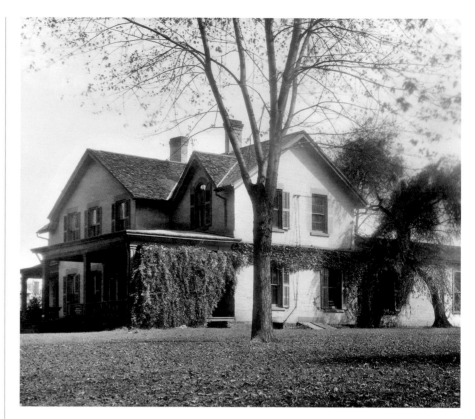

Allen Ford's 120-acre family estate was located in University Circle. A portion of it was sold in the early 1900s and became part of the medical center campus. According to Ford, "I was born in 1928 and, according to my father, the site [at University Hospitals] was where the cherry orchard stood on the family farm."

In Lakeside's 1899 annual report, Samuel Mather expressed pride in what had been accomplished and hope for what the institution could become, writing that those "most competent to judge" agreed that Lakeside Hospital was "undeniably and incomparably the best hospital west of the Alleghenies...We desire that its operation shall be commensurate with the character of its building, its equipment, and its opportunities, and that it shall be to the Middle States what Johns Hopkins' has been to the East—an inspiration and an example."

Years of growth and expansion followed. The annual report for 1911 described Lakeside as a community rather than merely a hospital, with its own post office; telephone exchange; school for nurses; separate residences for doctors, nurses, and orderlies; a sewing room where the nurses' uniforms were made; a grocery store; a garage; plants for producing ice and electricity; paint, machine, and carpentry shops; a brace room with a blacksmith's forge; and a soap manufacturing plant. Yet, despite near-constant renovations, additions, and improvements, the facility eventually outlived its usefulness and the growing presence of passing trains and factories, along with an unstable foundation, made the location increasingly unsuitable. Railroad tracks ran along the north side of the property. The Gund Brewery was next door. Otis Steel had a mill only

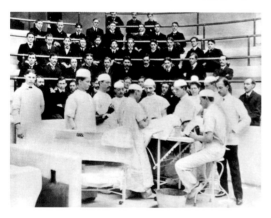

Surgery at old Lakeside Hospital in 1898. Before aseptic techniques became commonplace in American medicine, it was typical practice to leave windows open during surgical procedures. Surgeons and observers wore street clothes and smoking was permitted. Masks and gloves were not used consistently until after the 1900s.

Behind the Scenes: Old Lakeside Hospital

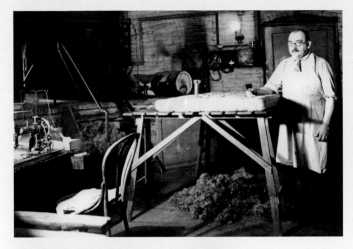

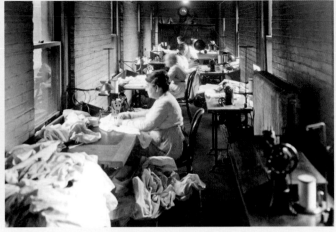

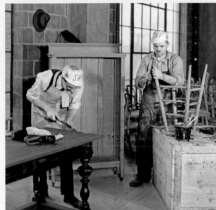

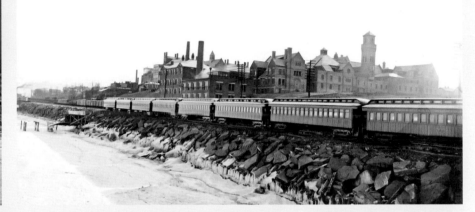

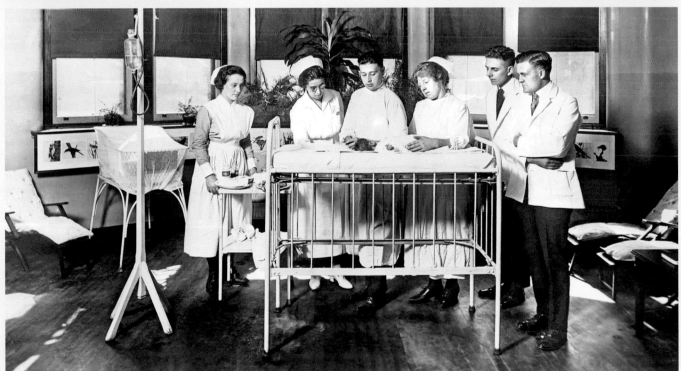

Top left: Mattress room, ca. 1910s. *Top right:* The sewing room, ca. 1910s. ***Middle left:*** Wooden furniture was made and repaired on site, 1928. ***Middle right:*** Old Lakeside Hospital with a view of the nearby train tracks that were so close to the building that staff had to contend with smoke and soot from the trains, ca. early 1900s. In a letter written by longtime nurse Olga Benderoff, RN, she recalled how her newspaper would shake so much when a train passed by that she couldn't read it.[9] ***Bottom:*** Old Lakeside Hospital provided pediatric care until the construction of Babies and Childrens Hospital in 1925.

12 blocks away. By 1914, problems with smoke, fumes, noise, vibrations, and grime prompted the decision to move east. But it would be 17 years before another hospital was funded and finished in University Circle.

Hospital Tour: Babies and Childrens, Maternity, and Rainbow Hospitals: 1925 – 1930

Hospitals had become central to the practice and study of medicine by the end of the 1920s. The new complex built for Babies and Childrens and Maternity hospitals opened in 1925, a year after the completion of Western Reserve University's new medical school, as part of the development of the academic medical center campus championed by Samuel Mather and other leading citizens.

Top: The new Babies and Childrens and Maternity hospitals, under construction, opened on their current site in University Circle in 1925. *Bottom left:* A pediatric dispensary at Babies and Childrens Hospital, ca. 1930s. *Bottom right:* Baby bath in the nursery of Maternity Hospital, ca. 1930s.

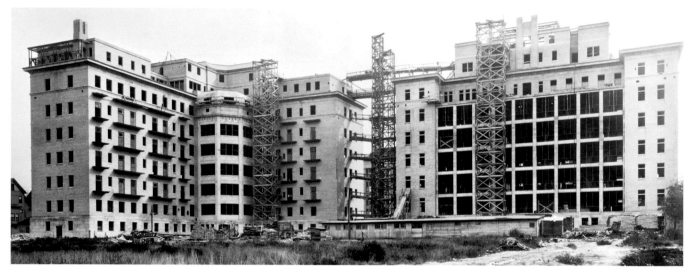

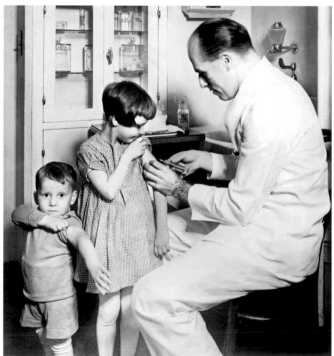

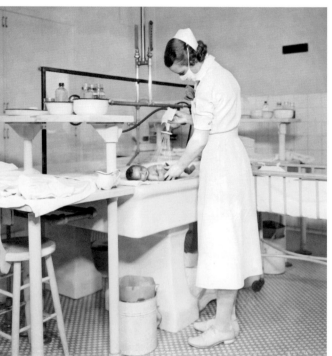

The hospitals paired novel amenities for patients and visitors with ideal conditions for doctors, nurses, and students. Remarking on the outstanding research facilities, Henry Gerstenberger, MD, the first Medical Director of Babies' Dispensary and Hospital, noted that laboratories adjoined the living quarters of physicians "so that they can arise at midnight to work if they wish."[10]

Maternity had a prenatal clinic "furnished," according to newspaper accounts, "with comfort and cheer," nurseries on every floor, and a "papa's room" where husbands could await the good news. "If the stork loiters on the way and papa is stuck for an all-day session he will find a kitchenet [sic]…where he can cook himself a snack or lunch."[11] At Babies and Childrens, little ones were bathed on "drain boards," like those found beside kitchen sinks, fitted with electric heating pads to keep them warm. These features mark the beginning of the family-centered, patient-sensitive practices that would follow in years to come, from extending visiting hours for new fathers and allowing them to be present during labor and delivery, to rooms with an extra bed in today's pediatric intensive care unit so parents can stay overnight.

A kitchen in Maternity provided meals for both hospitals, with food transported from one to the other via passages in a sub-basement. Those tunnels also made it possible to transfer premature infants and newborns needing medical care from Maternity to Babies and Childrens, which had a special "preemie" suite for seven babies, without stepping outside the building. Infants over 1 month old were sent downtown to Lakeside Hospital for surgery. Babies and Childrens was the first hospital in the city devoted entirely to the care of children under age 14, and the first

This "bambino" plaque adorned the main entrance to Babies and Childrens Hospital, 1925. The American Academy of Pediatrics later adopted the plaque as its logo.

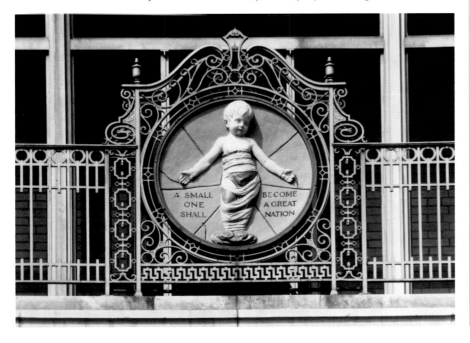

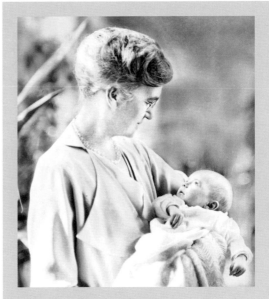

Superintendent, Calvina MacDonald, ca. 1930s.

Pioneer

Calvina MacDonald started as an obstetrical nurse at Maternity Hospital in 1909. A leader in maternal care, influential nurse trainer, and advocate for women and babies, she helped plan the layout of the new hospital, asking residents to drive her to University Circle during its construction to monitor the progress. The hospital was later renamed MacDonald House, honoring her 19 years of service. Today, its official designation is University Hospitals MacDonald Women's Hospital. It remains dedicated to women's health and is the only hospital of its kind in Ohio.

Nature's Power to Heal

A faith in Mother Nature's healing effects influenced the design and layout of all the hospitals that joined to become University Hospitals. Old Lakeside Hospital, positioned on a bluff overlooking Lake Erie, featured porches and solariums so patients could benefit from the view, sunshine, and clean breezes coming off the water. The new Lakeside Hospital in University Circle had an H-shaped footprint, reported a 1932 article, "so planned as to give the maximum of outside exposure to rooms…[O]ne feels that all the sunshine of Cleveland has been caught."[12] There were open-air wards on the roof of Babies and Childrens Hospital in University Circle until 1929, when the space was enclosed and put to other uses. It also had screened-in porches running along the front and back of the six-story building, as did Maternity Hospital. Rainbow Hospital on Green Road was also planned to "secure maximum benefits of fresh air and direct sun ray treatment," key parts of the institution's therapeutic model for convalescing children.[13]

Enthusiasm for nature's benefits waned as more modern and effective medicines and treatments became readily available. But, a renewed respect for the restorative power of being outside, exposed to sunlight and natural beauty, is evidenced in two recent additions for patients, families, and visitors on the University Hospitals Cleveland Medical Center campus.

The Mary and Al Schneider Healing Garden at the main entrance to University Hospitals Seidman Cancer Center was created in 2011 in memory of Mary and Albert Schneider by their son, Robert, and his wife, Cindy. The small park is a year-round oasis of scent and color, decorated with metal and granite sculptures, curving paths, and places to sit. Large windows provide a view of it from many areas inside UH Seidman. Similarly, a portion of a 2011 gift from Chuck and Char Fowler, in memory of their daughter Angie, who was diagnosed with cancer as a teenager, made it possible to convert the roof of the Leonard and Joan Horvitz Tower into a wheelchair-accessible garden at the top of University Hospitals Rainbow Babies & Children's Hospital. "There are pieces of sculpture, sun umbrellas, benches, fake grass to roll on, real plants, and trees," says Char. "Angie would have loved it." The addition of a glass-enclosed "sky lounge," named in honor of donors Theresia and Stuart Kline, provides an all-season spot.

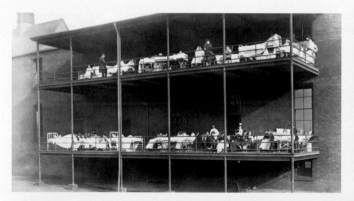
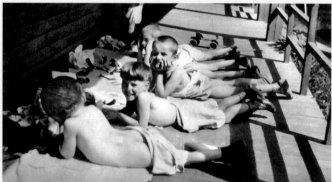

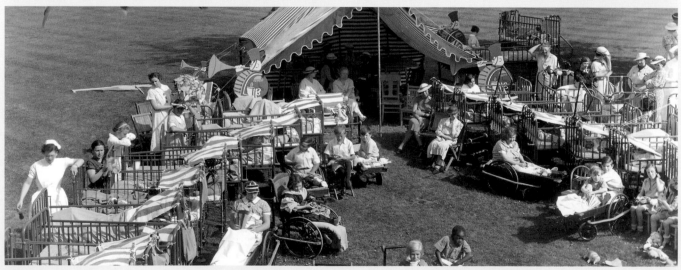

Top left: Old Lakeside Hospital sun porches, 1905. *Top right:* Rainbow Hospital, ca. 1930s. ***Bottom:*** Early on, Rainbow Hospital practitioners understood the therapeutic importance for pediatric patients to be outside, ca. 1950s.

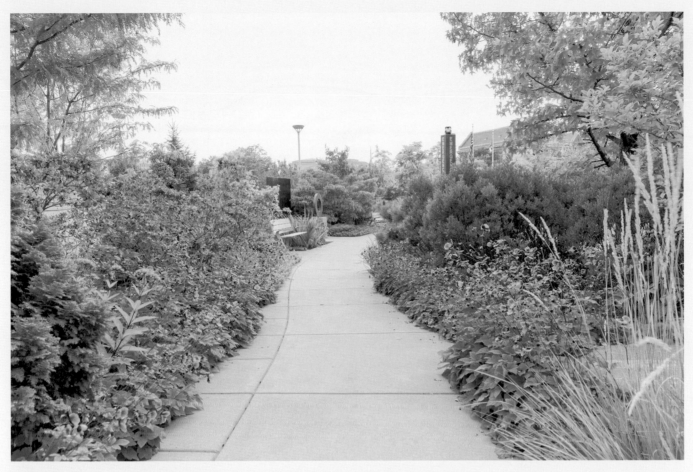

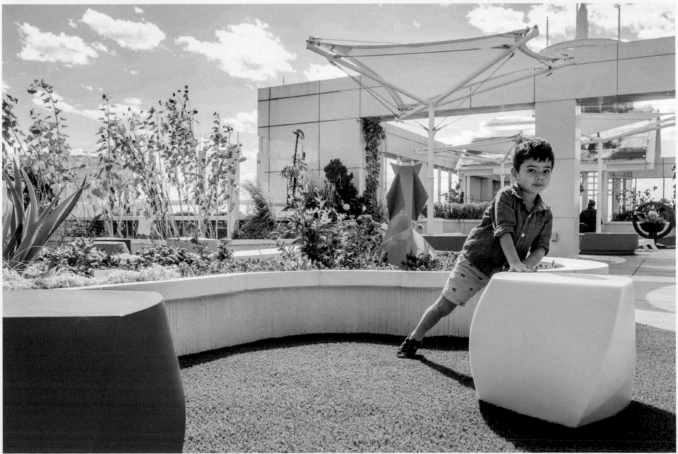

Top: Mary and Al Schneider Healing Garden at University Hospitals Seidman Cancer Center, 2015. *Bottom:* Rooftop garden at Angie Fowler Adolescent & Young Adult Cancer Institute.

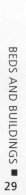

It's a Fact

Abram Garfield, son of U.S. President James Garfield, was the architect for three buildings on the medical center campus: Babies and Childrens Hospital (as well as its previous facility on East 35th Street), Maternity Hospital, and the Institute of Pathology, completed in 1929. When Lakeside Hospital's big, bronze front doors swung open, the institute, located right next door, was an invaluable resource for all of the members of University Hospitals and the Western Reserve University schools of medicine, nursing, and dentistry. In addition to laboratories, classrooms, and workspaces of various kinds, the building had its own morgue and chapel, stable, studios for a medical illustrator and photographer, and a specimen museum. John Carter, MD, Director of the Institute from 1966 to 1981, wrote that the institute "embraced anatomic, clinical and experimental pathology and immunology with teaching and service functions all under one roof…[S]taff members were expected to devote a substantial amount of their time to research." Integrating all these components, according to Dr. Carter, was revolutionary for its time.

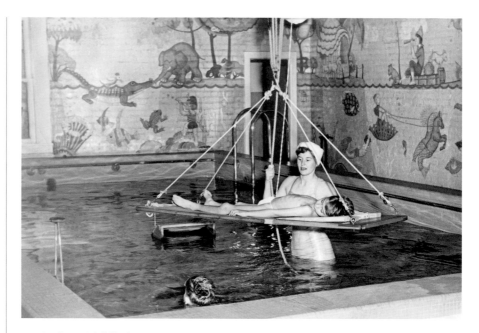

Despite financial difficulties precipitated by the Depression, Rainbow Hospital built a pool for physical therapy in 1934, paid for by the local Shriners chapter. It was named in honor of President Franklin Delano Roosevelt, who had been diagnosed with polio in 1921. Roosevelt's son James came to Cleveland for the dedication ceremony.

in the country to designate a ward strictly for youngsters with measles, whooping cough, diphtheria, and other common and highly contagious diseases, with a separate kitchen, entrance, elevator, and staircase.

Lakeside, Babies and Childrens, and Maternity hospitals joined to incorporate as University Hospitals of Cleveland in 1925. Two years later, Rainbow Hospital joined, but its trustees had no interest in relocating to the growing academic medical center campus in University Circle. Rainbow instead chose to erect its new facility on a 13-acre site on Green Road in South Euclid. Patient referrals would continue to come primarily from Lakeside and Babies and Childrens physicians, while pediatric, orthopedic, and surgical faculty and residents from the Western Reserve University School of Medicine would still oversee patient care. Because many of the children suffered from conditions that made walking difficult or impossible, it was a single-story building. According to *The Cleveland Press*, "Every effort has been made to get rid of the 'hospitalic' atmosphere, and the new building [at Rainbow] resembles a large country home more than what it really is. Besides space for actual treatment, there are recreation rooms, screened sleeping porches, and classrooms for the school."[14]

Hospital Tour: Lakeside Hospital and the Medical Center Campus, 1931 – 1968

It is fitting that Samuel Mather was present when the cornerstone was laid for the new Lakeside Hospital on the University Circle campus

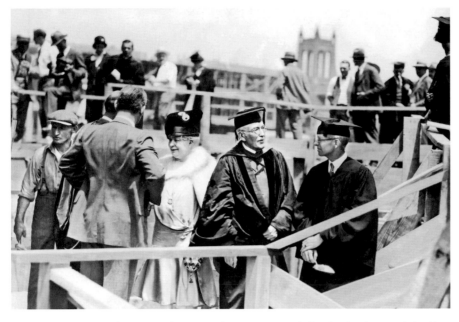

Samuel Mather (center) in cap and gown at the cornerstone dedication for the new Lakeside Hospital on June 13, 1929. The same day, philanthropists Leonard C. Hanna, Jr. and Arthur Baldwin laid the cornerstones for the Leonard C. Hanna House and the Nursing dormitories, respectively.

and at the opening ceremonies attended by leading medical experts, educators, scientists, and dignitaries from Cleveland and around the country. No single individual played a greater part in bringing about these events, which marked the final step in establishing the academic medical center.

Lakeside was impressive in scale, equipment, and efficiency. In combination with the Leonard C. Hanna House, an attached ward exclusively for private patients, there were 379 beds, a full complement of laboratories situated in close proximity to patients, operating suites, and therapy rooms. Noteworthy "extras" included scrub rooms, a radium plant, a centrally wired electrocardiograph station, and amphitheater seats equipped with earphones so physicians in the pit could communicate with students. Every doctor had an assigned number listed on electric "call boards" located near the elevators. They flashed to let doctors know that switchboard operators had someone on the line for them. Newspaper stories extolled the virtues of special lights that did not cast shadows in the operating rooms and reduced glare and eyestrain for lab workers. Pneumatic tubes eliminated the need for messengers and long walks through the medical complex. The system moved patient charts, memos, prescriptions, and even small packages quickly and efficiently around buildings and from one hospital to another using the power of compressed air. The dietary department was outfitted with a mechanical potato peeler, electric dishwasher, and heated food carts for transporting patient meals from the basement kitchens.

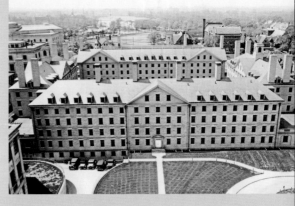

Lakeside Hospital dormitories, 1931.

It's a Fact

Four newly constructed residence halls, arranged in a quadrangle, opened simultaneously with Lakeside Hospital in 1931. The dormitories, funded by Samuel Mather, provided housing for nurses, residents, engineers, laundresses, cooks, gardeners, watchmen, and domestic workers.

Each residence "house" was named in honor of women who played key roles in the development of University Hospitals: Flora Stone Mather, philanthropist and wife of Samuel Mather; nursing pioneers Isabel Hampton Robb and Isabel Wetmore Lowman; and health care activist Kate Hanna Harvey, who was also a board member of Lakeside Hospital, Babies' Dispensary, and UH.

Dormitory life in the 1930s and '40s was robust with social activities ranging from group horseback-riding excursions and classical music nights to playing badminton in the Mather gymnasium and pool in the billiards room. Other activities included book clubs, folk dancing nights, a drama group, and bridge.

The buildings were demolished in 2007 and replaced with the new Center for Emergency Medicine as part of the Vision 2010 initiative.

The rapid advance of medical technology caused equipment and buildings to quickly grow obsolete. Frank Chapman, Lakeside's Director when the hospital opened, told a newspaper reporter that all the instruments and fixtures from the downtown building had been left behind or "traded in" like used cars. "Obsolescence in medical equipment is as rapid as in the automotive field," he said. "X-ray equipment is old in three years, old-fashioned in five. There is $200,000 worth of diagnostic and medical fittings in the new structure, much of which may have to be replaced in a few years." He also highlighted the utility stations on every floor, stating that never before in medical construction history had all the supplies needed for nursing activity, including washing, sterilizing, and dispensing of linens and medications, been assembled in one specially designated and supervised room.

Chapman noted that the medical center was taking a lesson from industry, reducing overhead by consolidating laundry, dietary, and housekeeping services for all three hospitals.[15] The very same kind of thinking has guided the more recent shift to a more cost-efficient regional hospital system, rather than single, independent facilities, with the University Hospitals Cleveland Medical Center campus serving as the hub of highly specialized care for complex cases.

Steam shovels had already carved out the massive hole for Lakeside's foundation when the stock market crashed in 1929, kicking off an economic depression that would impact the hospital group, the city, and the country for almost a decade. The outpatient departments logged 84,000 clinical visits during six months in 1931, and 88 percent of patients received care at no charge. A change from prior practice, patients could make appointments and see the same physician if returning for further treatment of the same condition. This marked a significant change in hospital policy and an innovation in the delivery of health care.

University Hospitals' employee Sergeant John Markley started as a night watchman for the nurses' dormitory in 1930 and became protective services supervisor the next year. Among his duties was managing the hospitals' gas station, where employees could purchase fuel at reduced rates. He also made sure that four cars used by the obstetrics staff for home

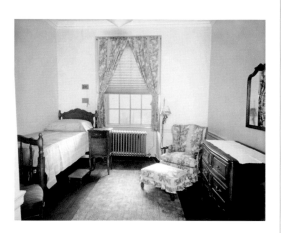

A private room in new Lakeside Hospital, ca. 1930s.

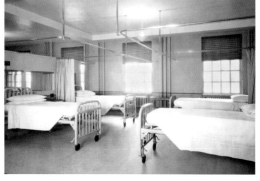

Patient ward in Lakeside Hospital, ca. 1930s.

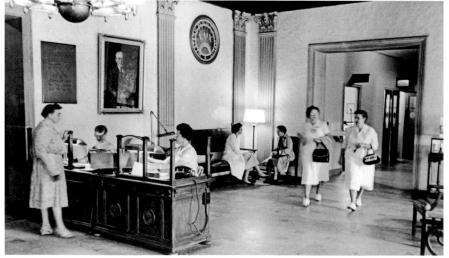

Today, visitors still enter this elegant marble-floored lobby, as it appeared in the 1950s, at Lakeside Hospital.

deliveries always had full tanks and were ready to go any hour of the day or night. "The old days weren't easy," Markley reminisced upon his retirement in 1958. "It was during the Depression and wages were extremely low—if you were lucky enough to have a job—but one thing can be said about that era, we didn't have any parking problems!"[16]

The year 1932 was tough. Income from patient fees and the endowment continued to diminish. More and more people needed free care. Budgets, wages, and staff were cut. But 1933 was even worse. After decades of growth in the city's industrial sector and the wealth of jobs that came with it, an estimated 50 percent of industrial workers in Cleveland were unemployed. UH was compelled to make further adjustments. Operations were only performed five days a week at Lakeside, and some wards were closed. After transferring their patients to Lakeside and Hanna House, Maternity and Babies and Childrens hospitals were forced to close for two years because of the Great Depression.

Lester Black recalled how Lakeside doctors saved the life of his wife, Gertha, in 1934, but being out of work and unemployed for years, he was unable to pay the $150 for her care. "Boy, did we have bills," he said. "We put off the hospital bill because we knew it was a big one, and I wanted to pay it all at one time." On December 16, 1957, Lester showed up at the hospital cashier's office and handed over all their savings to clear the debt. For the Blacks, "the Depression was finally over."[17]

Innovative financing options for how to pay for medical care evolved from these hard times. UH instituted an all-inclusive, flat-rate bargain plan in 1932 that covered medical, pediatric, surgical, obstetrical, tonsil, and adenoid services; cytoscopic examinations of the bladder

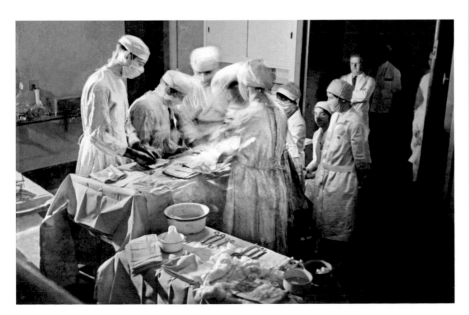

Chief of Surgery Elliot Cutler, MD, and cardiac surgeon Claude Beck, MD, performed the first operation at new Lakeside Hospital in 1931.

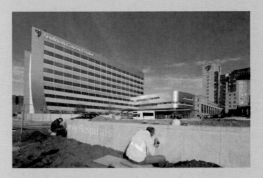

Vision 2010 gave University Hospitals Cleveland Medical Center a front-door make-over, 2011.

Game Changers

University Hospitals has a history of pursuing major building and improvement projects through economic downturns. A depression that lasted from 1893 to 1898 did not stop construction of old Lakeside Hospital downtown. Its successor in University Circle was completed in 1931, despite the Great Depression that began almost exactly a year after the groundbreaking. During the recession that began in 2007, the organization once again carried on with its strategic growth plan, Vision 2010. The major investment in new facilities was made possible, as in previous periods of economic challenge, by administrators' and trustees' resolve and resilience, a desire to serve the community that had so often supported UH in the past, and the generosity of major donors. In fact, the downturn actually made more local workers available for hire. "Other large projects in the city were put on hold," says Steven Standley, UH Chief Administrative Officer, "but we kept going and we kept people employed."

The Hospital as a City

Gerold Frank, a feature writer for *The Cleveland News*, spent a day exploring new Lakeside Hospital's basement in 1936. He described it as an "Underground City." Without ever going up to another floor, he had a physical at the health clinic, found relief for foot pain in the physiotherapy room, played squash, took a shower in the men's locker room, got his suit pressed at the tailor shop, had a haircut and shave in the barbershop, ate lunch in one of the staff cafeterias, and viewed the mechanical and maintenance facilities. A tour of the tunnels, some with electric trains running through them, took him under Euclid Avenue and Severance Hall to Flora Stone Mather College, a half-mile walk from Lakeside.

Frank finished his day down below with dinner and billiards in the company of Director Robert Bishop, MD, Samuel Mather's son-in-law and University Hospitals' first Chief Administrator. Frank quoted him in his story. "I sometimes wonder," Dr. Bishop said, "…if the people of this community really see the picture of this hospital center in its entirety…Here, on the one side we have the university, training and preparing young men and young women for a high professional service to the community. Here, on the other side, we have the hospital unit, furnishing the means for this service and continuing it in terms of the community's need. I'm proud of what we have here. I think the city should be, too."[18]

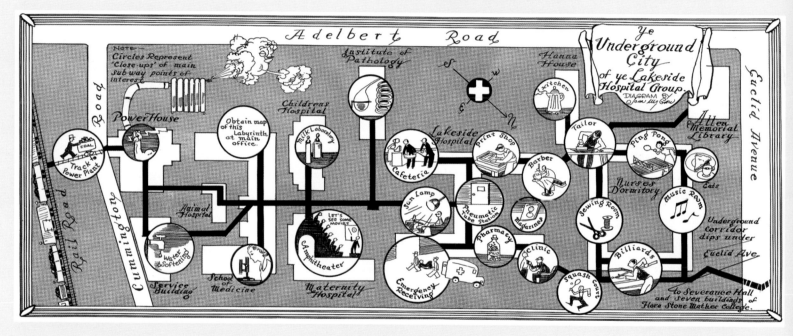

A map of the "Underground City" located in new Lakeside Hospital's basement, 1936.

and urinary tract; and 72 hours of inpatient diagnostic procedures. The plan also covered room and board, nursing care, operations, and certain drugs. There were, of course, many rules, restrictions, and exceptions, among them the requirement that fees be paid in advance in cash, but it was considered quite progressive for its time and a great asset for members of the community.

A next step in tackling the problem was conceived by John Mannix in 1934 when he was Assistant Administrator of UH. He founded the Cleveland Hospital Service Association. It created the first group hospitalization plan in the United States, which became the model for Blue Cross and Blue Shield. Individuals paid 60 cents a month, in many cases through their employers, and were "covered" for three weeks of ward service in any of the 13 participating hospitals. One year later, 13,340 Clevelanders had enrolled in the plan and member hospitals had been reimbursed for treating 600 patients.

Post-war Development

World War II brought shortages of staff, equipment, and supplies. But the post-war years marked a period of expansion and improvements to meet the increasing demands for modern hospital services. In 1956, another specialty hospital was added to the campus. The Howard M. Hanna Memorial Pavilion was both an inpatient and outpatient psychiatric unit and among only a few in the country connected to a general hospital. It was a valuable educational asset for students of Western Reserve University's medical, nursing, and applied social science schools. According to the late L. Douglas Lenkoski, MD, former Chief of Staff and Director of the Department of Psychiatry at University Hospitals and Case Western Reserve University School of Medicine, who retired in 1992 after 32 years, making The Hanna Pavilion part of an academic medical center reflected a new way of thinking. "It was very exciting," he recalled, "and evidence that psychiatry would stay close to the rest of medicine, which I felt was very important."

The five story, 92-bed Hanna Pavilion replaced a small psychiatric ward in Lakeside Hospital, a measure of the increasing importance of the Department of Psychiatry, established in 1946, and

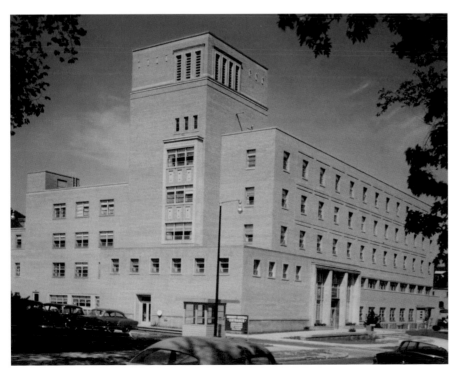
Howard M. Hanna Memorial Pavilion, 1956.

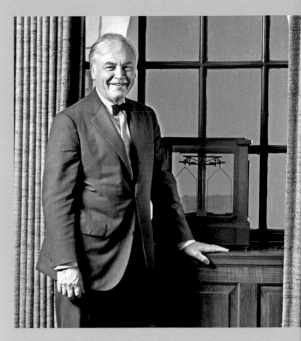
Former University Hospitals President and CEO Scott Inkley, MD, 1982.

I Work Here

Scott Inkley, MD, a pulmonary specialist, came to UH as an intern in 1945 and never left. By the time he retired in 1986, he had served as Chief of Staff and then President and CEO. He was the first hospital administrator to have the CEO title. Known for his ever-present bowtie, which he has said he wore because it never got in the way when he was bending over patients and didn't dip into his soup, he recalls that the doctors' dining room at Lakeside was much more than a place to eat. "People from the medical school came over to the hospital for lunch. A little Scottish lady ran it and told everyone where to sit. She got doctors mingling with faculty and scientists and that improved the communication between them. You got to know people you might never have met, and the discussions were very interesting. We talked about our work, things we saw, and exchanged ideas in ways that were beneficial for everybody."

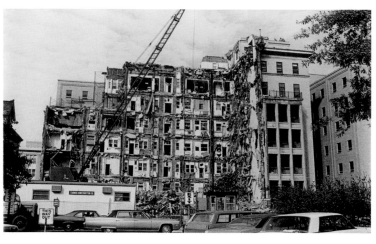

"The first hit of the steel ball loosened two bricks," remembers long-time University Hospitals Rainbow Babies & Children's Hospital physician Avroy Fanaroff, MD, when describing the demolition of Babies and Childrens Hospital. "It was very well-constructed, very solid."

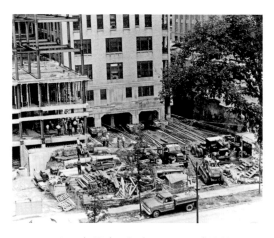

It took 12 days in the summer of 1969 to complete and "a total pulling force of more than 4 million pounds" to inch Babies and Childrens Hospital's original 30-million-pound structure 80 feet.[20]

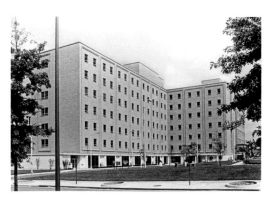

The new Rainbow Babies and Childrens Hospital, 1971. This view is now obscured by the Leonard and Joan Horvitz Tower.

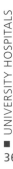

of the specialty itself. It was one of only a handful of facilities in the nation to set aside an area specifically for disturbed children. The pediatric floor featured a main corridor wide enough to accommodate tricycle traffic and a playroom that opened onto an outdoor deck equipped with a "splash shower."[19] Reorganized in 1966, the Children's Unit coordinated care and treatment provided by pediatricians, child psychiatrists and psychologists, social workers, psychiatric nurses, occupational therapists, and school teachers. The approach was unique in the Midwest. The unit closed in 1989, reflecting a statewide decline in beds for children diagnosed with mental illness. But in 2008, in response to an unmet need in the city, a therapeutic 12-bed inpatient pediatric and adolescent psychiatry unit opened on the third floor of University Hospitals Rainbow Babies & Children's Hospital, made possible through a $5 million gift from the Elisabeth Severance Prentiss Foundation.

The combination of private insurance companies cutting back on coverage for all inpatient care at psychiatric hospitals in the 1990s and the introduction of new medications and different approaches to treatment of mental health issues resulted in shorter and less frequent hospital stays. These factors influenced the decision to demolish Hanna Pavilion in 2009 to make way for major new construction on the medical center campus. Inpatient and outpatient psychiatric services were relocated and expanded to a state-of-the-art facility at University Hospitals Richmond Medical Center.

Similar forces to those that determined Hanna Pavilion's fate were at work when Rainbow Hospital's Board agreed to leave South Euclid and move to University Circle. It was a difficult but necessary decision, and one advocated by Charles Herndon, MD, Director of Orthopedic Surgery at Rainbow from 1953 to 1982 and Director of the Division of Orthopedics at UH. In addition to advances in orthopedic surgery, children's health had improved thanks to the development of vaccines, antibiotics, access to better food, clean milk and water, and public sanitation measures. "Rainbow Hospital…is the happy victim of medical progress. Little more than a third of its 82 beds are occupied by afflicted youngsters. The Salk polio vaccine is credited by Miss Elizabeth Rosenberg, [Rainbow's] director, as one of the major reasons for its emptiness. Polio victims were long its chief patients."[21] Fewer cases of malnutrition and rickets, polio, bone and joint tuberculosis, rheumatic fever, and other illnesses meant less demand for a place where youngsters could stay for months. Instead, those with crippling conditions needed more access to the specialists and resources only a major hospital could provide.

Hospital Tour: Rainbow Babies and Childrens Hospital, 1971

The medical landscape was changing, and like Rainbow Hospital, Babies and Childrens had to respond. New and different procedures required more modern facilities. Rather than renovate the old building, the two institutions agreed to join forces and erect a facility that they would share.

Constructing the new Rainbow Babies and Childrens Hospital involved an extraordinary feat of engineering. To make space for the north/south wing and ensure that children could continue to receive care during construction, the old Babies and Childrens Hospital was moved off its foundation and repositioned. "Tons of force, miles of cable, barrels of sweat and hours of frustration were poured into the move of the largest building ever to be transferred intact from one location to another." Remarkably "not a pane of glass was cracked."[22]

Patients moving into the new Rainbow Babies and Childrens Hospital, 1971

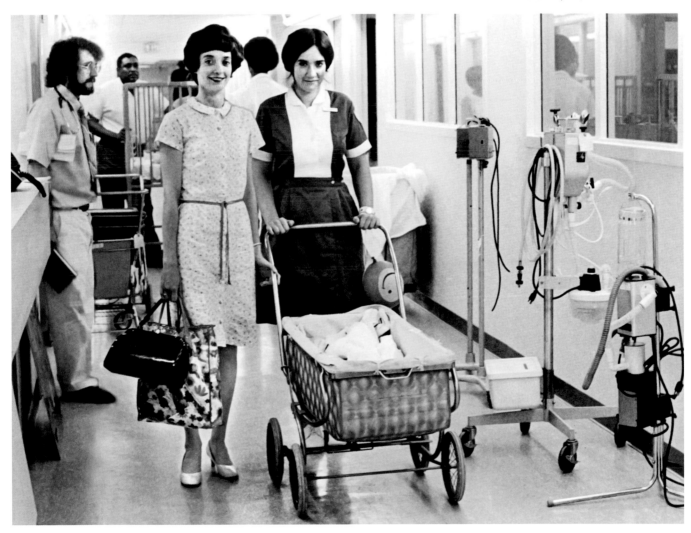

Avroy Fanaroff, MD, former Director of Neonatology for University Hospitals Rainbow Babies & Children's Hospital, arrived at UH as a fellow in 1969 and has vivid recollections of the event. "They dug under the foundations and put in rollers, which flattened from the weight. A steel cable attached to four World War II Army trucks [and to the building's footers] snapped like twine. They had to go to eight trucks and add more cables, but they did it. The remarkable thing was that we went back

Left: The Robert H. Bishop Building was built during the 1960s. This view is now only visible from the Atrium on the University Hospitals Cleveland Medical Center campus. ***Bottom:*** At one time there were tennis courts in the quadrangle where the Atrium is now located. The 18,000-square-foot Atrium officially opened in December 1989.

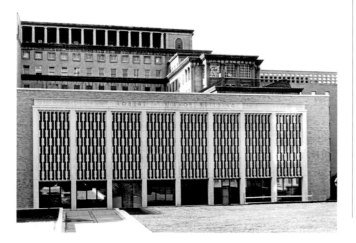

into our offices and not a book had fallen off a shelf. The utilities were back on within a few hours."

The old building was torn down after the new hospital began admitting patients to the eight-story, 220-bed facility in September 1971. The youngest and sickest patients were put on the upper floors. Resident staff and student quarters were also located there. Physical therapy, hydrotherapy, occupational therapy, and a pediatric dental clinic were housed in the basement, and a pediatric "walk-in" clinic was located on the ground floor. Patients were divided by age on the fourth and fifth floors, and those with infectious diseases were treated on the sixth. Rainbow was a separate division on the third floor for care and rehabilitation of boys and girls with orthopedic and cardiovascular problems and other conditions requiring extended stays in the hospital. The two hospitals took the final step to becoming fully integrated by forming a single board of trustees in 1974 for Rainbow Babies and Childrens.

Decades of Expansion and Change

The new hospital for pediatric patients was only one part of a major $54.8 million University Hospitals

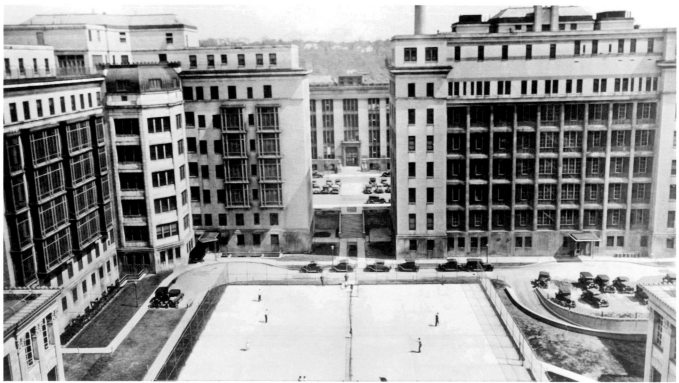

medical center development program. The Robert H. Bishop Building, containing operating rooms, radiology services, and a new cafeteria, opened in 1967. An Ambulatory Care building and renovations to Lakeside Hospital and the Institute of Pathology were in the planning stages. New construction, additions, refurbishing, and repurposing continued throughout the 1970s, '80s, and '90s.

The UH Health Center opened on the University Circle campus in 1984, reflecting the new emphasis on outpatient care. "When we built it, the duration of hospital stays was going down," explained former President and CEO Scott Inkley, MD. "We were able to do more things on an ambulatory basis. This was easier on patients and on the pocketbook, but it was also a better way to deal with many problems." Renamed the Harry J. Bolwell Health Center in 1986 in honor of a former board chair and longtime Trustee, it was expanded again in 1990.

James Block, MD, succeeded Dr. Inkley as UH's President and CEO from 1986 to 1992. During his tenure, many areas of the medical center got a facelift. Enclosing the quadrangle between the hospitals was part of the overhaul. The new Atrium included a gift and flower shop and a food court. "When I came, it was a huge empty space filled with grass and mud," recalls Dr. Block, a pediatrician by training. "The Atrium created a beautiful, open, sky-lit space that connected the hospital buildings and reinforced the idea that UH's many institutions are really one family. It became a destination and gathering place for patients, visitors, and staff."

Alfred and Norma Lerner Tower and the Samuel Mather Pavilion were dedicated in February 1994. Guests at the gala event, attended by keynote speaker Colin Powell, then Chairman of the Joint Chiefs of Staff, told *The Plain Dealer* that the lobby felt like "a posh hotel."[23] Polished granite, maple and cherry paneling, a curving staircase, soft area lighting, comfortable and intimate seating areas, and original artwork on the walls countered the image of a hospital as a cold, impersonal place. The interior layout, finishes, and furnishings were meant to put people at ease and make the sometimes long hours waiting for a friend or family member more pleasant.

History was repeating itself. In 1931, when Lakeside and Hanna House opened, they too

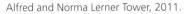

Alfred and Norma Lerner Tower, 2011.

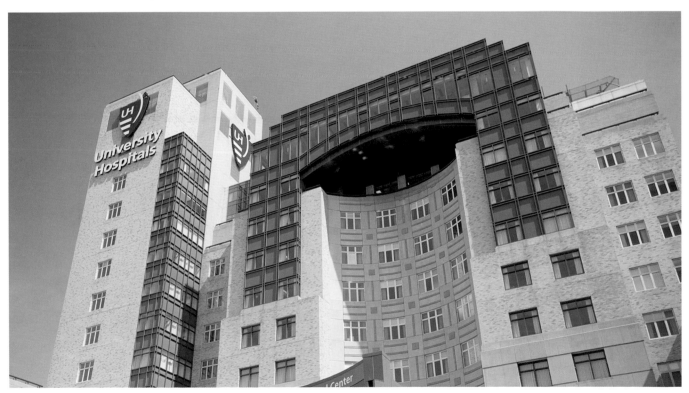

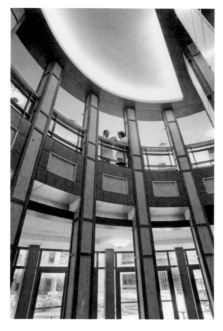

The design of Alfred and Norma Lerner Tower and Mather Pavilion won a Vista Award from the American Hospital Association, an organization founded in 1899 by Lakeside Hospital's first Superintendent, James Seward Knowles. The building created a new main entrance for University Hospitals and served as the cornerstone of the next phase of modernization and campus expansion projects. *Bottom:* The Leonard and Joan Horvitz Tower was made possible by longtime UH supporters, the Horvitz family.

were praised for their non-utilitarian appearance. Written accounts compared them to a deluxe hotel for the décor in the lobby, waiting areas, and private rooms; the oak-paneled library; and the presence of a beauty salon and barbershop, cafeteria, candy store, and newsstand. "The new Lakeside Hospital is de-institutionalized as far as possible," said Frank Chapman, Director. "We see strong therapeutic value in genial housing for patients, in a radio in each room, in garden picture wallpaper, in solariums, the walnut furniture, chintz upholstery, and ecru hangings."[24]

The campus skyline was once again dramatically altered with the completion of the Leonard and Joan Horvitz Tower, an eight-story addition that was constructed in front of the old Rainbow Babies and Childrens building and became its new "face." The 190-bed facility almost doubled the hospital's square footage and was considered among the most technologically-advanced and family-oriented in the nation when the ribbon was cut on April 5, 1997.

Many design ideas came from members of the Family Advisory Council, composed of young patients, their parents, and staff members who suggested ways to make the hospital a more pleasant and welcoming place. Single and double rooms replaced those meant for four. Parents could sleep near their children on pullout beds. There was an area for performances and parties. Counters were low enough to give kids a view over them. *The Plain Dealer* described it as "a friendly affirmative environment" embodying "the revolution sweeping health care facilities,

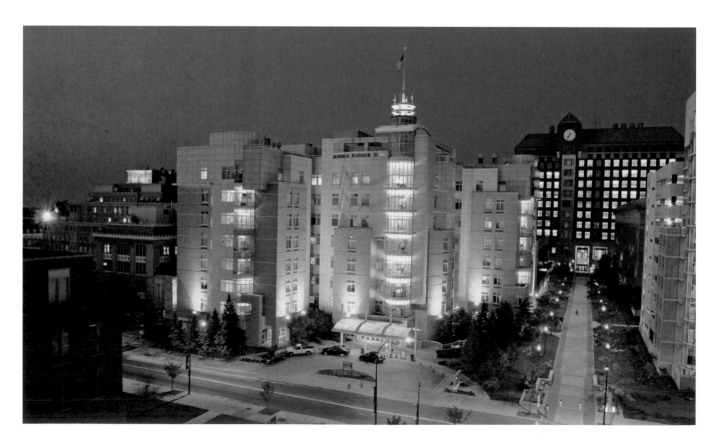

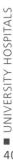

particularly children's hospitals" at that time. "The result is a building that tries to take the pain out of being in a place no one wants to go."[25]

Nancy Gorenshek, RN, got involved in planning and purchasing for Hanna House, Mather Pavilion, and the Lerner and Horvitz towers. "As assistant director of nursing for the med/surgical unit, I understood what patients needed as well as what was necessary for staff to do their jobs well." In 1898, the most common reason students at old Lakeside gave for dropping out of the nurse training program was that their feet hurt, and the situation had not improved much when Gorenshek wore a pedometer almost 100 years later. She discovered that during an eight-hour shift, she had covered 10 miles because of how inefficiently the floor was designed. "It was on Lakeside 20. The space was as big as a football field. You had to walk long distances just to get a patient their meds. There was a lot of wasted time." Gorenshek wanted to avoid that in the layout of these new facilities. "I worked with the architects on the final arrangement of certain spaces, negotiated with suppliers to allow personnel to use and evaluate products, and participated in the selection of furnishings."

Healing Environments for the 21st Century

Continuing the long tradition of investment in this community and in the people who live here is a measure of the organization's enduring belief in its future. Recent additions to the health system include University Hospitals Ahuja Medical Center in Beachwood. The main campus now includes the Center for Emergency Medicine and Marcy R. Horvitz Pediatric Emergency Center, the Quentin & Elisabeth Alexander Level IIIc Neonatal Intensive Care Unit inside University Hospitals Rainbow Babies & Children's Hospital, and University Hospitals Seidman Cancer Center, Northeast Ohio's first freestanding cancer hospital. All were part of Vision 2010, a five-year strategic plan to position the organization for the future. It represented a commitment to deliver the best and most advanced care to patients throughout Northeast Ohio and provide physicians, nurses, researchers, and technicians with model workplaces.

Sensitivity for the entire patient and staff experience informed the designs for UH Ahuja and UH

The Center for Emergency Medicine is a $41 million, 60,000-square-foot facility three times larger than the overcrowded one built in the 1970s that it replaced. It includes the Marcy R. Horvitz Pediatric Emergency Center and is the only Level I pediatric trauma center in the region.

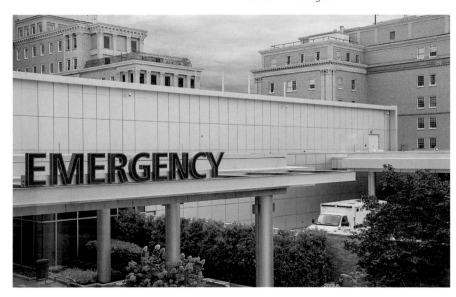

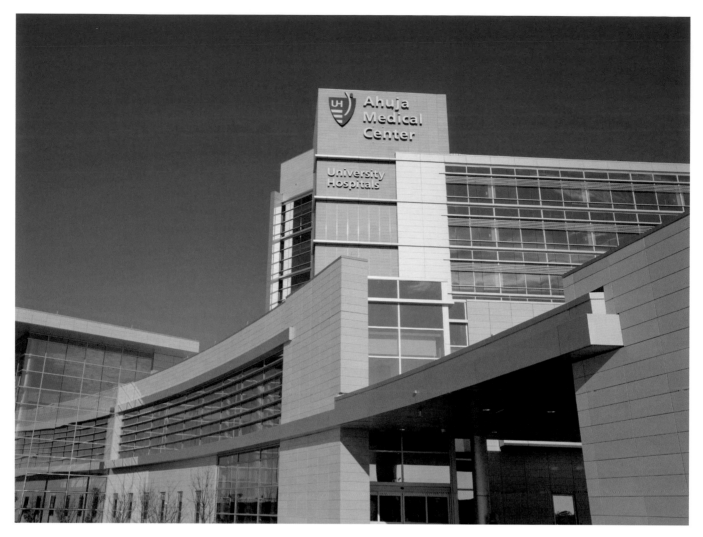

Situated on a 53-acre campus, the beautiful 60,000-square-foot University Hospitals Ahuja Medical Center consists of a seven-story hospital and Kathy Risman Pavilion for outpatient care. The pavilion was named in recognition of Bob, Eleanore, and Kathy Risman's contribution to advancing the goals of Vision 2010.

Seidman. Both opened in 2011, and both integrate the best, most sophisticated diagnostic and treatment technologies with a positive, people-focused atmosphere.

Winner of numerous design awards, UH Ahuja has been called "a true showpiece of modern architecture" that blends with masterfully landscaped grounds.[26] The medical center brings leading-edge diagnostic, treatment, and emergency services as well as preventive care, previously found only at University Hospitals Cleveland Medical Center, to Greater Cleveland's eastern suburbs. It is an outpost for clinical centers, including UH Harrington Heart & Vascular Institute, UH Neurological Institute, UH Digestive Health Institute, UH Urology Institute, and UH Seidman. The UH Fertility Center at UH Ahuja serves as the hub for fertility services throughout the system.

The Ahuja family's generosity played a key role in making much of this possible. In 2006, their $30 million contribution to University Hospitals' fundraising campaign was the largest single gift in the hospital's history. "I wish no one would have to go to the hospital," says Monte Ahuja. "But if you do, you won't find a better place in terms of quality, comfort, and care."

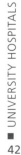

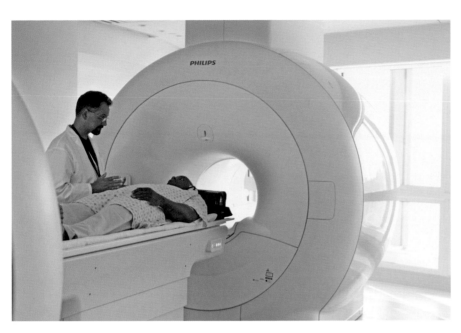

The Department of Radiology at University Hospitals Cleveland Medical Center partners with Philips Healthcare, which has one of its largest North American manufacturing facilities in Cleveland, to test some of the company's newest, most innovative imaging equipment such as this PET/MRI scanner.

UH Seidman is a 10-story hospital named in recognition of philanthropists Jane and Lee Seidman and their $42 million gift to Vision 2010. *U.S. News & World Report* ranks it among the top 50 hospitals in the country for cancer care. It was the first cancer hospital in the country to have an intraoperative MRI suite that provides surgeons with real-time images during procedures, contributing to better outcomes and reducing complications. It was also the first clinical setting in the United States and one of only four in the world to install a Philips PET/MRI (positron emission tomography/magnetic resonance imaging system) in a clinical setting. The technology generates enhanced digital images to pinpoint tumor locations more precisely than other diagnostic equipment.

"Our cancer care has always provided highly innovative treatment options in a context of patient-focused and compassionate care," says retired President of UH Seidman, Nathan Levitan, MD, "and with our new building, we've created an environment that is consonant with our model of care." Among the best features, notes Dr. Levitan, a hematology and oncology specialist, is that now all inpatient and outpatient cancer services are conveniently consolidated within a single facility with patient-care spaces that are comfortable and filled with natural light. Ann Pinkerton Ranney experienced the benefits of that environment firsthand. "When I was a patient at Seidman," said the Lifetime Trustee who served on the UH board and various committees for 28 years, "the most remarkable thing was the windows in my room. All that daylight pouring in made me feel so much better.

It's a Fact

George Crile, MD, who began his medical career at old Lakeside Hospital and became the hospital's Chief of Surgery, founded the Cleveland Clinic with three other physicians in 1921. The presence of both University Hospitals and Cleveland Clinic has transformed the city of Cleveland into a health care hub for the region, the country, and the world. Much is made of the rivalry between the two institutions. However, James Schulak, MD, a transplant surgeon who retired from UH in 2013, says, "Doctors at UH and the Clinic are great friends, often collaborating on both research projects and medical publications."

Former UH board chair Alfred Rankin Jr. is convinced the situation pushes both to be better and that is good for the city and all who live here. "The fact that we have these two institutions competing against each other has led to a determination by both of them to be very good. In addition, it has meant that there's enough scale that we've become a large research community in total."

The Case Comprehensive Cancer Center illustrates Rankin's view. This partnership supports cancer-related clinical research efforts at Case Western Reserve University where it is based, UH Cleveland Medical Center, and Cleveland Clinic. It is one of only 49 Comprehensive Cancer Centers in the nation designated by the National Cancer Institutes, and among 27 from this group elected to institutional membership in the National Comprehensive Cancer Network®, which sets standards for exceptional care, coordinated services, and guidelines for patient management.

Beds and Buildings Timeline

1868 Wilson Street Hospital opened on Cleveland's lakefront at Wilson Street near Clinton Street (later Davenport Street near East 18th Street).

1875 Wilson Street Hospital leased the Marine Hospital building on Erie Street (later East 9th Street) and Lake Street (later Lakeside Avenue). It operated as Cleveland City Hospital until 1888, when it was renamed Lakeside Hospital.

1891 Rainbow Cottage opened at East 105th Street and Lakeshore Boulevard in a rented farmhouse.

1891 Maternity Home of Cleveland, later named Maternity Hospital, opened at 58 Huron Road in downtown Cleveland.

1898 Lakeside Hospital reopened in a newly-constructed campus across the street from Marine Hospital on Lake Street between East 12th and East 14th streets.

1898 Maternity Hospital moved to a house at Carnegie Avenue (then called East Prospect) and East 65th Street.

1901 Rainbow Cottage moved to a new building in South Euclid, near the intersection of Richmond and Farnhurst roads.

1904 Rainbow Cottage was destroyed by a fire.

1905 Rainbow Cottage relocated to Green Road in South Euclid in the rented Novak Villa house and property.

1906 Maternity Hospital moved to a home on East 55th Street near Quincy Avenue.

1906 Infants' Clinic opened at the Central Friendly Inn at the corner of Broadway and Central Avenue (across the street from Progressive Field). The name soon changed to Babies' Dispensary and Hospital.

1907 Babies' Dispensary and Hospital relocated to 2500 East 35th Street, between Woodland and Scovill avenues.

1911 Babies' Dispensary and Hospital built a new facility on its existing property at East 35th Street.

1912 Maternity Hospital moved to a former sanitarium at 3765 Cedar Avenue.

1914 The new building for Rainbow Hospital for Crippled and Convalescent Children, formerly Rainbow Cottage, opened.

1925 Newly-built Babies and Childrens and Maternity hospitals opened as part of the new University Hospitals Medical Center campus.

1928 Rainbow Hospital for Crippled and Convalescent Children, informally referred to as "Rainbow Hospital" built a new facility on its South Euclid property.

1931 The "new" Lakeside Hospital opened in University Circle. Leonard C. Hanna House and the nursing dormitories opened.

1956 Howard M. Hanna Pavilion for psychiatric care opened.

1962 Joseph T. Wearn Laboratory for Medical Research opened.

1967 Robert H. Bishop Building opened.

1971 Rainbow Babies and Childrens Hospital opened. The former Rainbow Hospital property in South Euclid was later redeveloped into UH University Suburban Health Center.

1978 George M. Humphrey Building opened.

1984 University Hospitals Health Center opened; it was renamed the Harry J. Bolwell Health Center in 1986.

1994 Alfred and Norma Lerner Tower and the Samuel Mather Pavilion opened.

1997 Leonard and Joan Horvitz Tower of University Hospitals Rainbow Babies & Children's Hospital opened.

2003 Iris S. and Bert L. Wolstein Research Building opened as a joint project between University Hospitals and Case Western Reserve University.

2011 University Hospitals Ahuja Medical Center opened.

2011 University Hospitals Seidman Cancer Center opened.

2011 The Center for Emergency Medicine and the Marcy R. Horvitz Pediatric Emergency Center opened.

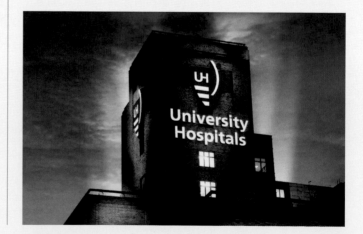

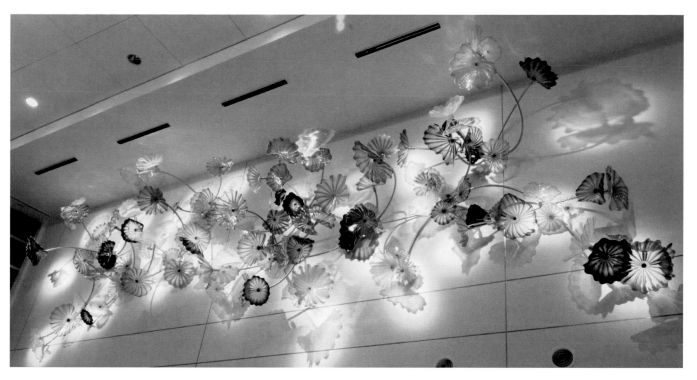

Six hundred works of art are prominently featured at both University Hospitals Seidman Cancer Center and University Hospitals Ahuja Medical Center. This 2010 installation by Dale Chihuly was commissioned specifically for UH Ahuja and is part of a 2,500-piece collection at University Hospitals begun by founding art curator Trudy Wiesenberger. Research shows that art-rich surroundings can enhance physical, mental, and emotional recovery, as well as improve workplace satisfaction.[27] Dale Chihuly, *Ahuja Azure, Citron and Amber Persian Wall*, 2010, 137 x 432 x 75", University Hospitals Ahuja Medical Center, Ohio.

I never planned to be there myself. But when I was, I realized just how important that feature is."

Another case in point is UH Seidman's Radiation Oncology Center. While it is located in a sub-basement area with lead-lined walls, the architects created a shaft that lets sunlight into the waiting area. It is the very opposite of what is expected in the anteroom of a place where people with cancer undergo advanced targeted procedures such as intraoperative radiation therapy, CyberKnife®, and Gamma Knife®.

Terryl Homes Koeth, MS, RN, former Director of Patient and Community Programs at UH Seidman, was Co-Chair of the Patient and Family Advisory Council. "We organized focus groups," she says, "to talk to people about what they felt was important and what should go in the new building. This approach is sweeping the country, but it is not new for UH. Rainbow Babies & Children's did it 20 years ago when we built Horvitz Tower."

These hospital buildings, old and new, serve as landmarks on people's personal journeys. They look at them and remember what happened there. "This is where my baby was born." "I had my operation here." "I got the good news there." "This is where my mother passed." "That was my room when I was sick." "This is where I worked for 25 years."

Mary Buell had a memory like that. She was diagnosed with a rare form of lymphoma when she was 30 and went through multiple rounds of chemotherapy and then a stem cell transplant. She spent a great deal of time at UH Seidman and grew close to the staff on her floor. She was there the day she turned 31 and feeling very down. "A nurse told me to get up out of bed and look out the window," she recalled. "All my caregivers—even those who had the day off—were lined up outside, in the rain, on the sidewalk, across the street. Each person was holding a sign with one letter on it. Together they spelled out 'Happy Birthday Mary.' Then they flipped them over, and the other side said 'Strong like Buell.' It was awesome." ▼

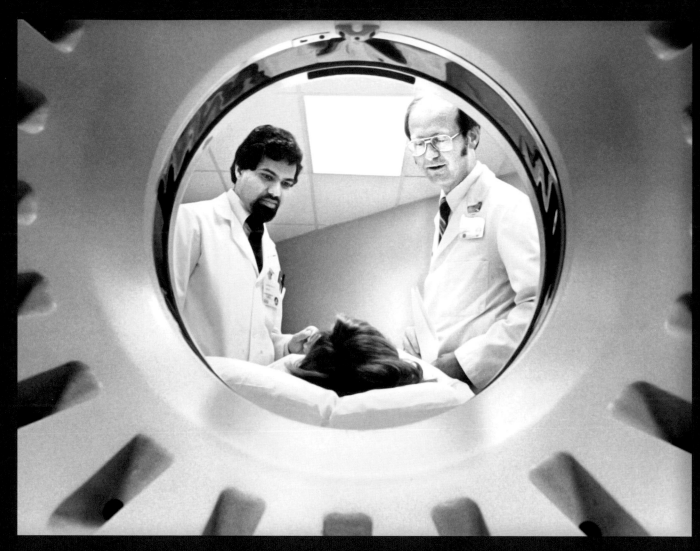

Interventional radiologist John Haaga, MD (right), and a colleague peer into a CT scanning machine in preparation for a pain relieving procedure, ca. 1980s. It is one of many image-guided therapies that have dramatically evolved over the years, often providing an alternative to surgery and new approaches for diagnosing, treating, and monitoring various conditions.

Purpose and Promise

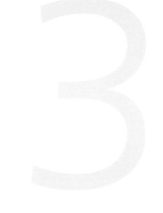

"We are always reflecting on how we can do better and give better care. When I look back at our history and our predecessors, they shared that same philosophy. We must ask ourselves, 'How do we evolve and change to do that?'"

– Patricia DePompei, MSN, RN, President, University Hospitals Rainbow Babies & Children's Hospital and University Hospitals MacDonald Women's Hospital

E rin Crane was pregnant when a large mass was discovered on her kidney. "The question was whether to wait until after I gave birth or have surgery right away," she explained. "There were risks associated with both options." She was seeing a urologist who had never done the procedure on a pregnant woman. "My husband and I were emotional wrecks. There were a lot of unknowns. We were scared and didn't know what to do." So the couple decided to get a second opinion. "We saw Dr. Lee Ponsky at University Hospitals. He was so reassuring and confident. Instead of focusing on the problem, the first thing he told us was that the baby and I were both going to be fine. He listed all the factors in our favor and explained what he could do." Dr. Ponsky, Director of the Urologic Oncology Center, successfully performed Crane's surgery laparoscopically through a small incision at 23 weeks. "It couldn't have gone better. I delivered a 9-pound 3-ounce girl at 39 weeks. Access to an expert was critical for us. I feel very lucky to have been his patient."

Techniques like the ones used to help Erin Crane reflect the great strides made in surgery over recent decades. Nothing even remotely similar to this was available or imaginable when Wilson Street Hospital opened in 1868. Crane's success story is one of thousands at UH. These triumphs, as well as the many unavoidable setbacks that were part of the

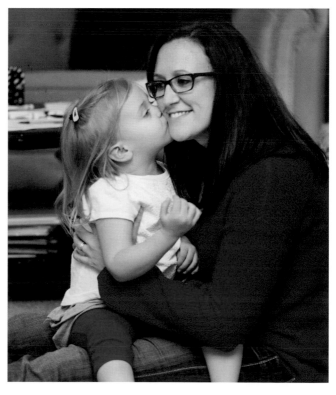

Erin Crane (right) enjoying a tender moment with her daughter, 2017.

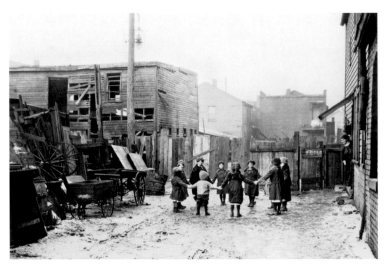

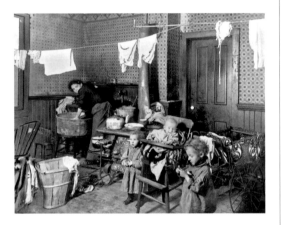

Dirty, overcrowded slums in Cleveland were ideal breeding grounds for communicable illnesses, ca. early 1900s.

An immigrant home in Cleveland, ca. early 1900s.

process necessary to achieve them, embody the essence of UH and all that it does. It is first and foremost an organization of people whose primary purpose is to diagnose and treat illnesses and injuries, alleviate suffering, repair defects, bring life into this world, and provide comfort for those who are at the end of it. While these are the primary functions of any hospital, UH has performed them exceptionally well for the last 150 years. Additionally, as an academic medical center, UH consistently integrates and adopts the best and latest advances in care. The hospital generates new knowledge by supporting those who push boundaries and explore the frontiers of medicine, and it teaches and trains others to become excellent clinicians, caregivers, and scientists. Together, these elements define UH and are the source of its strength as a medical institution and its stature in the community, the country, and the world.

The hospital was established in response to the city's pressing need for health care following the Civil War. Cleveland's population doubled from 1840 to 1850, doubled again from 1850 to 1860, and was in the process of doubling yet again by 1870. This dramatic growth, in combination with the rise of heavy industry during the Civil War, led to crowded and unsanitary living conditions. Among the ailments afflicting the 71 patients at Wilson Street in its first year were diseases such as tuberculosis, dysentery, and rheumatic fever, which flourished in this environment. Patients who could afford it received private care at home, and because doctors had few effective treatments or tools at their disposal at this time, hospitals were typically viewed as places where poor people went to die. However, as scientific and technical advances improved medical care, people began to view hospitals in a positive light. Reviewing Lakeside Hospital's performance in 1900, *The Plain Dealer* commented, "The dread of hospitals felt a dozen years ago by the most intelligent people is being rapidly broken down. People realize the benefits to be obtained by hospital treatment, and those who would once have shuddered at the mere thought of ever being sent to such a place are apt to say, 'When I'm sick just send me to a hospital. They know how to look after people there.'"[1]

In the 1900s, the medical staff at old Lakeside was organized into four departments: medical, surgical, gynecological, and pathology. Today, UH has more than 20 departments, more than a dozen cross-disciplinary institutes, and more than 70 medical and surgical specialties ranging from allergy and immunology to urology. Physicians treat every part of the human body and functional system from head to toe and from heart to mind. No single history of the organization can give each division its due,

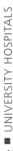

acknowledge every outstanding physician who has practiced at UH, or mention all the pioneering achievements during the past 150 years. What ties the specialties together is the incredible progress that has been made at UH to improve the practice and delivery of medicine. Some highlights from that history serve as a representation for all of the fields where UH has excelled, innovated, and made significant contributions.

Moving the Needle: Kidney Transplants

Organ transplants are fairly common procedures today, with tens of thousands of transplants taking place annually, but that is primarily due to the decades of research and experimental surgeries that led to today's successful outcomes. The first kidney transplant performed at University Hospitals in 1958 by surgeons Charles Hubay, MD, and Lester Persky, MD, was a last-resort, emergency procedure to save a child's life. At the time, there had been only five successful kidney transplants in the country, and those were cases where an identical twin sibling was the donor, making organ rejection less likely to occur. The procedure performed at UH was extremely experimental. Sadly, it was not successful, and the child did not survive. At that time, doctors still did not fully comprehend the workings of the body's immune system, and it would take years of research to better understand the mechanism of organ rejection and develop the necessary immunosuppressant drugs and surgical techniques to improve survival rates.

The formal kidney transplant program at UH began in 1968, and by 1970, nine kidney transplants had been performed, with five more people waiting for donor organs. The following year, the UH transplant team, using the first kidney donation to cross international borders, gave a little Cleveland girl a second chance.

Delphine Lamb's kidneys had begun to fail when she was 2½ years old. By the time she was 11, her kidneys had been removed, and she needed dialysis at UH three times a week, where she was hooked up to a machine for eight hours each visit. On December 22, 1971, her parents received a phone call telling them to bring their daughter to the hospital because a suitable donor organ had been found. The kidney came from a Toronto teen killed in an accident. That tragedy became an early surprise Christmas gift for Lamb and her family. The surgery took three hours, and she returned home on January 7. The surgery led to a good outcome for Delphine, giving her an additional 25 years of life. Inspired by their good fortune, her parents registered to be organ donors.[2]

Another successful transplant recipient, Harry Vincent, made a full recovery after his kidney transplant at UH in 1973. Three years later, he rode his bicycle 1,000 miles from Cleveland to Cincinnati and back

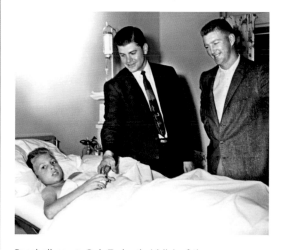

Baseball greats Bob Turley (middle) of the New York Yankees and Herb Score (right) of the Cleveland Indians visited the first kidney transplant recipient in Cleveland in 1958. Score was a patient at University Hospitals in 1957 when he was hit in the eye by a line drive off the bat of a New York Yankees hitter and immediately taken to Lakeside Hospital.

From Flu to AIDS: Responding to Epidemics

Highly contagious diseases were rampant in American cities in the late 19th and early 20th centuries. Scarlet fever, measles, and tuberculosis posed serious challenges to hospitals because controlling the spread of infection was difficult. Cleveland experienced an outbreak of smallpox that began in 1898, causing citywide panic. The smallpox vaccine administered at the onset of the epidemic was discovered to be impure and not entirely effective, creating public distrust and fear of the vaccine. The city was left to respond to the crisis by isolating victims and disinfecting their homes. When it was discovered that a woman admitted to Lakeside Hospital had smallpox, she was immediately quarantined until she could be moved to what was commonly referred to as "the pest house." Following her departure, "[t]here was a grand cleaning out in the ward after Mrs. Windbush was taken away. Nurses and doctors hurried to and fro squirting formaldehyde around promiscuously."[3] A student nurse at Lakeside made headlines when she volunteered to care for a smallpox patient and died several weeks after contracting the disease.[4] In 1902, at the peak of the epidemic with 1,248 identified cases, the city was finally able to secure a safe and effective vaccination campaign, and by 1905, there were zero cases of smallpox in Cleveland.[5]

An influenza pandemic in 1918 caused tens of millions of deaths across the globe, more than the total number killed in World War I. Despite bans on public gatherings and quarantines, it proved almost unstoppable, ultimately affecting a fifth of the world's population. The virus spread through Cleveland's communities in little more than two months, leaving behind a death rate higher than that of New York City or Chicago. From late September 1918 to February 1919, 3.5 percent of the city's population contracted influenza, and many of them further developed pneumonia. Of those infected, 16 percent died.[6]

To accommodate the large number of sick individuals, Lakeside converted numerous areas into isolation wards for influenza cases, including a separate one just for staff members who fell ill. By January 1, 1919, Lakeside had admitted 573 influenza cases, and 131 of those patients died from influenza or from associated complications. During the crisis, the hospital superintendent received a letter from the Red Cross Influenza Committee stating that Lakeside had done more than any other local hospital to meet the needs of the community.[7]

Another epidemic occurred in 1921, afflicting Clevelanders with an outbreak of diphtheria, a bacterial infection spread

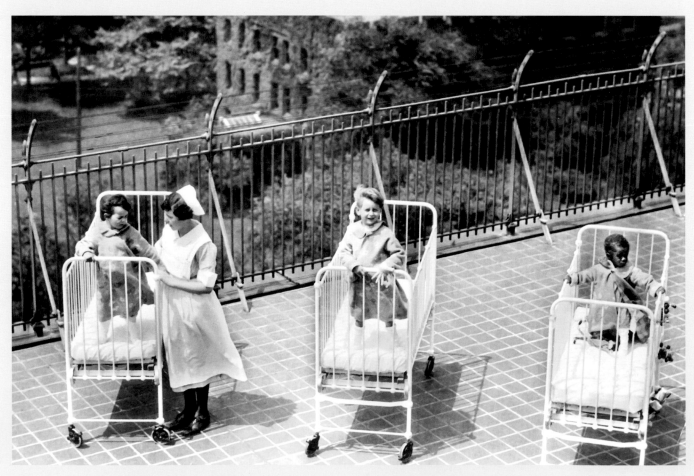

Tuberculosis ward on the rooftop of Babies and Childrens Hospital, ca. mid–late 1920s.

through personal contact. Children were more susceptible to contracting diphtheria, and one in every 10 children infected with the disease died.[8] In response, Babies' Dispensary and Hospital launched a massive effort to vaccinate Cleveland children ages 6 months to 6 years for free. The public was still suspicious of vaccines, despite the fact that they had almost completely eradicated smallpox in the previous decade, and the campaign required outreach to parents about the benefits of immunization. The effort proved to be very successful. "Prevention through vaccination is declared by Dr. Robert Lockhart, [Cuyahoga] county health officer, to be responsible for the low death rate among persons suffering from diphtheria in the year ended Oct. 1, 1921."[9]

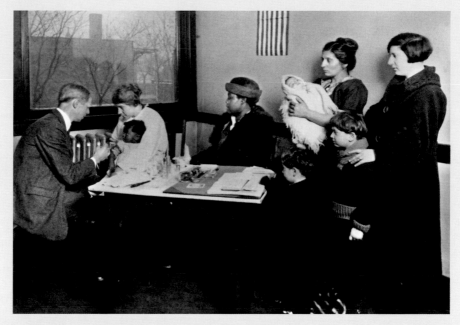

Babies' Dispensary and Hospital organized a city-wide campaign promoting the importance of vaccinations against diphtheria, 1921.

In modern times, acquired immune deficiency syndrome, more commonly referred to as AIDS, became the focus of many infectious disease experts at University Hospitals. In 1983, Michael Lederman, MD, now Associate Director of the Center for AIDS Research at UH, and Oscar Ratnoff, MD, longtime Chief of Hematology and Oncology, identified that the risk of AIDS-related immune deficiency in otherwise healthy men with hemophilia was due to the transmission of contaminated blood. As the number of Clevelanders infected with human immunodeficiency virus (HIV) grew, a special immunology unit was established at UH in 1985 to meet their primary care needs. It was the first comprehensive HIV clinic in Ohio and one of the first in the Midwest to combine clinical care with HIV research. In the ensuing decades, Dr. Lederman made other important discoveries that contributed to a better understanding of the disease and the effectiveness of specific therapies.

Renamed the John T. Carey Special Immunology Unit in 1997 in memory of its former director, the clinic provided primary medical services to the growing number of Clevelanders with HIV infection. One physician remembered the compassion UH staff brought to the task: "I was a medical student and resident in the late '80s and early '90s at the height of the 'AIDS scare.' Our floors were filled with patients with many opportunistic infections, and we all struggled to care for them with the limited resources we had. Not many patients survived those times, but I hope we made their suffering a little more tolerable. I remember one particular patient who seemed to have a new AIDS-related syndrome weekly. I would just sit, talk to him, and hold his hand. He continually expressed his gratitude

that we did not treat him as a 'disease' or a leper. He saw that we all knew he was a human first and treated him accordingly."[10]

UH's effort to confront the AIDS epidemic was facilitated by important research partnerships established in 1987. UH and Case Western Reserve University became founding members of the AIDS Clinical Trials Unit (ACTU). Sponsored by the National Institutes of Health, it was, at the time, the world's largest network of AIDS-related clinical trials. Through this ACTU membership, UH scientists have access to the Microbicide Trials Network, which works to provide new prevention tools for HIV-negative people who are at risk for infection. Additionally, UH and Case Western Reserve University joined forces with Makerere University in Uganda to conduct AIDS research and provide patient care. The partnership helped drive Uganda's leadership response to the emerging AIDS epidemic in Africa.

Grace McComsey, MD, Medical Director of Clinical Research Unit Services and Division Chief of Pediatric Infectious Diseases and Rheumatology at University Hospitals Cleveland Medical Center, and Associate Chief Scientific Officer for the UH system, studies the impact of the disease and HIV therapies on children, a group that has received less attention than adults have. A vocal advocate of the benefits of early screening and treatment, especially for infants, she pursued the field due to experiences she had early on in her career. "During my training, we lost five HIV kids. One was a 10-year-old. I saw him wasting and wasting and then dying. He was a hemophiliac and got [AIDS] through a blood transfusion. It just broke my heart…I wanted to make a difference."[11]

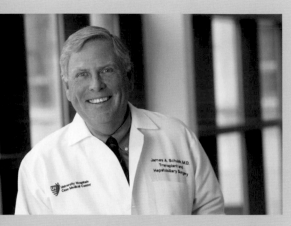

Transplant surgeon James Schulak, MD, 2013.

Pioneer

Nationally-esteemed abdominal transplant surgeon James Schulak, MD, joined the staff at University Hospitals in 1985 and played a leading role in expanding kidney transplantation and establishing new transplant programs for the liver and the pancreas as the Director of the Transplant Institute. He performed the first triple-organ transplant in Ohio in 1991 on a 38-year-old patient with cystic fibrosis. The patient was dying of liver disease, undergoing dialysis for kidney failure, and had diabetes. Other physicians thought he was too sick to undergo the procedure. After determining the young man's lungs were healthy enough to survive at least another five years, Dr. Schulak decided to perform the surgery, which took 12 hours. Approximately 10 years later, the patient's first kidney transplant failed, and Dr. Schulak performed a second kidney transplant, which functioned normally until the patient's death, 17 years after the original transplant operation. Now retired, Dr. Schulak oversaw more than 3,000 abdominal organ transplants during his 28-year career.

to increase awareness of the need for organ donation and demonstrate the success of the procedure. The trip, dubbed "Recycle Yourself," included three other cyclists and took four weeks to complete. Vincent received another kidney transplant in 1984 and continued to bicycle; in 1996, he bicycled from Los Angeles to Baltimore, and in 1998, he pedaled to Columbus to take part in the 1998 U.S. Transplant Games. He also bicycled daily to his job. After earning a nursing degree in 1985, he became a nurse practitioner at UH, where he worked until he died in 2005.[12]

By the end of 1998, 1,271 kidney transplants had been performed at UH, and surgeons were also transplanting the heart, pancreas, liver, and lungs in both adults and children. In 1999, UH performed the first live-donor pediatric liver transplant in northern Ohio utilizing a partial liver graft donated by a mother to her ill daughter. Additionally, the transplant team, led at the time by Christopher Siegel, MD, PhD, conducted Ohio's first "Domino" liver transplant, a rare type of transplant in which a person with familial amyloidosis, a life-threatening enzyme defect, donated their otherwise healthy liver and in turn received a liver from a deceased donor, thus saving two lives. Today, all of the solid-organ transplant programs are part of the University Hospitals Transplant Institute.

Moving the Needle: Diabetes

Among the top 10 causes of death in the United States, diabetes is unfortunately on the rise in the American populace. University Hospitals has been helping people with this chronic condition to live longer, healthier lives since the early 1920s when insulin was first accepted as an effective treatment. Lakeside Hospital was among a select group of hospitals around the country to receive a grant from the Rockefeller Institute for Medical Research to cover the cost of insulin for patients unable to pay for it and educate physicians on the value of the new drug and how to use it. The $10,000 award made front-page news in *The Plain Dealer* on June 20, 1923.

UH physicians have been actively engaged in research in this emerging field, improving care for those suffering from the chronic condition in the decades that followed. The hospital participated in a national study launched in 1960 called the University Group Diabetes Program under the leadership of Max Miller, MD, then Program Director of the UH Clinical Research Center. It was among the earliest randomized multicenter clinical trials to determine whether lowering blood sugar in diabetic patients would protect against the serious complications of the disease. Dr. Miller was also a contributor to

Progress

Improvements in health care have been steady but unpredictable, ranging from slow and almost imperceptible advances to astounding and seemingly sudden leaps forward. Every new idea did not prove to be as beneficial as its proponents hoped, sending physician-scientists and educators back to the drawing board. But cumulatively, the steady medical triumphs of the past 150 years have increased not only the human lifespan, but also the quality of life for everyone. University Hospitals has been at the forefront of these changes throughout its history. How UH can best help those in need was—and remains—a constantly evolving paradigm.

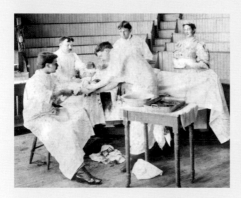
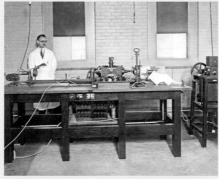
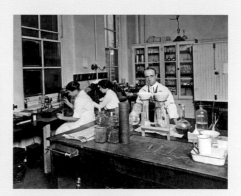
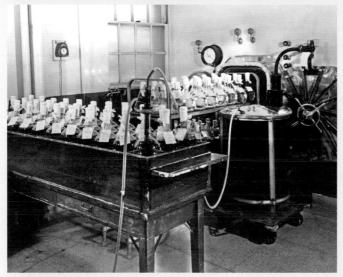
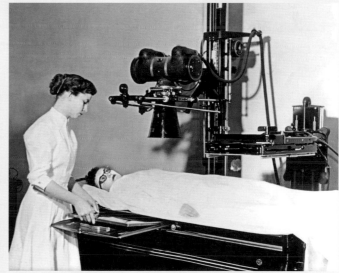
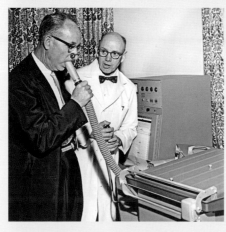
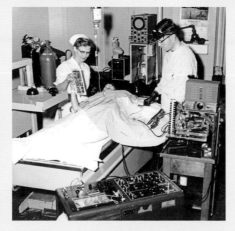
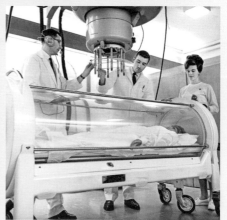

Top row: (left) Earliest known photo of an operating room at Lakeside Hospital, 1895; *(middle)* This electrocardiogram was at the leading edge of technology, ca. 1910s; *(right)* Old Lakeside Hospital pathology laboratory, ca. 1920s.
Middle row: (left) Anesthesiology instruments at Lakeside Hospital, ca. 1930s; *(right)* X-ray equipment, ca. 1940s.
Bottom row: (left) Cardiology heart testing equipment, ca. 1950s; *(middle)* First cardiac catheterization unit at Lakeside Hospital, 1955; *(right)* Radiology hyperbaric chamber, 1967.

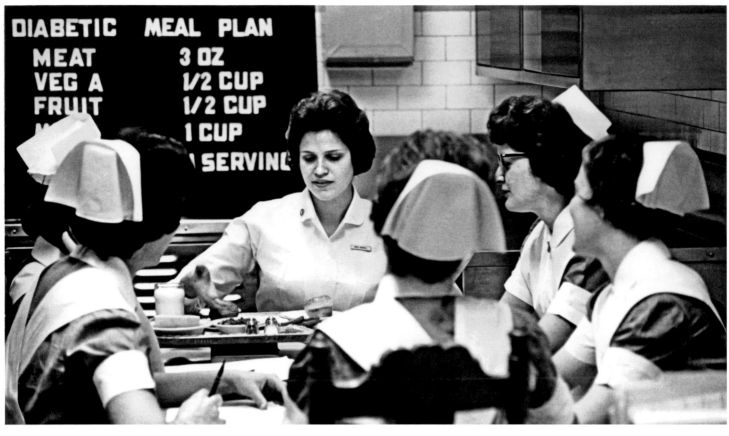

Diabetic meal planning, ca. 1960s.

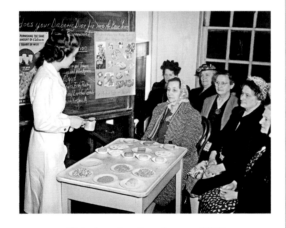

Diabetes education class, ca. 1940s.

studies that were among the first to demonstrate that obesity was a primary risk factor for type 2 diabetes when he observed extremely high insulin levels in many of his obese patients. In 1965, UH was awarded a grant from the U.S. Public Health Service to fund a project undertaken jointly by the hospital's medicine, nursing, and dietary staff focused on programmed instruction for diabetic patients that included education about their disease, treatment, and how to care for themselves. In 1967, Babies and Childrens Hospital began holding classes for parents of diabetic children, teaching them how to administer insulin injections, manage diets, and provide their youngsters with emotional as well as practical support.

Research conducted in the 1970s by biochemist Bernard Landau, MD, Chair of the Endocrinology Division at UH, furthered the understanding of diabetes and how to manage it by demonstrating a link between appetite, obesity, and insulin resistance in humans. Diabetes research at UH received a boost in 1973 with a $500,000 gift from Mary Blossom Lee, daughter of former UH board member Dudley Blossom, who had lived with diabetes since early childhood and had supported diabetes research around the country for decades. In 2000, the UH Board established the Mary Blossom Lee Chair to advance medical research on the causes, treatment, and consequences of diabetes.

The Diabetes Control and Complications Trial (DCCT), launched by the U.S. National Institute of Diabetes and Digestive and Kidney

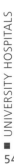

Diseases, ran from 1983 to 1993. UH participated in this landmark clinical trial across the United States and Canada that ultimately showed for the first time that lowering blood sugar in type 1 diabetes significantly lowered the risk of developing diabetes-related vision problems, kidney failure, and nerve damage. Paul McGuigan became a study participant in 1986, two years after he was diagnosed with type 1 diabetes. His experience inspired McGuigan, who had a painting company at the time, to enroll in nursing school. "When I finished, Dr. William Dahms, one of the [endocrinology] doctors who followed me in the study, asked me to cover for a UH nurse on maternity leave. I'm still at UH coordinating research studies in pediatric endocrinology."

UH endocrinologist Saul Genuth, MD, played a leadership role in the DCCT as study-wide co-chair and in an extension study called the Epidemiology of Diabetes Interventions and Complications (EDIC), which began in 1994 and is still ongoing. University Hospitals Rainbow Babies & Children's Hospital is the national coordinating center for the project. Findings from the study confirmed that lowering blood sugar prevents heart attacks and strokes and established that after 6.5 years of intensive blood sugar control, individuals are protected against heart attacks and other complications for at least another 18 years and most recently, that overall mortality with intensive therapy was similar to the general population.

In 2016, UH pediatric endocrinologist Rose Gubitosi-Klug, MD, PhD, who currently serves as lead investigator of the ongoing study, authored a review of 30 years' worth of findings from the combined DCCT/EDIC studies. The data provided significant insights about type 1 diabetes and the long-term complications associated with it, emphasizing current standards and guidelines for treating patients with the disease.[13]

In 1971, Chair of Orthopedic Surgery, Charles Herndon, MD, the first full-time orthopedic surgeon at University Hospitals, and the orthopedic surgical team worked with the Construction and Planning Department to create a bio-clean operating enclosure dubbed the "glass house" to reduce the risk of infection during joint replacement surgery. It was installed in an operating suite at Lakeside Hospital. Special attire designed and made by Sewing Room staff, including helmets covered by hoods with a clear, plastic faceplate, was worn. The helmets were equipped with earphones, a vacuum system for exhaled air, and transmitters.

Moving the Needle: Hip Replacements

Hip replacements have been one of the most common orthopedic surgeries performed at University Hospitals for more than four decades, largely due to the development of safe and durable prostheses. Charles Herndon, MD, who became chair of the Department of Orthopedics in 1953, performed the first total hip replacement at UH in 1970.

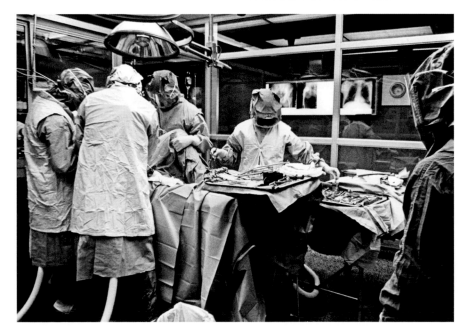

One-time orthopedic patient Jean Garbett (shown above in 1973 and below today) is also a volunteer veteran of 42 years having logged the most donated hours in the history of University Hospitals. In her 80s, she continues to volunteer at the hospital twice a week. She was the inaugural recipient of a new service award named in her honor in 2014.

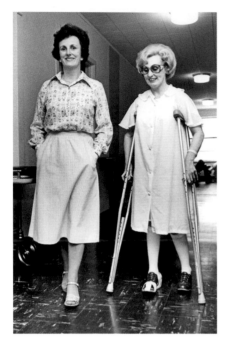

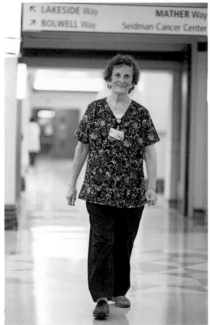

Jean Garbett became part of the joint replacement revolution after traditional surgical repair of both of her hips at UH failed. The 37-year-old homemaker and mother of two had spent five months in the hospital recovering from that first surgery. "They finally sent me home in January 1971 with a wheelchair and crutches," she recalls. "I was completely unable to walk on my own."

A few months later, she elected to have total hip replacement surgery and was among the first 100 people to receive the procedure at UH. Orthopedic surgeon John Makley, MD, performed the surgery, which was a resounding success. Garbett got back on her feet and has not slowed down since. She has volunteered at UH for more than four decades, visiting patients to tell her story. "When I started, very few people had the surgery," she states. "Because I had been through it and everything turned out so well, I could ease their concerns before and after the operation."

In the past 10 years, minimally invasive technology has transformed virtually every aspect of hip replacement surgery. Cathy Peltz was a beneficiary of these improvements. In 2016, she had her hip replaced with only a three-inch incision at University Hospitals Elyria Medical Center where she works in Information Services. The 62-year-old went home two days after her surgery and returned to work four weeks later. William Stanfield, MD, was her surgeon.

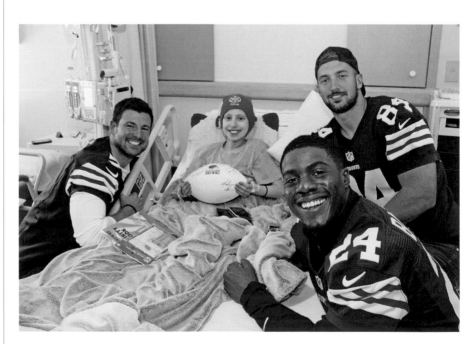

For years, visits from Cleveland's professional athletes have raised the spirits of children at University Hospitals Rainbow Babies & Children's Hospital. In 2014, University Hospitals became the official health care provider for the Cleveland Browns with James Voos, MD, as head team physician. Dr. Voos also serves as Chairman of the Department of Orthopedics and the Jack and Mary Herrick Endowed Director of Sports Medicine, an expanding specialty that includes performance enhancement for players; injury prevention; and treatment, nutrition, sleep, cardio-fitness, and concussion care. "Our sports programs are developed at the professional level and then translated to youth athletes so they experience the same benefit and expertise as the pros," says Dr. Voos.

When he completed his orthopedic training in 1997, hip replacement patients typically spent five days in the hospital followed by inpatient rehabilitation in a nursing home. At the time, most hip replacements involved a 10- to 12-inch incision. "My attending physicians taught me to make as big an incision as needed," explained Dr. Stanfield, as larger incisions made it easier to place the new hip. With today's minimally invasive approach, there is less damage to the muscles and soft tissue, allowing for "earlier mobilization, improved outcomes, and less pain."

Peltz's speedy recovery was enhanced by her participation in a program offered through the hospital's Center for Bone & Joint Reconstruction. Nicknamed "Joint Camp," it is a team approach to care and wellness before and after surgery. Patients are part of small groups that support each other from pre-op to post-surgical rehabilitation. Peltz received her outpatient physical therapy at Rehabilitation Services & Sports Medicine at University Hospitals Avon Health Center.

Moving the Needle: Cochlear Implants

Severe or profound hearing loss affects more than two million people in the United States. For most, the condition is the result of degeneration or malfunction of sensory cells in the cochlea (inner ear) due to illness, injury, or hereditary factors. Traditional hearing aids, which amplify sound, cannot help under these conditions. However, a medical device called a cochlear implant can help because it bypasses the damaged portion of the inner ear, stimulating the auditory nerve electronically so it can provide sound signals to the brain. It cannot fully reproduce normal sound, but the brain adapts with time and rehabilitation. Recipients experience improvement in understanding speech and speaking capability.

As a sophomore in high school in the mid-1990s, Ryan Lekan developed Ménière's disease, a chronic inner ear problem, and with it, moderate hearing loss. Despite this impediment, he graduated from high school, earned a teaching degree and a master's in educational technology, got married, and had two children. Around 2005, a second flare-up led to the loss of almost all hearing in one ear, and Lekan had to trade his teaching job for an administrative position. By 2010, he was nearly deaf. "I couldn't hear the TV. I couldn't hear my kids. Basic conversation was a struggle. At family parties, I'd surf on my smartphone to avoid conversation. I felt miserable and excluded from the world."

At the recommendation of Cliff Megerian, MD, former Chairman, Department of Otolaryngology Head and Neck Surgery, and Chair, Auditory Surgery and Hearing Sciences, Lekan underwent cochlear

It's a Fact

The cochlear implant program at University Hospitals focused on children when it began in 1995, but within two years the procedure was also available to adults. In 2011, 75 cochlear implant recipients attended a concert at Severance Hall performed by students from the Cleveland Institute of Music to mark the 600th cochlear implant performed at the hospital. Some youngsters in the audience had never heard live music before. The evening was titled, "A Celebration of Hearing with an Evening of Music."

Life-Changing Stories

Furthering medical progress to improve patients' lives is the hallmark of University Hospitals. Patients come to UH every day and put their trust in the skill of its physicians, nurses, and staff. It is these stories that best reinforce UH's reputation for excellence, with patients often going home much better off than when they arrived.

• • •

Gabriela Hubbard was only 3 years old in 1995 when doctors at Rainbow Babies and Childrens Hospital told her parents she was suffering from ALL—acute lymphoblastic leukemia. It is a fast-spreading cancer that produces rapid and abnormal growth of white blood cells. The diagnosis was the start of two years of tests, transfusions, chemotherapy, doctors' appointments, and hospitalizations.

"We spent many nights in the hospital. It was practically my first home. I finally completed treatment while I was in kindergarten," says Hubbard. Other kids, she recalls, had their favorite doll or toy for show-and-tell, but not Hubbard. "I brought in my Broviac [a type of catheter]." But, it wasn't all hardship and misery. "I got to meet Miss USA and wear her crown, I met Celine Dion, and I represented Ohio for

Children's Miracle Network. Not many 5 year-olds can say the same. I attended many telethons and even made commercials for Rainbow."

According to John Letterio, MD, Division Chief, Pediatric Hematology and Oncology at University Hospitals Rainbow Babies & Children's Hospital, a child diagnosed with this disease in 1960 had a less than 10 percent chance of being a long-term survivor. Today, the survival rate for children with standard risk ALL is 98 percent. "To see that kind of success is amazing," he says. "This disease was once almost incurable in every case, and now, we tell parents that their child will likely go on to live a happy life."

In the intervening years, doctors learned a great deal about this type of cancer, which has many sub-types, and the most effective forms of treatment to put it in remission and prevent recurrence.

Hubbard's recovery was complete and lasting, and the experience of being a UH patient at such a young age had a significant impact on her, too. "At the age of 22," she reports, "I graduated from Cleveland State with a bachelor's degree in health science and landed my first job at University Hospitals Seidman Cancer Center. I guess it was just meant to be."

• • •

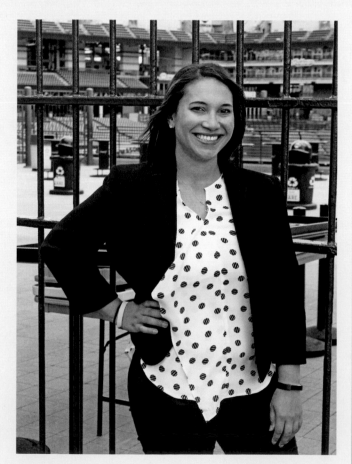

Gabriela Hubbard, 2017.

Julie and Chris Ilcin knew before they were married that the possibility of having a baby was slim because of earlier gynecological problems Julie had experienced with endometriosis, a common cause of infertility where endometrial tissue grows outside of the uterus. In 2006, their desire to have a family brought them to the University Hospitals infertility program where the couple was advised that their best option would be to use an egg donor. Julie's sister agreed to fill that role under the care of James Liu, MD, Chairman of Obstetrics and Gynecology.

After two complicated pregnancies, both resulting in the loss of the baby, Julie gave birth to a beautiful daughter in 2010. The baby spent a few days in the hospital and went home with her parents on February 14. "She was the best Valentine's gift I could ever receive," said Julie.

As recently as 40 years ago, the Ilcins' happy ending would not have been possible. The first baby conceived through in-vitro fertilization (IVF) in the United States was born in 1981 and created a sensation across the country. UH played a part in growing this rapidly changing field of medicine. James Goldfarb, MD, Director of University Hospitals Fertility Center, first came to UH in 1973 to complete his medical training and, while working at other area hospitals, is credited

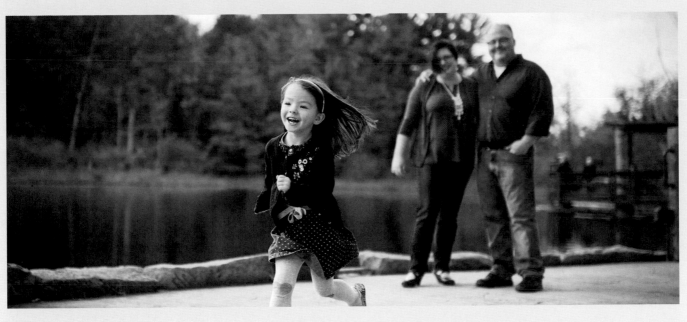

The Ilcins with their daughter, 2014.

with achieving Ohio's first birth via IVF in 1983 and the world's first surrogate IVF birth in 1986. Dr. Goldfarb returned to UH in 1989 and again in 2010 in his current role.

Landmark achievements like these are part of the extraordinary story of modern medical innovation, but for the Ilcins and the many other couples who come to UH for assistance, it is personal. "The doctors here gave us our family. They were 100 percent part of the journey, not just the outcome," said Julie.

• • •

Gayle Waxon endured debilitating seizures for 25 years beginning when she was 19. The seizures became more frequent as she got older, sometimes occurring twice a month or as frequently as four times a day. Waxon once had an episode while driving and lost control of her car. Her husband and children worried about her constantly. "I tried every medication available," Waxon recalls, "and had seen numerous specialists who could not pinpoint the exact part of the brain where the seizures originated."

In 2010, an MRI finally revealed pea-sized tumors in her brain, but she was warned that the surgery to remove them could leave her with permanent memory loss or the inability to speak, so she did nothing. There were no other options for Waxon until she read about a very different kind of brain surgery being performed at University Hospitals called multiple hippocampal transection. A series of very small, shallow cuts are made in the left temporal lobe. The technique severs the seizure-producing circuits without disrupting the neural pathways related to memory and speech.

At the time, UH was the only hospital in the United States where the procedure, brought from Japan by Hans

Lüders, MD, PhD, then Director of the Epilepsy Center, and neurosurgeon Robert Maciunas, MD, was available. Waxon contacted Dr. Lüders, and he introduced her to a man who had undergone the procedure. "After talking to him about his experience, I said, 'Sign me up!'"

Following extensive assessment, Waxon was deemed a good candidate for the procedure. Jonathan Miller, MD, Director, Functional & Restorative Neurosurgery Center, performed her surgery in October 2011. Waxon's seizures have since dramatically decreased, and she did not suffer from neural deficits as a result of the operation. "I'm a new Gayle, a new mom, a better wife, and a different person," she said. "I can do anything I want. Every time I think about UH and what the doctors did for me, I smile."

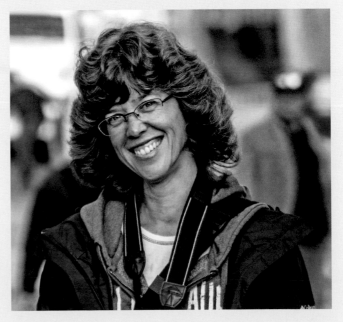

Gayle Waxon, 2012.

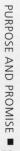

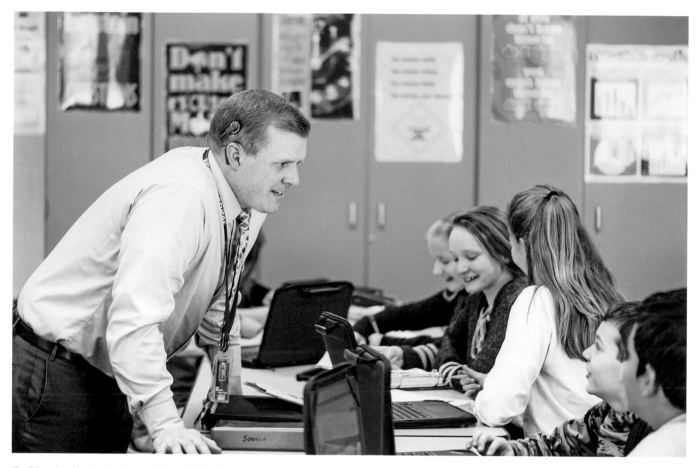

Cochlear implant patient Ryan Lekan, 2016. Ryan received an implant in his other ear in 2018.

implantation. He describes the activation of the device as "amazing." While his hearing is not 100 percent, it is greatly improved. He can communicate with his family and friends again and no longer feels isolated.

"I often wonder why I had any doubts about having the surgery. My hearing aids were frustrating and didn't sound as full as my cochlear implant. And, with the new advances in cochlear technology, I can wirelessly stream music, phone conversations, and TV. It's amazing," says Lekan.

Dr. Megerian, who currently serves as the President of UH Physician Network and System Institutes, is a nationally-recognized leader in the use of cochlear implants to treat hearing-impaired children. He was a driving force in establishing the Cochlear Implant Program at University Hospitals Rainbow Babies & Children's Hospital. In 2012, University Hospitals Ear, Nose & Throat Institute established an Audiology & Cochlear Implant Center which quickly became one of the world's foremost facilities for treating hearing-impaired

children and adults. In 2016, UH specialists implanted their 1,000th cochlear device.

John McGinty received one for his right ear in 2003 when he was 16 and a second one for his left ear in 2008. "When I first met Dr. Megerian," recalls McGinty, "he said I was a good candidate for this approach." While an implant could not restore full and normal function, it would allow him to hear specific sounds, consonants, and letter combinations and improve his ability to understand what people around him were saying.

"At first it was confusing," says McGinty. "It took a year of working with speech therapists and audiology specialists at UH to be able to distinguish one kind of sound from another and interpret what I was hearing." As much as he appreciates the chance to be a hearing person, McGinty also likes that the implant can be turned off as well. "I can opt into deafness. Silence can be a beautiful thing, too. Now, I have the best of both worlds."

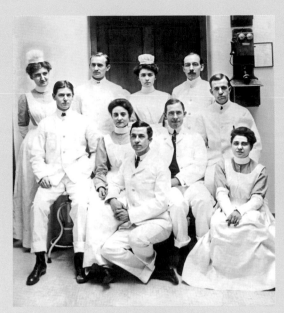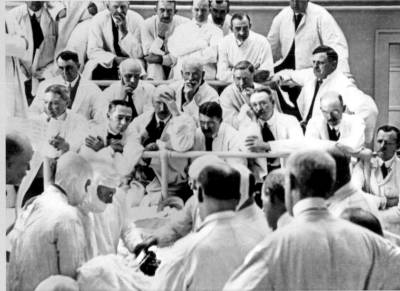

Left: Clinical investigation and teaching has been highly valued throughout University Hospitals' history. Medical students were taught by visiting staff on the faculty at Western Reserve Medical College, ca. 1900s. *Right:* Lakeside Hospital's large surgical amphitheater, one of the few of its kind in the country at the time, accommodated 250 students who could observe surgical procedures, ca. early 1900s.

Fulfilling the Promise: Educating the Next Generation

Teaching the next generation of health care providers is fundamental to the identity of an academic medical center and has been a defining force in the history of University Hospitals. It began with a relationship established between Lakeside Hospital and the Medical Department of Western Reserve University in the hospital's earliest days and has endured and evolved into the 21st century. John Morley, a UH lifetime trustee, observed that "there continues to be a great deal of synergy between the school and the hospital, and we will build on that for the future."

The collaboration between the hospital and the medical school began shortly after Wilson Street Hospital opened. Following the hospital's brief closure in 1868 because of a dispute among physicians, faculty members from the Medical Department at Western Reserve College were brought in by Hinman Hurlbut, president of the Wilson Street Hospital Board. Their students joined them soon after, and this arrangement continued and expanded when the move was made to the U.S. Marine Hospital property. Hinman Hurlbut then donated the funds to build an operating theater where

physicians could demonstrate surgical techniques to growing numbers of doctors-in-training. In 1895, the relationship between the two institutions was formalized with an agreement that came into effect when Lakeside opened its new facility in 1898. It was described by *The Plain Dealer* as "not so much a hospital as it is a great institution for the study, as well as the cure of disease."[14]

In the Lakeside annual report for 1907, Board President Samuel Mather commented, "Few hospitals have staffs comprising the names of so many physicians and surgeons of great skill and reputation in their professions, as has Lakeside; and their keen interest in the continued development and improvement of our work there, is manifested by their faithful devotion to all duties, and their wise counsel and advice ever at our service."

Decades later, Howard Dittrick, MD, a longtime Lakeside obstetrician, remembered the impact of his medical education and training at Lakeside during the 1900s. In particular, he credited two Lakeside physician mavericks who helped train him and other medical students. Gynecologist Hunter Robb, MD, "was deeply appreciative of his assistants, and like the other hospital chiefs, he was solicitous regarding their future. He encouraged research and medical

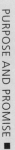

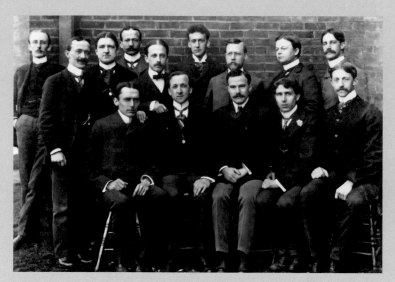

Old Lakeside Hospital house staff, ca. early 1900s.

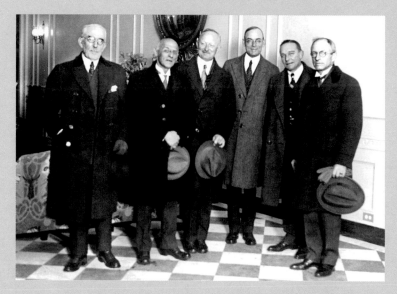

Longtime Board Chairman Samuel Mather (far left) and Abraham Flexner (second from left), at the dedication of Babies and Childrens Hospital, 1925.

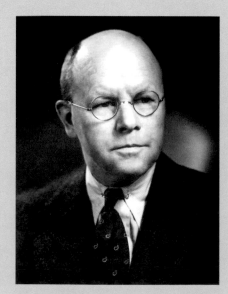

Joseph Treloar Wearn, MD, ca. 1950s.

writing, and even proffered financial assistance if the need arose." Dr. Dittrick also fondly remembered that Chief Surgeon Dudley Allen, MD, sitting on a table after a surgical procedure was completed, "would unbend and quite informally give his associates valuable clinical instruction. It was this characteristic that endeared him to his men."[15]

At the same time, medical education underwent a radical reform that was felt at Lakeside and elsewhere throughout the country. Previously, entry requirements, courses of study, and performance standards were inconsistent, and rigorous scholarship was often lacking for American doctors-in-training. There were numerous so-called medical schools in the United States that were merely diploma mills where students received a minimum of training and often little to no direct experience with patients. The need for consistent standards and quality medical education inspired the Flexner Report, a compilation of surveys from 150 medical schools published in 1910 that ultimately prompted the first major reform of medical education. Written by educator Abraham Flexner at the request of the Carnegie Foundation for the Advancement of Teaching, the report concluded that more formalized training was required in light of the rapid pace of scientific advances. Flexner felt that students should have a minimum of two years of college, with an emphasis on the sciences, to be accepted into a medical program. Additionally, Flexner recommended that medical students have access to laboratories and opportunities to work directly with patients in a hospital or clinic setting. Flexner visited Lakeside and the medical school of Western Reserve University in 1909 and praised the working relationship between the two, extolling it as a national model along with Johns Hopkins Hospital and Johns Hopkins School of Medicine in Baltimore.

The advancement of medical education in the United States took a giant leap forward when Joseph Treloar Wearn, MD, accepted a joint appointment as Professor of Medicine at the Western Reserve University School of Medicine and Director of Medicine at Lakeside in 1929. He later became dean of the medical school in 1945. At 5'4" in height, "Little Joe" had a big impact on teaching hospitals and medical education, launching a revolution in the instruction of physicians and

the curriculum of medical education in Cleveland that eventually spread around the country and the world.

Developed in collaboration with Thomas Hale Ham, MD, a hematologist and member of the medical school faculty, the innovative new curriculum was more holistic, interdisciplinary, and participatory for medical students than the curriculum previously taught. Students were treated as colleagues and were immersed in direct patient care as early as their first year of medical school. And, for the first time, the patient was viewed as a partner in the delivery of medical care and medical education. Describing the proposed changes in 1950, Wearn wrote, "By integration and co-ordination of the various departments, it is believed that a better job can be done in merging the art and science of medicine with the ultimate effect of better health for all."[16] The program was fully implemented at Western Reserve University and UH by 1952. The Western Reserve School of Medicine graduate and UH

Top left: Old Lakeside Hospital residents, ca. early 1900s. *Top right:* Babies and Childrens Hospital residents and faculty, 1945. *Bottom:* University Hospitals residents, 2016.

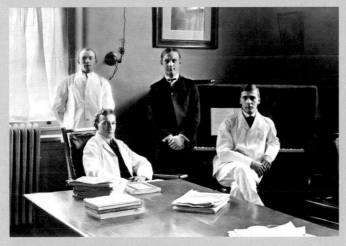

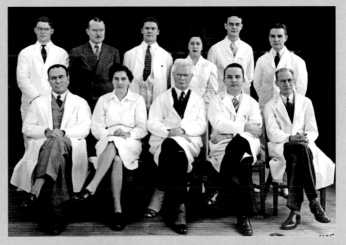

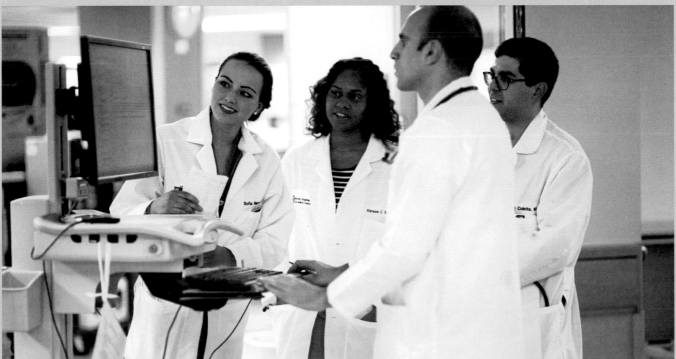

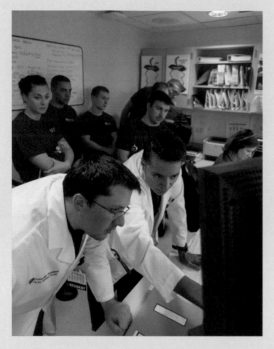

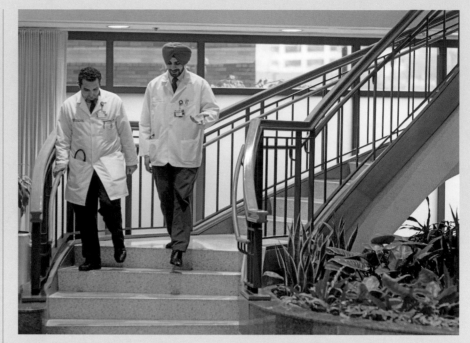

Left: The holistic approach to medical education at University Hospitals extends to the community it serves. The University Hospitals Emergency Medical Service Training & Disaster Preparedness Institute offers classes, lectures, and topic-specific symposiums for area firefighters, emergency medical technicians, paramedics, rescue teams, and hospital workers. These programs as well as continuing education opportunities are available online and through University Hospitals Ahuja, Bedford, Elyria, Geauga, Parma, and Samaritan medical centers. *Right:* Residents come to University Hospitals from around the country and the world to experience the team approach to physician training that was pioneered and developed at UH, 2016.

physician Carl Doershuk, MD, was among the first cohort of trainees to experience the new approach. "By breaking down departmental barriers...," Doershuk stated, "it got faculty and physicians working collaboratively rather than in isolation and that made for better clinical care and improved the quality of research."

For Jerome Liebman, MD, the new medical curriculum and training program made a profound impression and set a foundation for the rest of his career in medicine. Dr. Liebman arrived at UH in 1950 and became the first pediatric cardiologist in northern Ohio. "I was an intern, a senior resident, and then a fellow in pediatric cardiology," the late doctor recalled. "I had many wonderful mentors. Later, when I established the Division of Pediatric Cardiology and a training program, I became the mentor." One of the most important ideas the young Dr. Liebman learned at UH was to see the person in the bed as a teacher. "It was a new and different concept," he said. "Each patient we treated was part of our education, and the result was better care."

As the new curriculum became the established standard of health care delivery and medical education, it continued to shape the beliefs and behavior of students, physicians in training, and staff physicians. Remembering his years as an intern, resident, and fellow at Rainbow Babies and Childrens Hospital in the 1970s, Fred Rothstein, MD, former President of University Hospitals Cleveland Medical Center, said, "I learned as much from the nurses as I did from the faculty. Training the next generation of physicians, physician-scientists, and hopefully, physician leaders requires a team. Over the years, I was mentored and challenged by excellent and caring physicians who were exceptional role models. Working with them every day made me a better physician."

The proficiency of the medical and surgical professionals who train at UH is the result of the talent, education, and skills honed by both repetition and a steady infusion of the most up-to-date information. It is also a testament to the fact that UH has long attracted practitioners of the highest caliber. "We provide clinical care, we educate, and we do research," said Scott Inkley, MD, former Chief of Staff and former CEO of UH. "It's like the three legs of a stool. In this environment, I'm not sure who learns more, the students or the physician-teachers who must continue to learn and study. Being exposed to young people who have new and innovative ideas is not just a challenge—it's an opportunity."

In 1945, there were 40 residents at UH, and by 1960, that number had increased to 165. In 2016, UH trained 1,050 residents and fellows through 82 residency programs. Today's UH residents have taken the medical curriculum philosophy to a new level as they perfect their skills in the hospital and enhance that experience through community service. UH residents provide needed medical assistance to more than 30,000 underserved patients each year in the resident outpatient clinic and have the opportunity to work at Circle Health Services, formerly known as the Free Medical Clinic of Greater Cleveland, during a rotation in adolescent medicine. They also find innovative ways to address real-world problems. Advocacy projects designed by UH senior residents include a preventive health program for homeless children in Cleveland, an assessment of adolescent access to resources at a local rape crisis center, a study on youth violence, and development of a first-of-its-kind support packet to address the psychological needs of children who have a parent in prison. "We have a legacy of excellence in training physicians and physician-scientists," says Susan Nedorost, MD, Director, Graduate Medical Education at UH. "In our continuing education efforts, we're teaching residents and fellows about the benefits of working in teams and across disciplines. There is a tradition of that at UH and an enthusiasm for it." Many of these trainees will go on to assume leadership roles all over the country and the world, taking the UH approach and philosophy with them and earning recognition for their achievements and innovations.

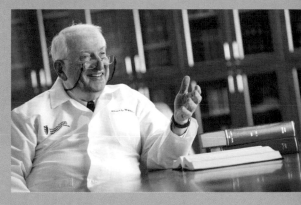

Albert Waldo, MD, PhD (Hon), 2012.

Pioneer

Albert Waldo, MD, PhD (Hon), moved to Cleveland in 1986. He was attracted to University Hospitals because it was a teaching hospital, had the technology available in the department of biomedical engineering needed to conduct his research in heart rhythm disorders, and the offer of an endowed chair at Case Western Reserve University School of Medicine. The Associate Chief of Cardiovascular Medicine for Academic Affairs at University Hospitals Cleveland Medical Center and at University Hospitals Harrington Heart & Vascular Institute, Dr. Waldo is an international authority on atrial fibrillation. His discovery of a concept called entrainment led to a better understanding of how to diagnose and treat arrhythmias, changing laboratory practices around the world. Having received several distinguished society awards, he is committed to the academic triad of patient care, research, and teaching. "The whole field has grown, and we have grown with it, leading the way in many respects. We've helped train many people from all over the world in cardiac electrophysiology," he says. "We helped them, and they will help others."

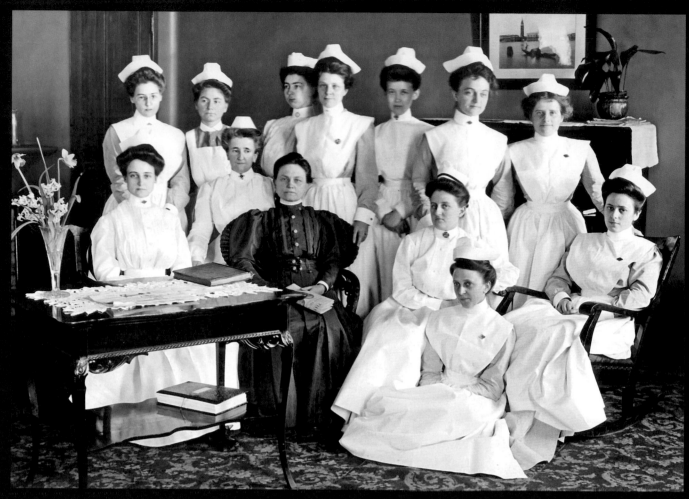

Nurses at Lakeside Hospital, 1905.

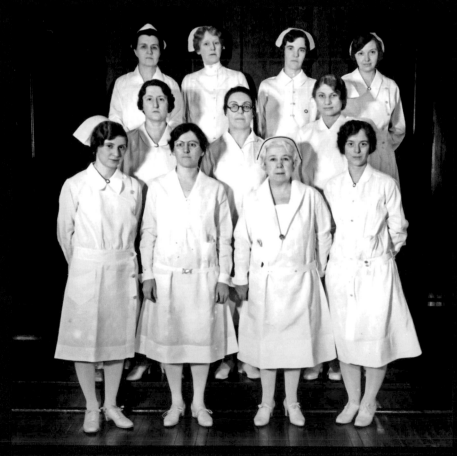

Staff nurses at Lakeside Hospital, 1931.

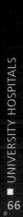

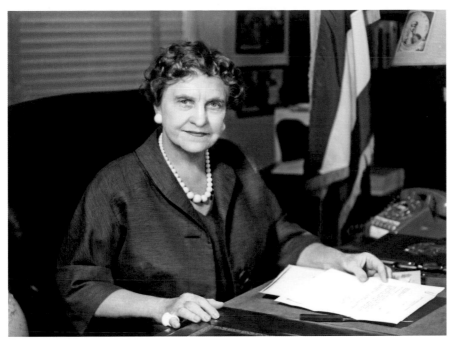

Francis Payne Bolton, ca. 1960s.

A Commitment to Nursing Excellence

The history of nursing as a profession traces the shift from providing kindness and basic comfort care to performing sophisticated, specialized medical duties once reserved for physicians. University Hospitals and its individual founding institutions have always been at the forefront of this transformational shift.

In 1868, nurses at Wilson Street Hospital had no formal schooling, as there were no nursing schools in America at the time. Nursing education as a discipline was first introduced in England in 1860 by Florence Nightingale, and the first American school was established at Bellevue Hospital in New York City in 1873. Lakeside Hospital launched a training school for nurses with the construction of the new hospital in 1898. According to Isabel Hampton Robb, a former nurse who developed the school's curriculum, the Lakeside Hospital Training School for Nurses was the first nursing school in the United States supported by private philanthropy to offer a full academic and clinical curriculum from the first day of its existence and the first to recognize that nurses needed rigorous academic training to be partners with physicians in a hospital setting. This monumental achievement in nursing education was accomplished a full 11 years before the Flexner Report was published for the standardization of medical education.

In 1923, the Lakeside Training School for Nurses and the Department of Nursing Education at Western Reserve University consolidated to become a single and separate college within the university, one of the first of its kind in the nation. Frances Payne Bolton,

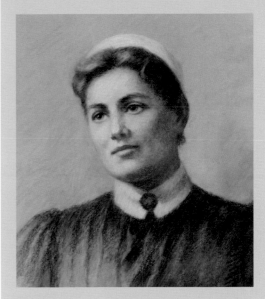

Pastel portrait of Isabel Hampton Robb, ca. 1890s.

Pioneer

Isabel Hampton Robb, an early proponent of nursing education and author, served as an advisor and lecturer for the Lakeside Training School for Nurses and was a member of Lakeside Hospital's Board of Managers. Robb had previously established and directed a nationally-renowned nursing program at Johns Hopkins Hospital that was regarded as the finest in the nation. Robb moved to Cleveland with her husband, Hunter Robb, MD, who joined the faculty at Lakeside. She was also a founder of the Cleveland Visiting Nurses Association, the American Nurses Association, and the *American Journal of Nurses*. In an article for *The Plain Dealer* about nursing and the opportunities it presented for women, Robb wrote, "Although modern nursing in America numbers but little over thirty years, its educational advancement has been remarkable."[17]

Robb was considered by many to be the American equivalent of Florence Nightingale as she transformed nursing from a vocation to a profession. The victim of a fatal streetcar accident in 1910, she was mourned by nurses throughout the country.

Professionalization of Nursing

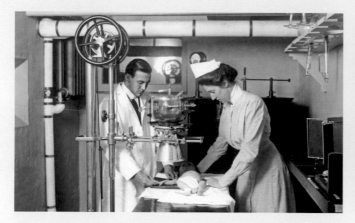

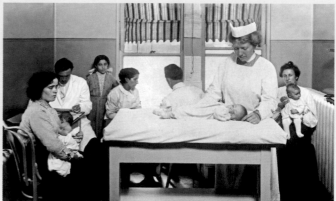

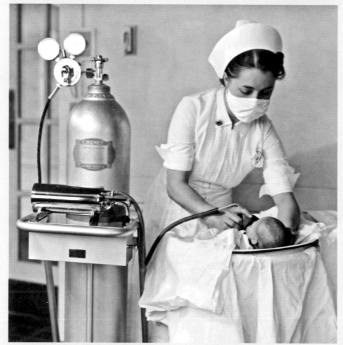

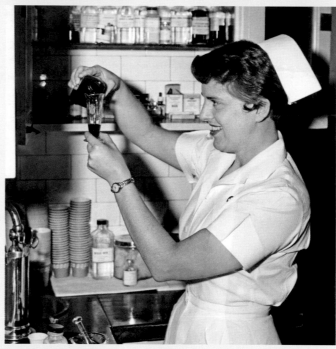

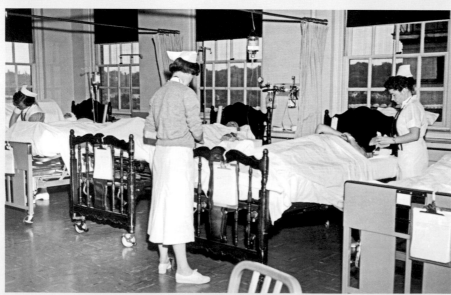

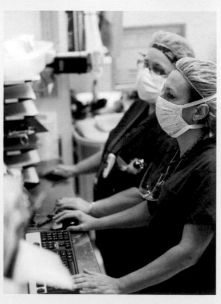

Top (left to right): Babies' Dispensary and Hospital X-ray, 1912; Babies' Dispensary and Hospital, ca. late 1910s. *Middle (left to right):* MacDonald House patient care, ca. late 1920s; Nurse preparing medicine, ca. late 1950s. *Bottom (left to right):* Lakeside Hospital Recovery Room, 1960; Nurses assist in the operating room at University Hospitals Ahuja Medical Center, 2016.

a member of Congress, health care reformer, member of Lakeside's Board of Managers, and hospital trustee, provided a $500,000 endowment gift. The school was renamed in her honor in 1935 as the Frances Payne Bolton School of Nursing at Western Reserve University.

The nursing school continued to have a close and cooperative relationship with the nursing service at UH. The "Experiment to Effect Change," which took place between 1966 and 1973, was a project to foster collaboration between the two. Its goals were to challenge nurses to find better ways to deliver patient care, educate students, and promote scholarly research. Rozella Schlotfeldt, PhD, the nursing school dean who spearheaded the initiative, drew inspiration from the clinical training medical students received. Nursing directors held joint appointments at the hospital and the school, and working nurses were seen as clinical experts. "The theory was that if the same people were responsible for patient care as well as the education of students, we should be able to narrow or close the gap between what's taught and what's practiced," explained former Chief Nursing Officer Charlene Phelps, MSN, RN, FAAN, who collaborated with Schlotfeldt.

Walter Pritchard, MD, Chief of Staff in the early 1970s, noted that the relationship between physicians and nurses changed as a result of the experiment. "Doctors, administrators, and nurses [sat] down together to determine what can help the patient...Respect [was] the key word...respect for the ability of a person who knows as much as you do about certain aspects, to carry out a vital part of the program." This view is in large part why UH has long been known as a "nurse's hospital." It is a place where physicians value nurses and perceive them as integral members of the health care team. Nurses at UH have the power to effect change and are offered opportunities for professional development and career advancement. "I have never been at a meeting where nurses didn't have a voice," says Nancy Haas, MPA, BSN, RN, former Director of Nursing Practice. "Shared governance has existed here for at least 30 years. [Nurses] are truly partners with physicians and other clinical staff."

UH nurses are also mentors. With 6,524 registered nurses, they help train close to 2,000 students annually from 70 nursing schools around the country. The guidance and hands-on experience these aspiring professionals receive embodies a progressive model, rooted in science and implemented throughout the system. It improves patient outcomes by integrating clinical practice with research, which enhances care planning and implementation; emphasizing relationship building with patients; and providing essential culturally-sensitive support for patients and their families. "There are skills you learn in

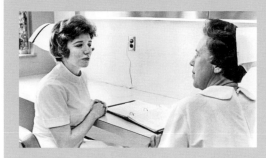

Charlene Phelps (left), MSN, RN, FAAN, 1971.

Game Changer

Charlene Phelps, MSN, RN, FAAN, who died in 2016, graduated from the Frances Payne Bolton School of Nursing master's program in 1965. She began her career at University Hospitals in 1962 as a staff nurse, completed her MSN, and returned to UH in 1971 as an assistant director of medical/surgical nursing in Hanna House. But her real job was to be a "fixer." To get nurses to spend more time at the bedside, she shifted responsibility for mixing medication, washing utensils, and managing laundry to other departments. She noticed that when nurses recorded vital signs or observations, they wrote notes on slips of paper, stuffed them in their pockets, and later entered the information on the patient's chart at the nurses' station. Phelps had boxes installed on patient room doors to hold charts so data could be recorded on the spot.

"It took almost 11 years for me to be satisfied we had all the systems in place we needed," Phelps recalled. "If you get caught up in the day to day, you can't make changes. I would take some time about once a month to be away from everything and think about where are we with this? How are we with that? What do we need? Because if you don't do that, [change] won't happen."

During her more than three decades at UH, Phelps held various administrative positions. At retirement, she was Chief Nursing Officer of UH Health System.

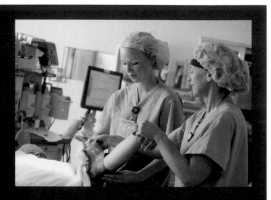

University Hospitals nurses at work, 2016.

It's a Fact

In 1981, one out of every three University Hospitals employees, totaling more than 1,600 people, was part of the Department of Nursing, representing the largest employee group in the institution. Registered nurses comprised more than half of this group, with a growing number holding master's degrees in specialized areas. Today, 43 percent of the UH employee population, approximately 10,600 people system-wide, staff the nursing department.

nursing school," says Mary Lou Kubu, RN, "But the art of caring for people compassionately you get from working with other nurses who understand what it means."

Nursing pioneer Isabel Hampton Robb gave a speech in 1898 at the opening of the Lakeside Hospital Training School for Nurses. Her words are as true now as the day they were spoken. She praised the trustees for "their broad mind and far seeing policy," which recognized that "patients can be taken care of only by intelligent and well-trained

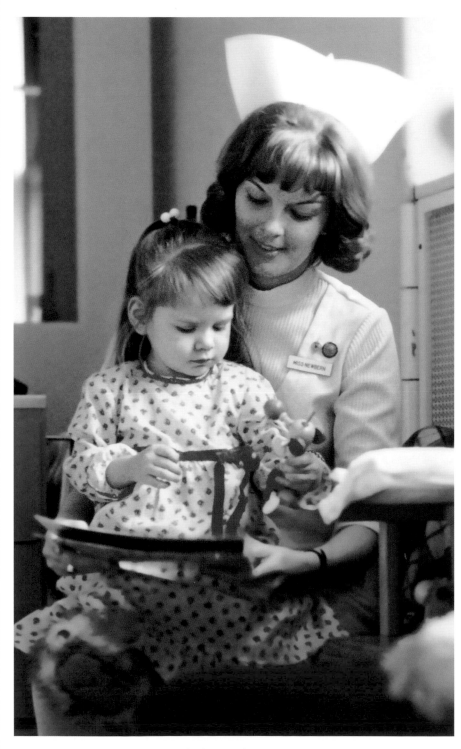

University Hospitals' staff have been the heart and soul of the patient experience for 150 years, ca. 1960s.

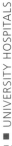

nurses," and proudly stated that the nursing profession was "not standing still...ever aiming at improvements upon older methods." Expanding on that thought, Catherine Koppelman, MSN, RN, former UH Chief Nursing Officer and Patient Experience Officer, said, "This is not just our history. It is the culture at UH, and it is something we must protect and preserve."

· · ·

University Hospitals doctors do their best to make patients better every day. Sadly, however, there is not always a happy ending. But, there is no end to trying. A hospital is a place where heartbreaking realities must be confronted because not every condition can be cured and not every injury can be successfully repaired. However, the tens of thousands of dedicated employees and volunteers who meet the needs of patients in many roles throughout the hospital system are committed to providing help and hope to all who come seeking care, 365 days a year, from early morning to the darkest hours of the night. They are motivated to know more, teach others, and alleviate suffering, each in their own way to advance the institutional mission. Collectively, they keep the massive organization functioning to help people improve the quality and length of their lives. ▼

"Our strength is in our people," says Steven Standley, UH Chief Administrative Officer. "That's what makes us exceptional. Of course, we aim to hire the best, most talented and competent employees. But, we're also looking for people who are passionate about UH and about what we do and the way we do it here."

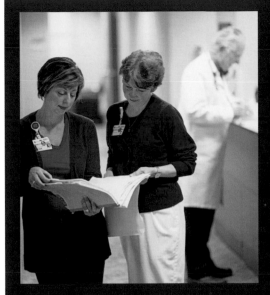

Nursing excellence is a hallmark of University Hospitals, 2016.

It's a Fact

In 1984, University Hospitals was named one of 41 original Magnet hospitals in a national historic study conducted by the American Academy of Nursing Task Force that analyzed characteristics of hospitals to determine why some were able to successfully recruit and retain nurses and have high-quality patient outcomes. As the program evolved, UH continued to achieve Magnet status, receiving the formal Magnet designation in 2006, which it has maintained ever since. The recognition, conferred by the American Nurses Association, is a measure of nursing excellence as determined by high-quality patient outcomes and satisfaction among nurses with the work environment and interdisciplinary professional collaboration. With only 8 percent of U.S. hospitals having earned this prestigious award, it is the highest form of external peer review.

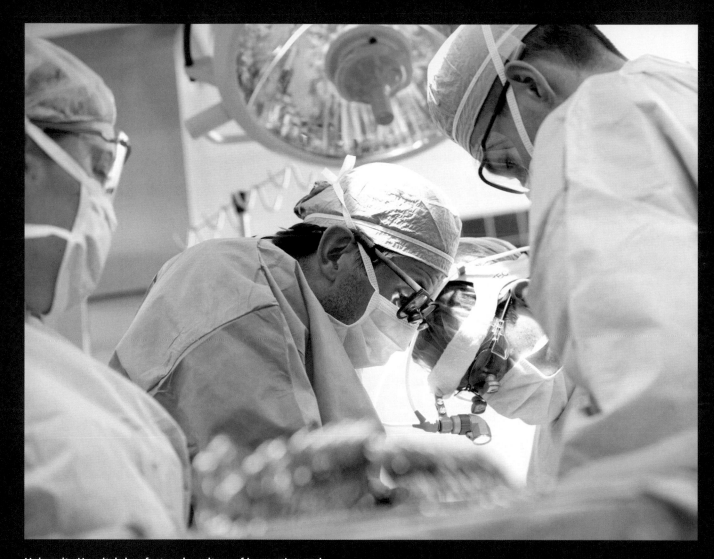

University Hospitals has fostered a culture of innovation and discovery in the laboratory, at the bedside, and in the operating room. In their personal quests to know more and improve outcomes for their patients, physicians, researchers, and nurses have helped advance medical science, clinical practice, and patient care around the world, ca. 2010s.

Breakthroughs

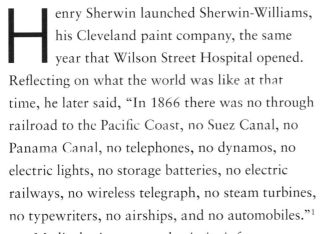

"We're constantly looking for ways to improve. Is this the best we can do? What could we change? How can we break new ground?"

– Avroy Fanaroff, MD, former Chairman of the Department of Pediatrics and former Division Chief of Neonatology, University Hospitals Rainbow Babies & Children's Hospital

Henry Sherwin launched Sherwin-Williams, his Cleveland paint company, the same year that Wilson Street Hospital opened. Reflecting on what the world was like at that time, he later said, "In 1866 there was no through railroad to the Pacific Coast, no Suez Canal, no Panama Canal, no telephones, no dynamos, no electric lights, no storage batteries, no electric railways, no wireless telegraph, no steam turbines, no typewriters, no airships, and no automobiles."[1]

Medical science was also in its infancy. Physicians had limited knowledge about the body; few tools beyond scalpels, scissors, saws, and stethoscopes; and a small arsenal of treatments and tonics. Aspirin, blood typing, and vaccines for cholera, rabies, typhoid, tetanus, diphtheria, and polio had yet to be discovered. Anesthesia and antibiotics were not available. Doctors could not see inside the body unless it was cut open. It is astounding to think how far health care, like the world Henry Sherwin described, has evolved since University Hospitals was founded.

UH has a 150-year commitment to scientific investigation and clinical innovation. Dudley

Peter Allen, MD, joined the medical staff of Lakeside Hospital in 1893 after returning from studies in Europe, and eventually became chief of surgery. He was among a small, select group of local physicians who brought the latest advances in scientific medicine, bacteriology, surgical technique, and equipment to Cleveland from England and the continent.

In an article about the founding of hospitals and the establishment of the medical school during the city's first 100 years, Dr. Allen wrote, "The great progress shown in these institutions gives a ground...for the positive expectation that within a few years to come still greater advancement may be looked for not so much in the increase in numbers of public institutions as in the work done by them, and it may confidently be predicted that the time is near at hand when Cleveland will occupy, if it may not already be said to occupy, a prominent position in the development of medicine in the United States."[2]

The best kind of medical care goes hand-in-hand with a spirit of inquiry. The hospital and Case Western Reserve University School of Medicine,

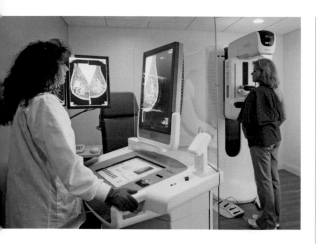

University Hospitals was the first health care provider in Northeast Ohio to offer tomosynthesis, advanced three-dimensional breast imaging, for the earliest detection of breast cancer. A study published in 2014, co-authored by Donna Plecha, MD, Director of Breast Imaging at UH Seidman Cancer Center, showed that this technology reduces false positives and finds significantly more invasive cancers.[3]

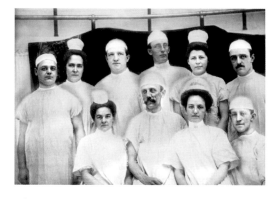

Lakeside Hospital chief surgeon Dudley Allen, MD, (first row, second from left) also served on the faculty of the Western Reserve University School of Medicine for 27 years, 17 of which were as head of the Department of Surgery. During his tenure, he helped to modernize and improve the medical profession, ca. 1900.

ranked among the top research medical schools in the country by *U.S. News & World Report*, have had a working relationship since the late 1800s. Initially, it was an arrangement that allowed students to round with doctors and apply what they learned in the classroom. Today, 24 departments and centers share the same physician faculty who care for patients, teach, and conduct research. These doctors have pioneered novel ideas, trailblazing approaches, leading-edge treatments, and breakthrough techniques. Some have set the standard of care in their field.

"An active program of research in a medical center has an influence beyond that of discovery," said the late Douglas Bond, MD, Director of Psychiatric Services at UH from 1946 to 1969 and former Dean of the university's School of Medicine. "It adds spark to routine, it adds a continuous criticism of the current practices, and above all, it means the restless searching for better ways to do things." Today, the UH Clinical Research Center, a collaboration with Case Western Reserve University School of Medicine, forms one of the largest biomedical research centers in Northeast Ohio, and one of the top 15 in the country. Much of what is happening in clinical research today is driven by applications that link basic lab science to the actual practice of medicine in the hospital and out in the community. It is called translational research. In 1996, UH established a center for clinical research and technology, but long before that, UH was one of the first five hospitals in the country to have a hospital-based clinical research unit where investigators could have subjects on a nursing floor. It was established at Lakeside Hospital in 1962, and a similar, smaller unit for children soon followed that continues today as the Dahms' Clinical Research Unit, a state-of-the-art facility named after nationally-recognized University Hospitals Rainbow Babies & Children's Hospital endocrinologist, William T. Dahms, MD. The Wearn Laboratory for Medical Research, a joint project of UH and Western Reserve University, was also inaugurated in 1962.

Sometimes clinical research leads to cures or revolutionizes how procedures are done, but more often it does not make headlines; it is about taking little steps forward and accumulating an understanding over time. At UH, exploration is a constant. In the first half of the 20th century, each decade had its defining discoveries and developments. By building on the past and with the help of improved instruments and methods of study, the pace of discovery quickened dramatically. There were significant achievements with every passing year, too many to highlight individually, but all meaningful in the forward march of medical science and the impact on people's lives.

Research Through the Decades

Discovery is an important part of healing, and clinical research is one of the fundamental tenets of an academic medical center such as University Hospitals. Due to pioneering work in UH laboratories, research studies, and clinical trials, numerous groundbreaking advancements in many medical disciplines have been achieved. Laboratories from the early 20th century were quite primitive compared to today's sophisticated, well-equipped versions, but the important work completed in them helped to modernize medicine.

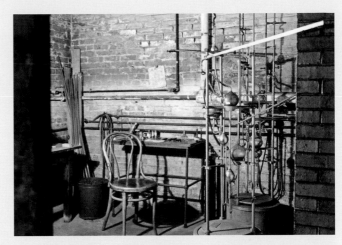

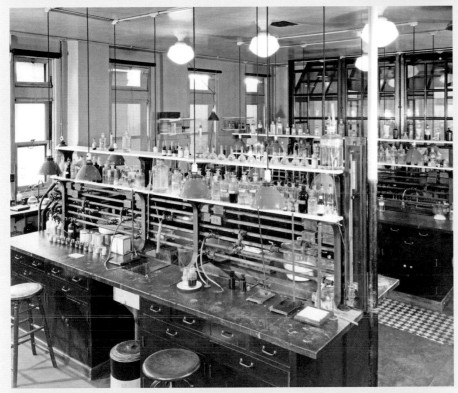

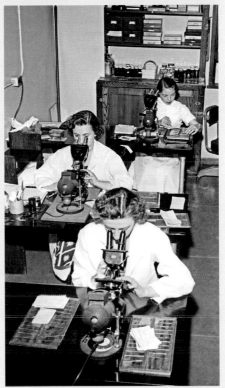

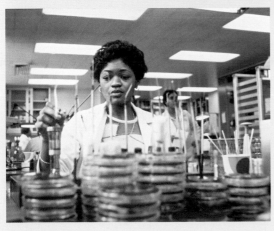

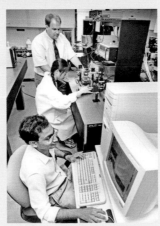

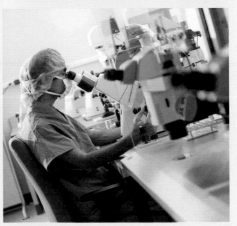

Top right: Research laboratory at Lakeside Hospital, ca. 1920s. *Middle left:* Babies and Childrens Hospital, ca. late 1920s/early 1930s. *Middle right*: Cytology laboratory, 1959. *Bottom left:* 1960s research laboratory. *Bottom center:* 1990s research laboratory. *Bottom right:* Modern laboratory, 2016.

Medical Advances: 1900 – 1929

Ronald Richard, President and CEO of the Cleveland Foundation, which began in 1914, describes the city of that era as "a hotbed of invention, entrepreneurship, and vision." Inventors pioneered technologies in electricity, chemicals, metals, paints, and machining.[4] It was also a period when physicians and nurses at Lakeside and Babies and Childrens hospitals made strides in three areas—anesthesia, goiter, and infant care—that would have enduring and widespread impacts for generations to come.

Anesthesia

In a collaboration that began in 1908, Lakeside Hospital surgeon George Crile, MD, and nurse Agatha Hodgins perfected the use of nitrous oxide-oxygen anesthesia. It was superior to ether and chloroform, the two most common methods of sedation used at the time, because it was safer and more effective. Lakeside became the first hospital in the world to manufacture its own nitrous oxide gas in 1910, piping it directly into operating rooms.

Dr. Crile, who had been researching surgical shock, selected Hodgins, Chief Nurse of the private patient pavilion, to train with him and be his full-time anesthetist. Described as a woman of inventive genius in her obituary, she played a key role in developing "many techniques, procedures, and appliances now used by anesthetists the world over…Working with [Graham W.] Clarke, inventor of the Ohio monovalve apparatus, Miss Hodgins also made notable contributions to the progressive improvement of the gas machine, forerunner of the efficient piece of equipment we know today."[5]

A facility for research in chemical warfare was quickly built in 1917 on old Lakeside's downtown grounds. It was deemed one of the best-equipped labs in the world for the study of cardio-respiratory conditions. Physician investigators worked with scientists from the U.S. War Department and professor and inventor, Roy Pearce, of the University of Illinois, to develop a more comfortable and protective gas mask. After lab testing on human subjects, the new devices were manufactured by BFGoodrich® in Akron.

Hodgins organized the Lakeside School of Anesthesia in 1915. It is believed to be the first formal training program of its kind in the country, established primarily for the training of nurse anesthetists. "Lakeside Hospital became the

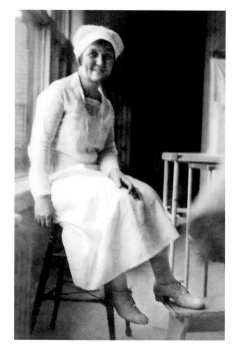
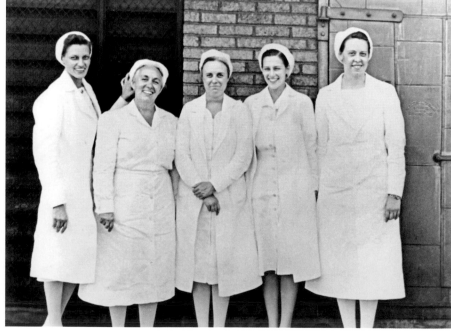

Left: Agatha Hodgins, ca. 1920s. *Right:* Nurse anesthetists, ca. late 1930s.

World War I

Before the United States officially entered WWI, George Crile, MD, Lakeside Hospital's Chief of Surgery, recruited volunteers for the first American medical group to provide medical care to Allied soldiers wounded in Europe. The war provided an unprecedented opportunity to continue his research into the effects of shock, blood transfusion, hemorrhage, and surgical treatment of traumatic injuries. The knowledge gathered from treating the wounded pushed surgical care forward and provided valuable information for military medical planners in future conflicts.

Nurse Agatha Hodgins, along with three Lakeside nurses, sailed to France as part of Dr. Crile's team in December 1914. Hodgins worked with surgeons in Paris at the Ambulance Americaine (the term for a French military hospital). Her fellow Clevelanders returned home after three months, but she stayed for an additional five months to instruct French medical personnel in the administration of nitrous oxide anesthesia. When the Lakeside Unit, including 44 Lakeside nurses and University Hospitals physicians, returned to France in 1917 to establish Base Hospital No. 4 in Rouen, Hodgins remained in Cleveland. It was deemed more important for her to continue teaching and preparing others to serve.

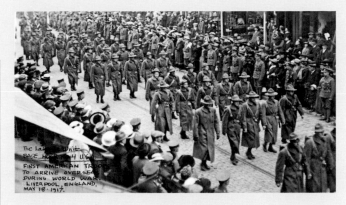

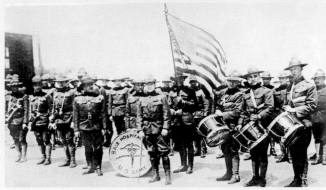

Top: Lakeside Unit Base Hospital No. 4 arrived in Liverpool, England, on May 18, 1917. *Bottom:* Officers and soldiers of Base Hospital No. 4, also known as the Lakeside Unit, arrived at the British Expeditionary Force's General Hospital No. 9 on May 25, 1917. While overseas, the unit treated 82,179 patients.

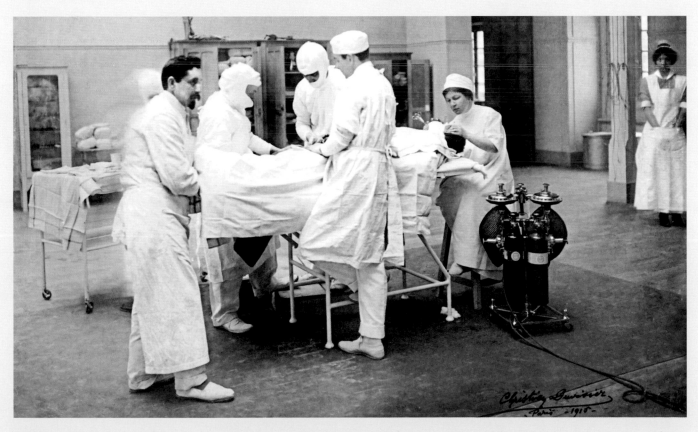

Lakeside Unit surgeons operating in France, 1915. Agatha Hodgins (far right at table) is shown using the Ohio monovalve, an apparatus used for the administration of nitrous oxide, oxygen, and ether. It was invented in Cleveland by Graham W. Clarke, a founder of the Ohio Chemical Co., with Hodgins' assistance. Lakeside Hospital was the world's first hospital to perfect the manufacture of nitrous oxide gas in 1910.

I Work Here

In 1966, there was a nationwide shortage of physicians specializing in obstetric anesthesia. To fill the void, a center for training them was established at MacDonald House (now University Hospitals MacDonald Women's Hospital). University Hospitals was among the first in the country to have a dedicated anesthesiology staff for maternity patients that could offer 24-hour coverage. It was one of the things that attracted Mary Ann Hulme, MSN, RNC, former nurse manager of Obstetrics, to join the staff as a Labor, Delivery, and Antepartum nurse in 1977. "There was no waiting for the surgical team. If a patient needed a C-section, you could do it right away."

mecca for students of the nitrous oxide technic [sic]. In this phase of development of anesthesia, Hodgins played a leading role. One now famous surgeon who went to Cleveland to learn the technic [sic] was admonished by his chief. 'George [Crile, MD,] will talk a lot, but you watch Agatha.'"[6] The school accepted students until 1953, with Hodgins serving as its director until 1933. She also founded the American Association of Nurse Anesthetists, gathering a group of alumnae on June 17, 1931, at Lakeside for the organization's first meeting.

Goiter Prevention

David Marine, MD, started his career at Lakeside Hospital as a pathology resident and in 1915 began his research into the cause and prevention of goiter, an enlargement of the thyroid gland and a common problem in the Great Lakes region of the country. He discovered that goiter was the result of iodine deficiency and launched the first large-scale trials of iodine supplementation, dubbed the "Akron Experiment," that ran from 1917 to 1922 with Akron schoolgirls. His study discredited the widely held belief that iodine was poisonous in small doses and revived interest in an idea from the 1830s that salt was an easy method to increase the public's intake of this essential nutrient. As a result of his work, in 1924 it became common practice for U.S. table salt producers to fortify salt with potassium iodide.

In 1950, there were only four documented cases of goiter among Akron students. Oliver Kimball, MD, was Dr. Marine's assistant. He once wrote, "Goitre [sic] prevention as practiced today is based entirely on the teachings of David Marine."[7] It was, and remains, an achievement of national and international significance, spreading around the globe through the efforts of the World Health Organization.

Infant Nutrition

Early in the 20th century, it was understood that human and cow's milk were nutritionally and compositionally different. When Babies' Dispensary and Hospital opened in 1911, its first Medical Director, Henry Gerstenberger, MD, began research to find the ideal liquid food when breastfeeding was not possible. His efforts reflected a dedication to the health of the city's poor and the well-being of children. Within two years, he developed a basic preparation that was better than anything else available, but it was not perfect and experiments continued.

Dr. Gerstenberger's original research partner was Harold Ruh, MD, a Babies' Dispensary physician. William Frohring, a young biochemist, joined the team in 1915, working nights while keeping his day job. That

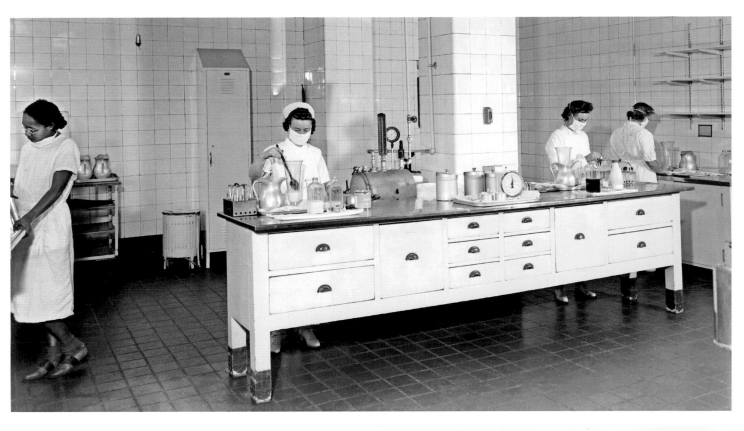

year they achieved their goal—a modified milk formula that was easily digestible and nutritionally balanced called S.M.A. (Synthetic Milk Adapted). The cod liver oil in it, naturally rich in vitamin D, provided the side benefit of protection against rickets, a common problem at the time for urban children. Clinical trials with more than 300 babies confirmed its value, and the findings were published in 1919.[8]

Initially the Babies' Dispensary kitchen prepared S.M.A., bottling close to 1,000 quarts a month for delivery to area doctors, who dispensed it by prescription. With demand increasing, Telling-Belle Vernon, the largest dairy company in Ohio, was licensed to manufacture and distribute it. Eight weeks after they assumed production, sales doubled. S.M.A. soon became available in both liquid and powdered form, and a 1922 news story reported that 900 babies in and around Cleveland were receiving it.[9]

Dr. Gerstenberger received a patent for the formula in 1923 and assigned the rights to Babies' Dispensary. The royalties, a major source of revenue for an endowment that funded research, also covered costs for a library, laboratory expenses, building renovations, and allowed pediatric residents in the early years to study in Europe. The revenues even helped to pay for patient bills and employee salaries. *Cleveland News* commented upon Dr. Gerstenberger's death

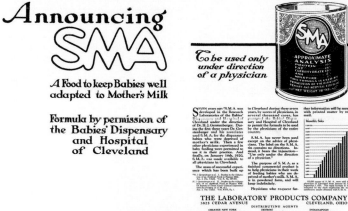

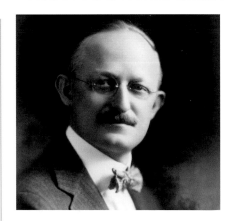

Top: Milk laboratory, Babies and Childrens Hospital, 1942. *Middle:* S.M.A. infant formula ad. The formula is still sold today under different brand names. *Bottom:* Henry Gerstenberger, MD, ca. 1920s.

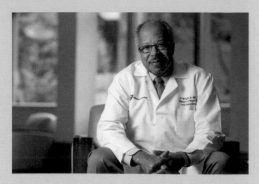

Jackson Wright, MD, PhD.

Game Changer

The results of the multi-site SPRINT (Systolic Blood Pressure Intervention Trial) study, the largest clinical research study on high blood pressure, were published with Jackson Wright, MD, PhD, Director of the Clinical Hypertension Program at University Hospitals, as lead author and co-principal investigator. The trial, funded by the National Institutes of Health (NIH), examined if lowering systolic blood pressure well below currently recommended levels reduces the risk of heart and kidney disease, stroke, and age-related decline in memory and thinking. The findings, published in *The New England Journal of Medicine* in 2015, were dramatic. Managing blood pressure to achieve a lower target in high-risk patients significantly reduced cardiovascular disease events and death from any cause, and yielded better health results overall.

Dr. Wright was also the lead author of the landmark NIH-sponsored Antihypertensive and Lipid-Lowering Treatment to Prevent Heart Attack Trial (ALLHAT) in 2002 involving 45,000 patients. As the largest antihypertensive treatment trial ever conducted, the study reported that thiazide-type diuretics (water pills) are at least as effective as the more costly drugs available at preventing cardiovascular disease and are recommended as the first option for treating high blood pressure.

in 1954, "Certainly we have no other citizen who could be credited with the saving of not one, or 100, but tens of thousands of children's lives, in nearly half a century of usefulness to his community."[10]

Medical Advances: 1930s – 1940s

The financial constraints resulting from the Great Depression, followed by manpower and material shortages as a result of WWII, impeded research and innovation during this period. Nonetheless, there were some notable achievements with long-lasting impact.

"We learn from the past as we continue to advance and lead change," says Fred Rothstein, MD, past President of University Hospitals Cleveland Medical Center. This view is especially true when thinking about the contributions of Harry Goldblatt, MD, and Claude Beck, MD, whose research had an indelible impact on medical understanding about cardiology and cardiovascular health, disease, and treatment.

Hypertension

Harry Goldblatt, MD, was a pathologist at Lakeside Hospital and a professor of pathology at Western Reserve University. His seminal experiments in the 1930s clarified the link between kidney function and high blood pressure. To support his research efforts, Dr. Goldblatt developed clamps that constricted the main renal artery, simulating what happens when blood flow to the kidneys is restricted. His findings, published in a 1934 issue of *The Journal of Experimental Medicine*, were the precursor to further research in Cleveland and around the world, leading to the development of effective methods for controlling high blood pressure and treating chronic hypertension, problems that today affect nearly one-third of all Americans.

Heart Disease

Claude Beck, MD, a major scientific and surgical pioneer of the 20th century with an international reputation, looms large in University Hospitals' history. He arrived in Cleveland in 1924 to train as a surgical research fellow. Within a few years, he became a resident surgeon at Lakeside Hospital and an instructor at Western Reserve University, where he organized the school's first surgical research lab. His interests originally focused on neurosurgery, earning him the title of tenured professor in that field. Over time, he expanded his focus to include the human heart, and in 1952, the university named him professor of cardiovascular surgery, a title never before conferred on a doctor in the United States.

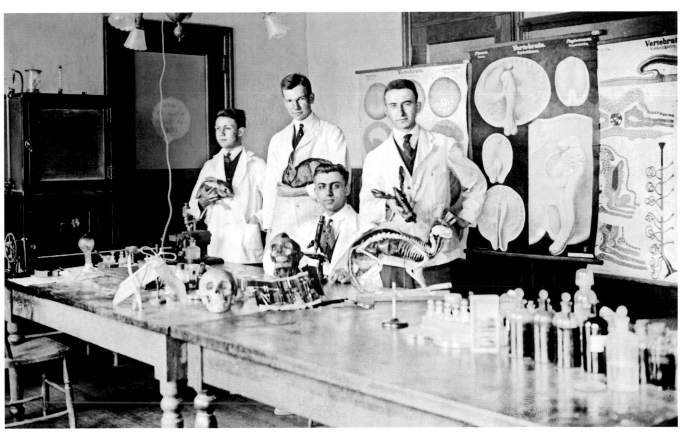

The laboratory of Claude Beck, MD, (back row, middle), was for many years the only one in the country entirely devoted to cardiac studies, ca. 1920s.

Dr. Beck was a leading expert in finding surgical solutions for coronary artery disease. In 1935, he performed a procedure, known as the Beck I, which provided an alternate blood supply to the heart via vessels in the chest muscles. This procedure marked "the first operation in the... world for the relief of angina pectoris, a heart ailment which in the past ha[d] been regarded as incurable and eventually fatal...Medical men believe that in all probability the operation will quickly become known as one of the most important medical discoveries of recent times."[11] In 1947, the improved Beck II procedure, which became the forerunner of what is known today as bypass surgery, employed a technique to improve circulation by rerouting blood away from a damaged artery through a vein graft that formed a new connection between the aorta and the heart.

This same year, Dr. Beck and his team accomplished a medical feat that had never successfully been done before: the defibrillation of a human heart. He combined direct manual cardiac massage while using a device that delivered an electric shock to restore a normal heart rhythm to revive heart attack victims. This approach grew out of the work of his colleague physiologist Carl Wiggers, a professor at Western Reserve University's medical school. While it was initially only possible to resuscitate a heart in an operating room when the chest was open and the heart exposed, it has become standard practice today due to education and relatively easy access to automated external defibrillators in public spaces. The pioneering impact of Beck's discovery is illustrated

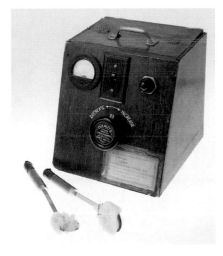

The open-chest defibrillator first used by Claude Beck, MD. He developed the device with his friend James Rand III, a Cleveland scientist and industrial designer, ca. 1930s.

by the story of Richard Heyard, age 14, whose "pulse suddenly stopped," "whose blood pressure could not be heard," and who was "apparently dead" near the end of a chest operation at Lakeside. "[He] was brought back to life by a new method of resuscitation employed by Dr. Claude S. Beck…the first of its kind in human beings in recorded medical history… It is believed that other hospitals will follow the example of University Hospitals by training their surgeons in this method."[12]

Medical Advances: 1950s – 1960s

What had been learned about treatment of battlefield injuries, blood preservation and transfusion, the mass production of penicillin, and radiation and atomic energy during WWII improved medical care in the United States in the decades immediately following the war. More medications and vaccines, including the Salk vaccine for polio, became available, and more funding for research from the federal government precipitated great strides in understanding various disorders and their management. Speaking about the value of basic scientific investigations, Alan Moritz, MD, Chairman of the Department of Pathology at University Hospitals until he retired in 1965, said, "We can never anticipate what new knowledge will lead to in its practical implications…from heretofore unrecognized, unsuspected facts about the mechanism of disease."[14]

Resuscitation

Claude Beck, MD, continued to spearhead advancements in lifesaving cardiac practices. The procedures he developed led to the ability to perform closed-chest cardiac resuscitations outside of the operating room. In the early 1950s, Dr. Beck and his colleagues developed what is today commonly referred to as CPR (cardiopulmonary resuscitation) and began teaching it to medical professionals. Working with the Cleveland Heart Society, more than 3,000 doctors and nurses were trained in less than 20 years. Against a backlash from the medical establishment who at the time felt only trained medical professionals should perform resuscitation, Dr. Beck led a targeted education campaign in 1963 to teach CPR to the layperson. CPR classes are still taught today to people of all ages and professions.

At a retirement luncheon in Dr. Beck's honor in 1965, Harris Shumaker Jr., MD, Chairman of the Department of Surgery at Indiana University School of Medicine and a cardiac and vascular surgeon of note, said, "Certainly no one has more effectively challenged the concept that death must be final than Claude Beck."[15]

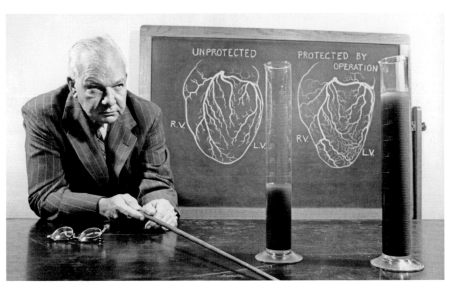

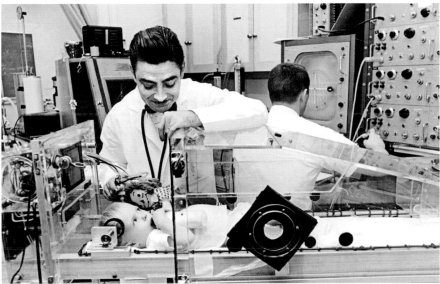

Top: The work of Claude Beck, MD, had both theoretical and practical applications that led to better diagnosis and new approaches for treating coronary artery disease, 1955. *Bottom:* Cystic fibrosis expert LeRoy Matthews, MD, 1966.

Cystic Fibrosis

In 1950, an infant with cystic fibrosis (CF) usually died within six months, and those who did survive were very sick and rarely lived past the age of three. It is an inherited, life-shortening disease characterized by over-production of thick, sticky mucus that impedes breathing, increases susceptibility to chronic infections in the lungs, and prevents the release of digestive enzymes from the pancreas, leading to malnutrition. In 1956, UH pediatrician LeRoy Matthew, MD, changed those odds when he developed a new approach to medical and home care. In 1961, *The Plain Dealer* credited Babies and Childrens Hospital with improving "[t]he lives of more than 100 children with cystic fibrosis…due to a new treatment program developed at [the hospital]," citing that "no baby has died there of cystic fibrosis since 1957."[16]

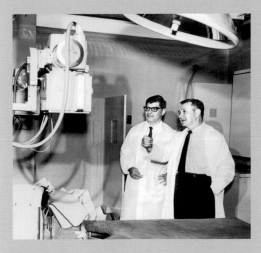

Radiologist Hymer Friedell, MD (right), ca. late 1960s.

Game Changer

Hymer Friedell, MD, joined University Hospitals in 1946 as the first Chair of the newly-created Department of Radiology. During the course of his 32-year career at the hospital, he pioneered the use of radioisotopes for diagnostic purposes and for cancer treatments. In the post-war era, it was believed that atomic energy could have a revolutionary effect on medical research, and due to his expertise in the field, Dr. Friedell was actively involved. He served as the Deputy Director of the Health Division of the Manhattan Project, commissioned by the government to collect data on the effects of radiation from the aftermath of the atomic bomb dropped on Hiroshima in August 1945. He also served on the Atomic Energy Commission's Advisory Committee on Isotope Distribution and established the Atomic Energy Medical Research Project at Western Reserve University to study the clinical use of radioisotopes. Additionally, in the early days of color television, Dr. Friedell was involved in a study sponsored by television manufacturers and the U.S. Public Health Service to determine the radiation risks, if any, from sitting too close to the TV. The study concluded the risk was extremely low.

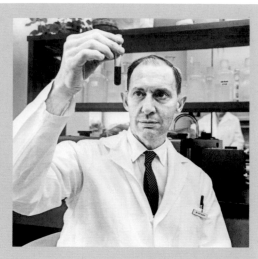

Oscar Ratnoff, MD, an international expert on blood coagulation, ca. 1970s.

Pioneer

The work conducted by Oscar Ratnoff, MD, from the late 1950s through the 1980s made important contributions to understanding the mechanisms of blood clotting, bleeding disorders, and the treatment of wounds. A profile on him published by the American Society of Hematology praised Dr. Ratnoff and his research for embodying the idea of translational research—applying science to real patient problems—"before the term was ever popularized." His formulation of the coagulation waterfall sequence to explain the various proteins involved in the blood clotting process was described as "a moment of chalkboard brilliance," and the profile noted that his observations, along with those of his colleagues, "provided the guiding light for research and education into the clotting process for decades to come" and "laid the foundations for today's research advances in the field."[17]

Dr. Matthews established the Cystic Fibrosis Center, dedicated to both the care of CF patients and the scientific study of the condition. Carl Doershuk, MD, joined him in 1960 as a fellow in pediatric pulmonology, and much of what they learned and put into practice with their patients shaped the care of CF patients worldwide and led to dramatic improvements in survival rates. Dr. Matthews' medical philosophy emphasized early intervention and prevention, and it involved a team of medical specialists, nurses, respiratory therapists, dietitians, and social workers.

"The importance of what Dr. Matthews did cannot be overstated," says Robert Stern, MD, a specialist in pediatric lung diseases who retired from University Hospitals Rainbow Babies & Children's Hospital in 2015. "At the time, few doctors wanted to work with these kids because it was seen as a lost cause—they wouldn't survive. He looked carefully and closely at each facet of the disease, followed his patients closely, treated all the symptoms, tracked improvement, and made progress." A diabetic, Dr. Matthews was so dedicated to his work that he often missed meals and had problems managing his blood sugar. "His patients kept candy bars on hand for him," recalls Dr. Stern.

Until the invention of the heparin lock in 1972 by Dr. Stern, CF patients spent long hours in the hospital hooked to an IV. His device, implanted in the arm, hand, or chest, provided a safe, reusable port for administering intravenous medications on an as-needed basis, giving patients freedom of movement. "It also meant IV therapy could be done at home," says Dr. Stern, "and this kept people out of the hospital."

Dr. Doershuk, who designed the first pulmonary function testing equipment for infants and children, succeeded Dr. Matthews, serving as Director of the Cystic Fibrosis Center from 1968 to 1998 and as Chief of the Pulmonary Division from 1969 to 1984. Chrissy Falleti, age 42, saw him regularly until he retired. "I've been a patient since I was 6 weeks old. My parents made the postural drainage treatments part of our daily routine, and Dr. Doershuk helped them find the balance between being protective and letting me be a normal, active kid.

A key protocol for treating cystic fibrosis was postural drainage. Developed by LeRoy Matthews, MD, the procedure involved clapping and vibrating the chest to loosen secretions in the lungs with the child in 13 different positions. Parents were taught how to perform the 45-minute procedure at home, ca. late 1950s.

Having CF wasn't so terrible to me growing up. I didn't have my first hospital admission until I was 16."

Chrissy was a gymnast from early childhood through high school, went to college, married, and works as a teacher. In 2006, she suffered a lung collapse. "This was a major setback, but then I had an opportunity to participate in the initial trials at UH for a new drug. It only works for CF people with specific kinds of gene mutations and is now approved. It has changed my life." Whatever the future holds for her, Chrissy considers herself a very fortunate person. "I've benefited from the treatments that started here and also helped advance treatment for others."

Today, the hospital's Cystic Fibrosis Center is the largest of its kind in Ohio, drawing patients from around the region. Because many who came to the CF Center for evaluation and treatment as youngsters live longer than the national average for those with this disease, there is a special unit at UH Rainbow Babies & Children's for adult patients. Reverend Anthony Cassese, who passed away in December 2014 at the remarkable age of 66 given his diagnosis, was one of these patients.

"I was diagnosed by Dr. Matthews and was one of the first children admitted to the new center," said Rev. Cassese. "When I was in fourth grade, he asked me what I wanted to be when I grow up. My answer was a priest. He said 'OK, and someday you'll preside at my funeral.' And I did."

Dr. Matthews' belief that Anthony could have a future had a powerful effect on the young boy and his parents. Although there were times when he was very sick, the combination of hope, home care, and regular hospital stays made it possible for Rev. Cassese, who was ordained in 1977, to pursue his dream, become pastor of a church, and lead a full and rich life. "I never expected to become a senior citizen. And, in my own small way, by giving blood and volunteering to be part of many studies here, I helped doctors improve treatment and get closer to finding a cure."

Michael Konstan, MD, succeeded Dr. Doershuk in 1998 as Director of the CF Center and remained in this role until he was appointed Chairman of the Department of Pediatrics at UH Rainbow Babies & Children's in 2010, a position also held by Dr. Matthews 25 years earlier. Dr. Konstan, who served as chairman for five years, and his team are internationally recognized for clinical research leading to novel therapies for CF.

Dr. Konstan was recruited to UH in 1985 by Pamela Davis, MD, PhD, who had recently been appointed Chief of the Pediatric Pulmonary Division at UH Rainbow Babies & Children's and is currently the Dean of Case Western Reserve University School of

Pioneer

Marvin Lough, MBA, RRT, FAARC, became Technical Director of the Pulmonary Function Laboratory at Babies and Childrens Hospital in 1964 and was responsible for directing a new pediatric respiratory therapy unit there. At the time, there were fewer than 200 registered respiratory therapists in the country, with only a handful trained to specialize in children. In the following years, Lough developed the first academic-based respiratory therapy training curriculum with a strong emphasis on the needs of children—a three-day course in pediatric respiratory therapy used at two local community colleges that drew professionals from all over the country—and authored the first textbook on pediatric respiratory therapy in collaboration with Carl Doershuk, MD, and Robert Stern, MD.

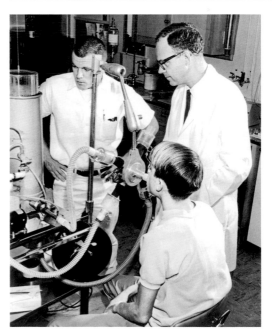

Carl Doershuk, MD (right), pioneers the first pulmonary function testing equipment used for infants and children, 1968.

Medicine. Dr. Konstan's early research focused on developing a therapy to treat the excessive inflammation in the lungs of CF patients. He found that ibuprofen, given in very high doses twice daily for four years, nearly halted the progression of lung disease in children with CF. His landmark article in *The New England Journal of Medicine* in 1995 established ibuprofen as the first effective—and still as of today the only—therapy to suppress the damaging inflammation in the CF lung.

Dr. Konstan subsequently turned his attention to therapies that treat the underlying cause of CF. He was instrumental in the design and implementation of the clinical studies that led to FDA approval of two drugs, Kalydeco and Orkambi, that target the abnormal gene product of CF. In 2016, Dr. Konstan published his findings of a clinical trial of Orkambi that he led that included over 1,000 CF patients from 15 countries. The drug improved lung function and decreased the need for IV antibiotics. According to Dr. Konstan, "It has the potential to benefit nearly 50 percent of the 70,000 people that suffer from CF worldwide."

"Our CF Center has been an innovator for 60 years," says Dr. Konstan, who was the first to hold the Austin Ricci Chair in Pediatric Pulmonary Care and Research, endowed by aviation entrepreneur and University Hospitals Cleveland Medical Center board member, Kenn Ricci, and named for his son. "The first 30 years were focused on defining

Achievements by Michael Konstan, MD, in cystic fibrosis drug development have revolutionized care for this disease around the world, 2008.

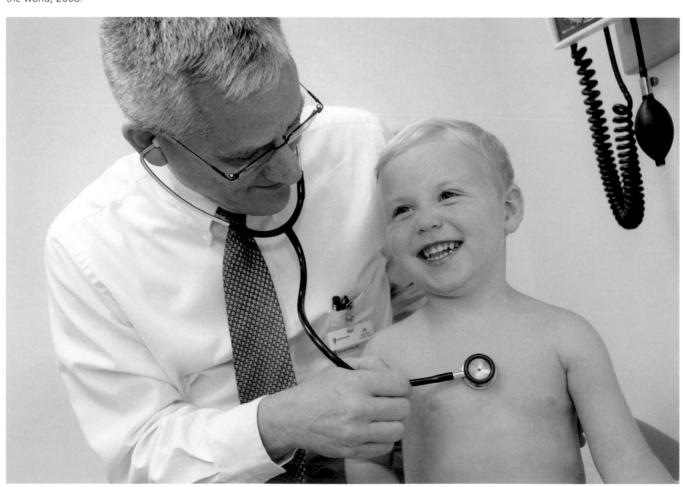

the disease, treating its consequences and complications." He adds, "The close collaboration between the physicians at UH and the scientists at the medical school is unique and has been key to the CF Center's success."

Blindness in Babies

A little-known but very important episode in the history of ophthalmology took place in Cleveland in the early 1950s, and a courageous decision by one doctor to stand by her findings had far-reaching effects on countless lives. University Hospitals was part of a cooperative nationwide study of the role of oxygen in retrolental fibroplasia (RLF), a condition prevalent in premature infants that can lead to blindness. Anita Gilger, MD, was in charge of examining the babies and collecting data.

Before joining the staff at Babies and Childrens Hospital in 1948, Dr. Gilger had conducted clinical research on the condition at Children's Hospital in Cincinnati. Preliminary findings from the new study corroborated her own earlier hypothesis: the high levels of oxygen commonly administered to all preemies were the cause of RLF. Evidence presented at a 1953 conference of ophthalmologists that she attended confirmed her conclusions. But the leaders of the joint study felt another year of observation was required before a definitive recommendation to change the practice could be made. "Doctor Anita Gilger faced an important decision. Should she wait until the official pronouncement from Committee headquarters…or should she, on her own initiative, request that oxygen be curtailed on all low-weight prematures in Greater Cleveland…realizing that if she were wrong, she might jeopardize the lives of many premature babies in Cleveland hospitals. That afternoon, after a conference with Doctor Lorand Johnson, professor of ophthalmology at Western Reserve University…she sent a telegram to all pediatricians cooperating with her in RLF research, strongly urging them to immediately stop high oxygen control." A year later, the Joint Committee made Dr. Gilger's recommendation official.

"Somewhere in Cleveland today are twenty children who can see the smile on their mother's faces and know the beauty of a sun-filled day." They owe their sight to the doctors and clinical researchers who found the answer to RLF and to a Cleveland woman, Dr. Anita Gilger.[18]

Medical Advances: 1970s

Big changes for University Hospitals began with Rainbow Hospital relocating to the University Circle campus in 1971 and the

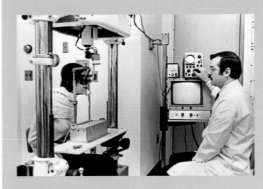

Opthalmology ultrasound, ca. 1970s.

It's a Fact

University Hospitals Chairman of the Division of Opthalmology, Charles Thomas, MD, performed the first successful corneal transplant in Northeast Ohio in 1945. The first to participate in the UH ophthalmology residency program established in 1937, Dr. Thomas also founded the Cleveland Eye Bank in 1958, which arranged for people to donate their eye tissue after death for transplantation so others might see. By 1970, approximately 90 percent of corneal transplants done locally each year were performed at UH by Dr. Thomas and his colleagues. The Eye Bank, now known as Eversight Ohio, serves all of the Cleveland-area hospitals. The division continues to advance the field of ophthalmology. Jonathan Lass, MD, University Hospitals Eye Institute's former Director; William Reinhart, MD; and Beth Ann Benetz, MA, CRA, FOPS, were investigators in a 2013 National Eye Institute multi-center corneal transplant study conducted for over more than a decade, called the Cornea Donor Study. It showed that donor age was not a significant factor in the success of corneal transplantation, a discovery that significantly expanded the pool of available tissue.

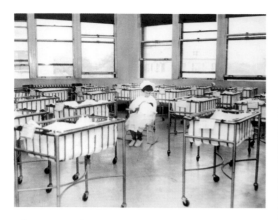

Infant care at the MacDonald House nursery in the late 1950s. This scene, common in most U.S. hospitals for decades, changed with the "open nursery" policy developed at University Hospitals which allowed both mothers and fathers to visit and touch their infants from the start to optimize bonding.

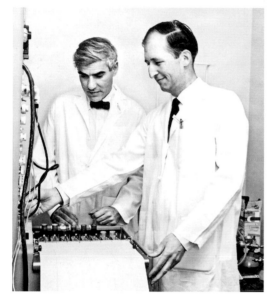

The findings of John Kennell, MD (right), and Marshall Klaus, MD, (left), on infant bonding laid the foundation for making family-centered care standard practice in premature nurseries and delivery rooms around the country, ca. 1970s.

establishment of a joint board of governance with Babies and Childrens Hospital in 1974. New thinking and major developments in tools and techniques at UH as well as in the larger medical world improved care, especially for newborns. Simultaneously, the feminist movement put women's needs in the spotlight. Health and well-being rather than sickness took center stage at UH in this decade.

Infant Bonding

Pediatrician John Kennell, MD, and neonatologist Marshall Klaus, MD, began studying the relationship between mothers and their newborns in the 1960s, using cameras to film mother and baby interactions at MacDonald House. In 1972, when Drs. Kennell and Klaus released their initial report, it was common to separate mothers and babies immediately after birth and have nurses provide all the care and feeding in the nurseries. The physicians concluded that this interfered with what they termed "bonding"—the formation of a deep emotional connection rooted, they believed, in the body's own hormonal chemistry—that takes place in the first few hours and days of a baby's life. This connectivity is sparked by parental feelings of warmth, intense love, devotion, and a sense of responsibility. Their ideas were applicable to healthy, premature, and ill babies and had a profound influence on maternity ward routines and the handling of newborns everywhere, creating a much more positive and humane experience for families.

That same year, the mothers living-in program for sick children became the parents living-in program. Cots and reclining chairs, showers, and kitchenettes were available for those who stayed overnight. "The father's support of the living-in program makes a world of difference to the child and the mother," said Dr. Kennell, associate pediatrician at University Hospitals whose collaboration on a 14-year study on child rearing (under the direction of renowned child care expert Benjamin Spock, MD) led to the development of the program. "Our studies have shown that even the best equipped hospital with the finest medical and nursing staff cannot meet the young child's emotional needs as well as his own parents [can]… [T]he child's emotional wellbeing is closely related to how well he responds to treatment."[19]

Drs. Klaus and Kennell co-authored a revolutionary book titled *Maternal Infant Bonding*, which explored the benefits of immediate close physical contact between mothers and babies and was published in 1976. This practice was eventually extended to include fathers, who they encouraged to be present during labor and delivery. In later years, the doctors revised their language about the bonding timetable, changing their description of the period right after birth from critical to sensitive, suggesting that it was not the only opportunity for parents to forge normal, lasting emotional ties with their babies.

When Northeast Ohio's first pediatric intensive care unit opened at Rainbow Babies and Childrens Hospital in 1977, special emphasis was placed on parent participation. Parents were encouraged to visit and help feed, dress, and entertain their child just as they would at home. Rainbow Babies and Childrens was also among the first hospitals in the country to welcome parents into the neonatal intensive care unit (NICU). Paula Forsythe, RN, a neonatal nurse, received a grant in 1992 to create three semi-private spaces for families to stay with their babies prior to discharge. The impact was so positive that all the rooms in today's NICU are set up for parents and babies to stay together around the clock.

When Avroy Fanaroff, MD, arrived as a pediatric resident and fellow in 1969, the NICU was primitive by today's standards. While it housed incubators to keep newborns warm, there were no monitors to continuously track blood pressure, heart rate, and respiration. He recalls that if a baby stopped breathing, indicated by a change in color, the doctor or nurse would stimulate the infant by pulling on a piece of string tied to his or her toe.

The quality of care dramatically improved as more sophisticated tools designed specifically for babies became available. In the early 1970s, a team of Rainbow Babies and Childrens neonatologists, including John Kattwinkel, MD, a research fellow with a degree in biomedical engineering, developed silicone nasal prongs for the

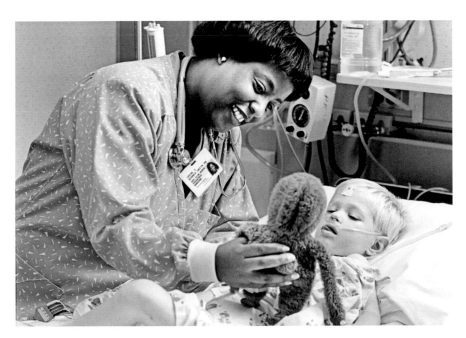

Pediatric Intensive Care Unit, ca. early 1980s.

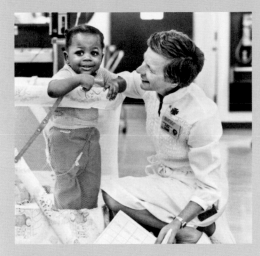

Dalia Zemaityte, MSN, RN, (right), was often referred to by her colleagues as the heart and soul of University Hospitals Rainbow Babies & Children's Hospital. She retired in 2012 after 52 years of service but continues to come in four days a week as a volunteer.

Game Changer

At University Hospitals Rainbow Babies & Children's Hospital, there is an emphasis on the importance of family involvement that began at Babies and Childrens Hospital in the late 1950s. Before, parents were given limited access to caring for their child while in the hospital. No individual deserves more credit for bringing about this shift in policy than Dalia Zemaityte, MSN, RN. In 1960, as Assistant Supervisor of Nursing for Babies and Childrens, she was a staunch supporter of efforts to provide for the emotional needs of children and establishing family-friendly practices, such as allowing parents to stay overnight and changing staff perceptions about the value of partnering with parents. In 1971, she was instrumental in the formation of one of the first Family Advisory Councils, in partnership with parents, in the country. "Implementing [all of] this was initially a challenge," Zemaityte says, "but I consider it the crown jewel of my work here. Now doctors and nurses can't imagine doing without all of the help parents provide by staying with their children, bathing, feeding, and playing with them."

The Evolution of the NICU

Intensive care options for newborns have improved dramatically over the past 50 years and University Hospitals helped lead the way. Babies went from sleeping in open cribs similar to those used for a healthy baby to enclosed incubators. In the early 1970s, University Hospitals opened its first neonatal intensive care unit (NICU) that included state-of-the-art monitoring equipment to track babies' vital signs and new technology to assist with respiration. University Hospitals Rainbow Babies & Children's Hospital was one of the first children's hospitals in the nation to welcome parents into the NICU.

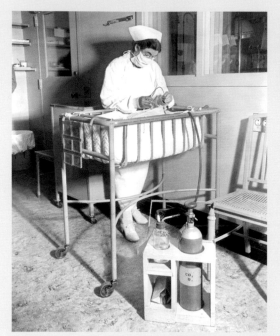 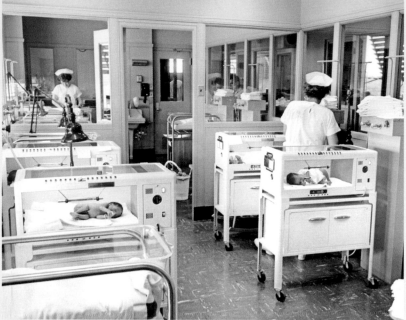

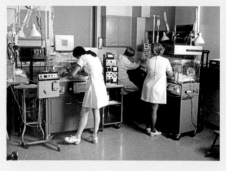 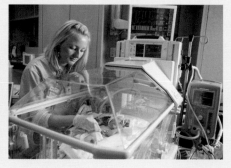 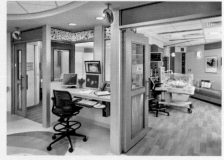

Top left: 1944. *Top right:* 1960. *Bottom (left to right):* First NICU at Rainbow Babies and Childrens Hospital, 1971; Modern NICU, 2000; The Quentin & Elisabeth Alexander Level IIIc Neonatal Intensive Care Unit, built in 2009, is considered a model for NICUs across the country and around the world.

application of continuous positive airway pressure in treating respiratory distress in preterm and near-term neonates. They are still in use today. "It was a major advance [to develop] a minimally invasive way to treat babies with respiratory failure and improve their oxygenation," says Dr. Fanaroff. "Eventually this [technology] was patented, and we received some income for many years that supported the educational program in the neonatal division."

Since UH Rainbow Babies & Children's founding, neonatologists have focused on refining and improving the quality of care for the most

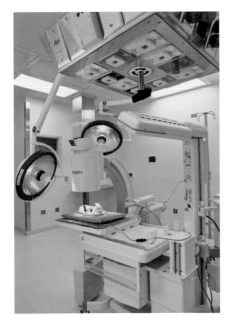

The Rainbow Flex surgical bed was developed in 2009 by a team at University Hospitals Rainbow Babies & Children's Hospital to keep babies warm and allow access from all four sides. The bed is a mobile unit that can be dispatched to operating rooms.

premature infants. Statistics are a measure of what has been achieved. In 1972, a baby who weighed only 2.25 pounds at birth had a 10 percent chance of survival at Rainbow Babies and Childrens. In 2012, the survival rate for a baby of that weight was 96 percent, a figure that is among the highest in the nation. "Over the last 20 years, we have seen improved survival at all birth weights and gestational ages, even for babies delivered at 23 and 24 weeks' gestation," says Michele Walsh, MD, MS, Division Chief of Neonatology. "It's small, but it's real." Dr. Walsh is quick to point out that the improvement in survival is a team effort at UH. "It's not any one intervention," she says. "It's the increasing sophistication of the high-risk OBs and neonatologists taking care of them. It's making sure that the moms get antenatal steroids before delivery. It's avoiding injuring the babies' lungs as much as possible and improving their nutritional status by using human milk. The more human milk we are able to get them, the more protected they are from severe infections, both in the bloodstream and in the intestines."

Heart Health

Unlike most physicians of the 1950s, University Hospitals cardiologist Herman Hellerstein, MD, did not advocate for bed rest and inactivity for those with heart disease. Instead, he prescribed a comprehensive lifestyle approach for the rehabilitation of cardiac patients and the prevention of future heart attacks. He advised people to lose weight, stop smoking, eat a healthy diet, and exercise regularly. His ideas were considered radical and controversial at the time.

Dr. Hellerstein launched a study in the early '60s that involved 300 Cleveland men between the ages of 40 and 50 who had either survived a heart attack or were predisposed to one. Participants engaged in calisthenics and conditioning classes to build up endurance, and played volleyball or basketball. They had their blood pressure, EKG, and heart rates checked regularly. Additionally, their wives were recruited to work with a dietitian to plan meals containing less saturated fat.

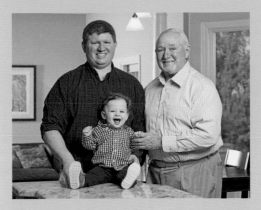

Three generations of Fanaroffs: Jonathan (left), Avroy (right), and Mason, 2013.

Family Ties

Avroy Fanaroff, MD, was only four days into his pediatric fellowship at Rainbow Babies and Childrens Hospital, when his wife, Roslyn, gave birth to their son, Jonathan. The baby spent his first three weeks in the very same neonatal intensive care unit (NICU) where his father worked. Co-Medical Director of the NICU since 2007 and a neonatologist like his father, Jonathan Fanaroff, MD, was part of the team that designed the Rainbow Flex, the world's first surgical bed specifically designed for the smallest newborns. He is involved in collaborations to develop and enhance noninvasive therapies to minimize pain and discomfort in neonates. One such intervention is a specialized incubator for MRI exams that keeps babies comfortable and able to sleep though the procedure, decreasing the need for anesthesia and sedation. The younger Dr. Fanaroff and his wife, Kristy, a neonatal nurse practitioner at University Hospitals Rainbow Babies & Children's, found that their drive to improve conditions for these tiny, fragile patients became even more personal in 2012 when their son, Mason, was born. He was also an early arrival, spending 30 days in the NICU where his father, mother, and grandfather have helped so many.

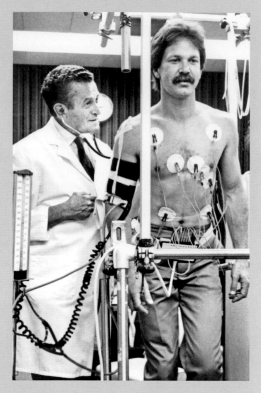

Cardiologist Herman Hellerstein, MD (left), 1985.

I Remember

"My dad experimented on us," recalls Elizabeth Hellerstein, MD, a pediatrician at University Hospitals and the youngest child of Herman Hellerstein, MD. "I grew up on skim milk and whole grains. We weren't allowed to have beef or ice cream. Nobody else I knew was eating like this in the '60s and '70s. We hiked and biked as a family instead of watching TV. He had a lab at the hospital, and when I went there with him, I played on the treadmill and the stationary bike. Sometimes, he'd even hook me up to get my vitals."

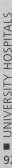
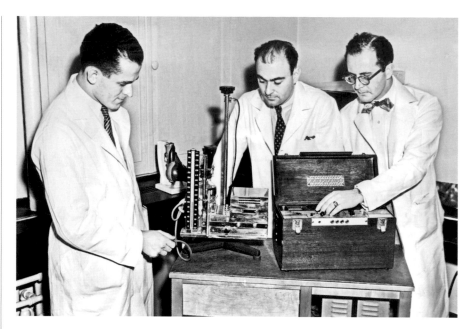

Herman Hellerstein, MD (far left), worked with a team from Western Reserve University School of Medicine to develop an automated, non-invasive technique to diagnose certain types of heart disorders by measuring cardiac output and lung function. It was also useful for assessing a patient's response to therapy and physical exercise, 1950.

"Dr. Hellerstein was my physician," said Cleveland legend and food columnist Maury Feren, a study participant who lived to be 100 years old. "He found signs of blockage in my arteries, and after I had bypass surgery, I joined his program and became one of his stars. He required I exercise three times a week. I biked, I jogged, I lifted weights, and he gathered data on me and everyone else to prove his theories."

Feren remained dedicated to a fitness regimen along with healthy eating long after the study. He did not stop going to the gym or playing tennis regularly until age 98. "Dr. Hellerstein saved my life and made it better," Feren says, "and he did the same for so many, many others."

In 1971, Dr. Hellerstein played an instrumental role in developing the ergometer, a stationary bicycle that measured pulse rate, heartbeat, and calorie consumption per minute. It was used to detect and evaluate a heart condition and could be calibrated to provide the correct level of challenge for rehabilitation.

By 1975, Dr. Hellerstein was no longer a lone voice in promoting diet and exercise as management tools for heart disease. The American Heart Association had come out in support of physical training programs for heart attack survivors, and cardiac rehab programs based on the principles he espoused began to proliferate around the country.

Medical Advances: 1980s – 1990s

As health care improved and people lived longer, questions about how to best respond to the needs of an aging population took on special importance. Shorter hospital stays and more outpatient procedures were becoming common. Computers and emerging imaging technology were providing physicians with more information than was previously available about what was happening inside the body. Old diagnostic and surgical techniques were being replaced or refined, and the availability of new materials and device technology was leading to better outcomes. Almost every aspect of medical care was changing with University Hospitals leading the way in many cases.

Geriatric Medicine

The Benjamin Rose Institute on Aging opened a rehabilitation hospital devoted to older patients in 1953 in University Circle on the University Hospitals campus, entering into an association with University Hospitals from 1957 to 1968. It was among the first facilities of its kind in the nation devoted to the care of elderly patients. Addressing the unique needs of this age group gained momentum at UH in 1981 with the opening of the Center for Assessment and Care of the Elderly, established with a $500,000 grant from Revco, one of the largest unrestricted corporate gifts in UH history at that time. The innovative program implemented a team approach to evaluating the medical, emotional, and social needs of older patients. It was renamed the Joseph M. Foley ElderHealth Center in 1987 and later the UH Foley ElderHealth Center to honor the man who played a key role in its establishment.

Many programs for seniors are now part of the multidisciplinary Center for Geriatric Medicine at UH. A special unit is devoted to Acute

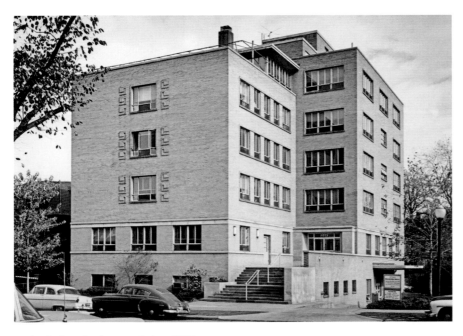

Benjamin Rose Institute on Aging, 1957.

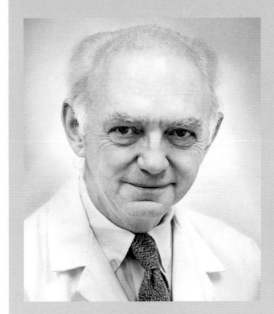

Joseph Foley, MD, 1981.

Pioneer

Joseph Foley, MD, was Chairman of the Department of Neurology at University Hospitals Cleveland Medical Center from 1961 to 1979. Robert Daroff, MD, who was recruited to replace Dr. Foley when he retired, describes him as a giant in American neurology. In 1980, Dr. Foley focused his attention on aging and care of the elderly. Speaking to an interviewer in 2008, the 92-year-old explained why. "I became interested in aging because of the research I was doing on diseases that are prominent in old age, particularly dementia and the movement disorders of old age. These are diseases that command attention because of their prevalence and impact. That research and the fact that there was a large group of patients who were, in effect, being ignored—was why [Dr. Amasa B.] Buzz Ford and I started University Hospitals' geriatric assessment center…We had to move it three times, and each time we moved, the facilities got bigger and better."[20]

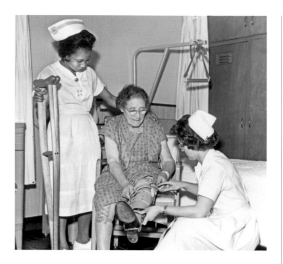

Geriatric care at Benjamin Rose, 1962.

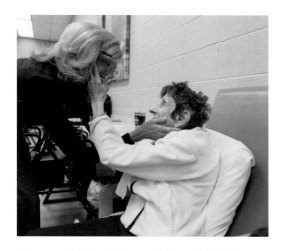

Elder care at University Hospitals Parma Medical Center's Senior Center, 2016.

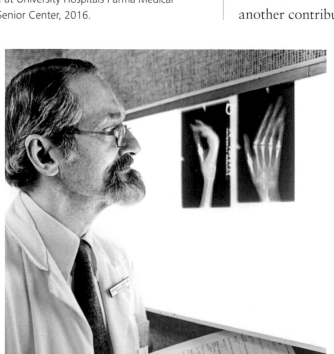

Kingsbury Heiple, MD, pioneered improvements of artificial finger joints (shown in X-ray), ca. 1980s.

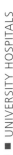
Care for the Elderly (ACE), an innovative concept for meeting the care needs of frail seniors that was developed at the hospital in 1994. Two UH medical centers, Bedford and Richmond, are the first in the region to have Senior Emergency Rooms. Today, Alzheimer's disease is the focus of drug trials, genetic studies, and clinical research on caregiving methods and outcomes for patients at the Brain Health & Memory Center at University Hospitals Neurological Institute.

Repairing Bones and Joints

In 1980, Kingsbury Heiple, MD, announced that after 15 months of experimentation with a revolutionary titanium and synthetic rubber joint he helped to develop, use of the fingers for those suffering from arthritis or crippling hand injuries could be restored. The news made headlines around the country. According to a newspaper article, "until recently, Heiple was the only orthopedic surgeon in the world implanting the new artificial joints," which would allow most patients to "acquire an excellent range of motion and finger function after 4 to 6 weeks of therapy sessions at University Hospitals' Rehabilitation Center."[21] Dr. Heiple was highly regarded for the research he conducted over a 30-year period gauging the stresses of daily activities on artificial weight-bearing body parts. He received a patent in 1987 for a cutting tool used to prepare a femur for an implantable prosthesis. Victor Goldberg, MD, who followed Dr. Heiple as Chair of Orthopedic Surgery at University Hospitals, is another contributor in this arena, recognized for his design modifications of hip and knee components that significantly improved modern joint replacement outcomes.

Like Dudley Allen, MD, more than a century before him, orthopedic surgeon Randall Marcus, MD, left Cleveland to study and brought advanced ideas back to UH. He learned a revolutionary new technique for treating fractures of the femur and tibia, developed in Germany and perfected in Seattle, which eliminated the need for traction and body casts and all the accompanying problems that come with being immobile for long periods of time in bed. "It was called intramedullary interlocking nails. In the operating room, we would make small incisions, insert stainless steel rods inside the hollow part of the bone, and line up complicated fractures...using an X-ray fluoroscope to guide us. Then, we could put the nails through the bone and the rod, locking the pieces into place," said Dr. Marcus.

Dr. Marcus was the first to perform the procedure in Ohio in 1982 on Ned Owens, who had been in a terrible motorcycle accident. "His [Ned's] right thigh bone was broken into several pieces and was penetrating the skin," remembers Dr. Marcus. "The left thigh bone was also severely shattered. I was able to fix both in one operation the night he came into the hospital. With excellent nursing care and physical therapy, he healed well and eventually went back to his full activities, including running. That would have been virtually impossible in the days before this technique." Interviewed for a magazine article 18 months later, Owens said, "I'm still getting used to the fact that my legs are normal. I thought I'd never walk again."[22] Former Chairman of the Department of Orthopedics, Dr. Marcus was granted a patent for the multi-use femoral intramedullary nail in 1986.

Another leading figure in the Department of Orthopedics was Henry Bohlman, MD. Viewed by colleagues around the world as the "father" of modern cervical spine surgery, he began his career at UH in 1972 and was Director of the hospital's Spine Institute at the time of his death in 2010. Dr. Bohlman also spent 27 years as Chief of the Acute Spinal Cord Injury Unit at the Louis Stokes Cleveland VA Medical Center. He made enduring contributions to the field through his innovations in anterior surgical techniques, repairing the spine by entering through the front of the body rather than the back and restoring mobility to paralyzed limbs. This technique avoids disturbing the spinal cord, spinal nerves, and neck muscles, revolutionizing treatment for injury and degenerative conditions in this region of the spine.

An advocate for the importance of long-term follow-up care, he saved all of his X-rays and notes and often said he "never discharged a patient" because he wanted to assess the effectiveness of procedures five, 10, 15, and even 20 years later.

Taking care of young patients with broken bones, skeletal deformities, bone infections, tuberculosis, polio, and bone tumors has been part of UH since sick and

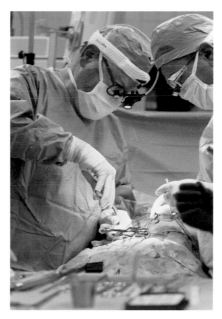

Orthopedic surgeon Henry Bohlman, MD (left), came into the public eye for procedures he performed on well-known sports figures: pro golfer and PGA Tour winner Garner Dickinson (1984); Cleveland Cavaliers center Brad Daugherty (1994); Baltimore Orioles pitcher Scott Kamieniecki (1998); and Orioles short stop and third baseman "Iron Man" Cal Ripken, who achieved the additional nine hits he needed to join the 3,000 club during the season following his surgery (1999).

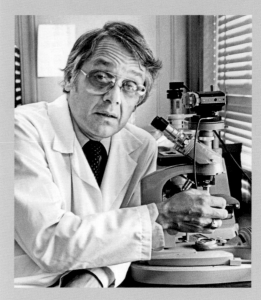

Roland Moskowitz, MD, ca. 1985.

Pioneer

Rheumatologist Roland Moskowitz, MD, former Director of the Rheumatology Clinical Research Unit at University Hospitals Cleveland Medical Center, was recognized around the world as a trailblazer in the clinical research, education, and treatment of osteoarthritis, which currently affects more than 22 million Americans. Until 1990, doctors believed that osteoarthritis was the natural result of old age and joint wear. However, Dr. Moskowitz discovered for the first time that the painful disease was linked to genetics. Dr. Moskowitz once remarked that the most exciting aspect of this finding was the prospect of recognizing who is at risk for osteoarthritis and that further study could lead to the development of measures to prevent joint breakdown.[23]

Dr. Moskowitz earned international recognition for his work when he received the President's Gold Medal Award from the American College of Rheumatology in 2000. "I have spent my career practicing medicine, teaching, and doing research," he said. "UH has been a very nurturing environment for what I wanted to do, and that made all my accomplishments possible."

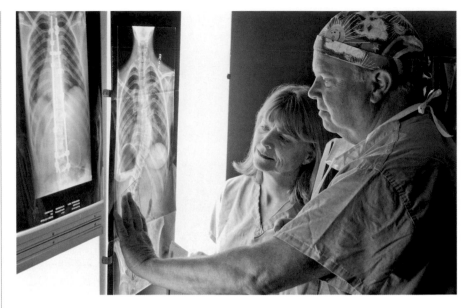

George Thompson, MD (right), began his career at University Hospitals in 1979 and became Director of Pediatric Orthopedics in 1987. A child Dr. Thompson treated for scoliosis wrote in a grateful patient letter, "My life has changed in so many ways after the surgery…Now, I am in no pain…My appearance has also changed in a major way…I see that my clothes fit better… I'm taller, and I feel as if I have a better attitude towards life."

injured children began coming to Rainbow Cottage to convalescence in the late 1800s. From the day it opened, the Department of Pediatric Orthopedic Surgery at University Hospitals Rainbow Babies & Children's Hospital quickly became one of the preeminent divisions in the United States. Under the direction of world-renowned orthopedic surgeon George Thompson, MD, the division has been a leader in the treatment of children's spinal and limb deformities, hip abnormalities, and trauma. Years ago, the standard of care for treating scoliosis was surgical correction of the spinal curvature, followed by five to six months in the hospital encased in a full body cast. The process often had to be repeated as a child grew. Today, pediatric orthopedic surgeons at UH Rainbow Babies & Children's Hospital are among the most experienced in the country at using an alternative approach: surgically-inserted growing rods. The technique is ideal for young patients with severe spinal deformities because the rods expand as the child develops.

Medical Advances: 2000 – 2018

The increasing focus at University Hospitals on translational research that brings together practicing physicians, laboratory scientists, and biomedical engineers has led to significant progress in the development of new products—drugs, therapies, technology, and devices—that help prolong and improve quality of life for people with serious injuries and illnesses. "In health care, our golden age is now," UH CEO Thomas F. Zenty III told an audience at Cleveland's City Club in 2015.

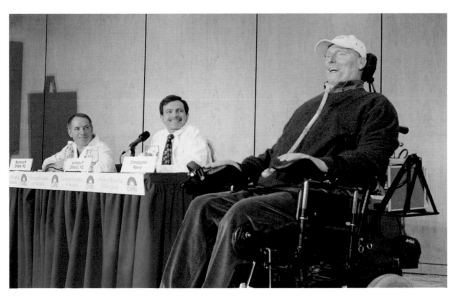

Hollywood actor Christopher Reeve, aka "Superman," was the second person in the world to receive the experimental diaphragmatic pacing system technology in 2003. For Reeve, who had suffered a severe spinal cord injury in an accident that left him a quadriplegic, it meant his quality of life improved for the better. At a news conference following the procedure, he spoke about the pleasure of being able to smell coffee, a result of breathing through his nose instead of the hole in his throat that connected him to a ventilator. The media coverage of Reeve's surgery put the procedure and the possibilities it offered into the national spotlight.

Respiratory Paralysis

One of the biggest challenges patients with paralysis face is the inability to breathe on their own without assistance. University Hospitals has been a pioneer in this arena, changing the quality of life for these patients for the better. In 1998, gastrointestinal surgeon Raymond Onders, MD, holder of the Margaret G. and Walter K. Remen Chair in Surgical Innovation, and colleagues at Case Western Reserve University, the Louis Stokes Cleveland VA Medical Center, and MetroHealth Medical Center created a device that enables individuals with severe paralysis or amyotrophic lateral sclerosis (ALS, or Lou Gehrig's disease) to breathe for periods of time without the aid of a mechanical ventilator. Known as the diaphragmatic pacing system (DPS) and rooted in research originally conducted by Michael Nochomovitz, MD, a former pulmonologist at UH, the small battery-powered device replaces awkward, noisy, heavy equipment. It stimulates the muscles and nerves that draw air into the lungs to contract via electrical impulses traveling through wire-like electrodes threaded through the abdomen. This strengthens the diaphragm and for some can lead to breathing with assistance from the new device.

DPS earned FDA approval in 2008, and the following year, Dr. Onders implanted the device in a wheelchair-bound 10-year-old boy, the youngest patient to date to receive it. The outpatient surgery lasted only 90 minutes. DPS is also now used to help patients with ALS. In 2013, Daniel Darkow, a 21-year-old college student, became the first

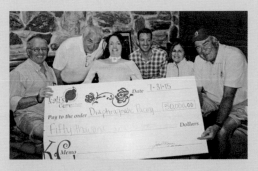

Diaphragmatic pacing system recipient Kali Pung (center), with Raymond Onders, MD (far left), and Pung's family: Mike Pung (father), Mike Pung (brother), and Alice Pung (mother), and family friend Frank Beckmann, 2015.

Pass It On

"I had a swimming accident in 2006, hit my head, and was paralyzed from the neck down," says Kali Pung. "My parents found out about DPS (diaphragmatic pacing system), and I was the 33rd patient to get the implant, which was still in clinical trials. I remember it was painful for the first five minutes. And then all of a sudden, I was breathing. It was a great feeling. Having the pacer changed everything. It's easier to talk. I'm healthier, less susceptible to pneumonia, and I've been able to be on an aggressive physical therapy plan."

"What happened to Kali was catastrophic," says her father, Mike. "The pacer has been a miracle."

Kali and her parents started Kali's Cure, a private foundation that supports those with spinal cord injuries and those working on treatments to help them. "We've raised almost $650,000 for Dr. Onders, his work, and even to purchase batteries for those who can't afford them," Kali says. "And, we don't plan to stop. What he's doing is absolutely amazing and benefits so many."

person with spinal muscular atrophy, a form of muscular dystrophy, to receive the diaphragmatic pacing system implant. He says that Dr. Onders' device "gave me back my life."[25]

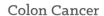

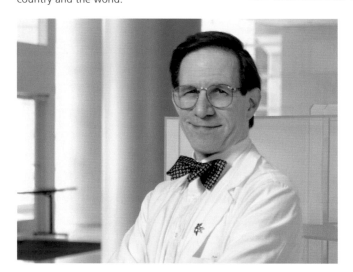

Colon Cancer

Colorectal cancer is the second leading cause of cancer-related deaths in the United States. The work of physician-scientist Sanford Markowitz, MD, PhD, is helping to change that statistic. The University Hospitals oncologist conducted the foundational research for a first-of-its-kind at-home colon cancer test. Dr. Markowitz's work pioneering stool DNA testing was the first to be licensed for commercial development and was instrumental in creating the Cologuard test. Approved by the Food and Drug Administration in 2014, this test is suitable for colon cancer screening in adults over 50 years old with an average risk of developing the disease. According to the American Cancer Society, which endorses the DNA-based screening tool, early detection saves lives, but most people avoid getting tested with a standard colonoscopy.[26] As an alternative, this test is simple, noninvasive, and, most important, effective at revealing the presence of cancers plus many precancerous growths.

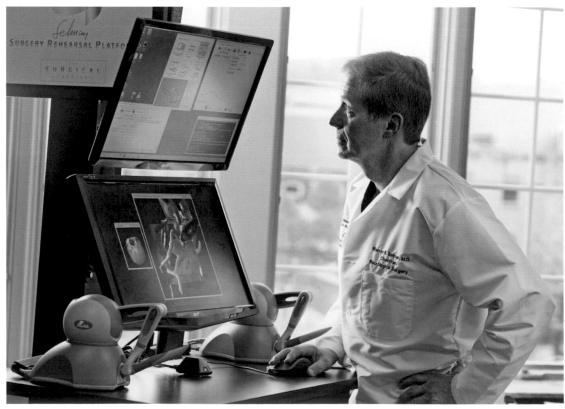

Dr. Markowitz cites his father's colon cancer as the motivating force for his investigations. Between 1995 and 2005, Dr. Markowitz discovered and elucidated the workings of a genetic "on/off switch" that he showed plays a key role in suppressing the development of cancerous colon tumors. Dr. Markowitz showed that genetic inactivation of this switch explains how and why colon cancers develop in Lynch syndrome, in which the disease arises at a young age and in multiple-related individuals. A DNA test Dr. Markowitz developed to distinguish Lynch versus non-Lynch-type colon cancers is widely used by hospital pathology laboratories worldwide for identifying individuals and families with this inherited cancer syndrome.

Former *CBS Evening News* anchor Katie Couric, who lost her husband to colon cancer in 1998, made a televised appeal to help Dr. Markowitz recruit families for his studies, and the Entertainment Industry Foundation National Colorectal Cancer Research Alliance, which she co-founded, provided added support. Following a visit to Dr. Markowitz's lab in June 2010, she called him and the physician-scientists he works with "the real heroes of our society," adding that they "are changing the face of cancer in this country. I can't think of a nobler endeavor than that."[27]

Brain Surgery

Simulation technology is transforming surgical practice and medical education, and Warren Selman, MD, Neurosurgeon-in-Chief at University Hospitals, is a key player in that revolution. In 2009, he teamed up with former Israeli Air Force officers who had expertise in flight simulators to develop a computer-based surgical rehearsal program, known as Surgical Theater technology. It uploads CT and MRI scans and other images of a patient's brain to generate a realistic, interactive onscreen 3-D model. With an accurate replica of what they will encounter during an operation, surgeons can experiment with different approaches until the right one for each patient is found. "It supports patient-specific surgery, improves efficiency and outcomes, and provides a collaborative training environment for medical colleagues to work together on cases as well as teach young physicians," Dr. Selman explains.

A portable iteration of the technology, called SNAP (Surgical Navigation Advanced Platform), earned FDA approval in 2014. It brings the surgical rehearsal platform into the operating room, making it possible for a surgeon to review, test, and plan every detail of a procedure both before and during the operation. In 2016, Dr. Selman and his colleagues took the simulation technology one step further, adding precision virtual reality. Through the use of virtual reality

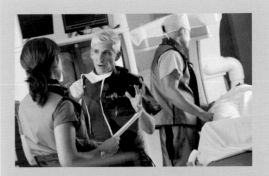

University Hospitals and Case Western Reserve University School of Medicine collaborated in 2006 to recruit Daniel Simon, MD, (center) to create a multidisciplinary team of cardiovascular medicine and surgery experts and physician-investigators at UH.

Game Changer

In a talk he gave in 1947, cardiac surgeon Claude Beck, MD, spoke about the need for an institute to encourage and support advances in coronary care. Fifty years later that dream began to take shape when four separate UH divisions—cardiology, cardiothoracic surgery, vascular surgery, and cardiac anesthesiology—joined together to form the Heart Institute. Today, it is called University Hospitals Harrington Heart & Vascular Institute. Marco Costa, MD, President of UH Harrington Heart & Vascular Institute, leads a group of 11 centers, each with a specific focus of inquiry, diagnosis, and treatment. UH Harrington Heart & Vascular Institute is the focal point for clinical, research, and educational activities related to heart and vascular disease at UH. Every UH medical center is home to a branch of UH Harrington Heart & Vascular Institute, bringing the highest caliber of heart care out into the community.

headsets, physicians can now virtually "fly" through their patient's brain or body. This enhanced viewing capability enables surgeons to work with even more precision and safety.

Heart Repair: Less Invasive, Better Outcomes

In the 1950s, people were dying of heart attacks, and medical interventions to manage them were limited or nonexistent. Physicians at the time were working to develop solutions, but they did not have the sophisticated technology and techniques that are available today. With the introduction of newer and safer interventions over the years, University Hospitals cardiologists and cardiac surgeons have been at the forefront of pioneering clinical advances and employing practice-altering changes in technology in this ever-expanding clinical arena. "Technology is completely changing the way we are treating disease, and the future will bring more changes, making treatments safer, more predictable, and more effective," says Daniel Simon, MD, University Hospitals Cleveland Medical Center President and former President of University Hospitals Harrington Heart & Vascular Institute.

In 2015, cardiologists and radiologists at UH Harrington Heart & Vascular Institute became the first health care professionals in the country to utilize a novel FDA-approved, non-invasive diagnostic tool

University Hospitals is a high-volume Center of Excellence and a training center for the minimally invasive TAVR approach, 2016.

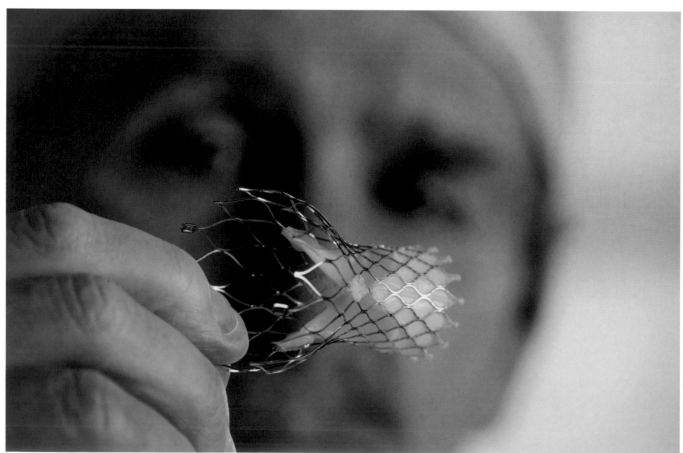

called fractional flow reserve computed tomography (FFRCT) to detect coronary artery disease, the leading killer of both men and women, and determine the right treatment plan for each patient. The highly accurate imaging technology, developed by HeartFlow, Inc., is like no other. It has the potential to replace exercise stress testing, providing detailed anatomical and functional information about the extent of coronary artery blockage and whether it is hindering blood flow to the heart. This modeling platform promises to improve overall accuracy while, at the same time, reduce radiation exposure and complications.

Another major technological advance for cardiac patients with aortic stenosis pioneered at UH is TAVR (transcatheter aortic valve replacement). TAVR, which is performed while the patient is awake and talking, offers a promising treatment alternative for aortic valve replacement, which in the past required open-heart surgery. "Valve replacement used to mean someone was in the hospital for 7 to 10 days, in rehab for two weeks, couldn't drive for six weeks, and didn't feel good for three months. Now, we discharge patients after TAVR in two days," notes Dr. Simon. UH is also one of a select number of institutions across the country to now offer TMVR (transcatheter mitral valve replacement) for patients with mitral regurgitation.

Among other clinical firsts, cardiac surgeons at UH Cleveland Medical Center performed the first durable biventricular assist device (BVAD) procedure in Ohio in 2015. Using a modified left ventricular assist device (LVAD), specialists were able to improve blood flow to both the left *and* right ventricles. In 2014, UH cardiologists treated a high-risk patient who had been rejected for a third open heart surgery elsewhere by implanting a new mitral valve using a valve-in-valve TAVR-like approach through a one-inch incision. The life-saving procedure had never before been performed in the U.S. Also in 2014, UH was the first hospital in Ohio to perform coronary angioplasty procedures using robotic-assisted technology for more precise placement of stents and balloons.

"UH is a national leader in the development of new and less invasive technologies in the cardiovascular space," says Soon Park, MD, Division Chief, Cardiac Surgery. "These innovations will be the dominant mode of treatment within five to ten years, addressing unmet clinical needs and making interventional cardiology a powerhouse of options for patients." ▼

It's a Fact

Four Nobel Prize winners spent time on staff or doing clinical training at University Hospitals.

- **Frederick C. Robbins, MD,** earned the shared prize in Physiology or Medicine for his work with poliomyelitis viruses that contributed to the development of the polio vaccine, 1954.
- **Alfred Gilman, MD, PhD,** earned the shared prize in Physiology or Medicine for the discovery of G proteins and their function in cell communication, 1994.
- **Ferid Murad, MD, PhD,** earned the shared prize in Physiology or Medicine for the discovery that nitric oxide functions as a signaling molecule in the cardiovascular system, 1998.
- **Peter Agre, MD,** earned the shared prize in Chemistry for the discovery of aquaporins, by which water molecules move through cell membranes, leading to a better understanding of many physiological processes and diseases, 2003.

"We can't promise cures," says neurosurgeon Andrew Sloan, MD. "No one can. But, with all our expertise, research, and clinical trials being conducted, there's always hope on the horizon."

Breakthroughs by the Decade

1900 – 1929

1900 William Corlett, MD, a dermatologist at Lakeside Hospital, was among a select group of physicians to test salvarsan, a new treatment for syphilis.

1906 George Crile, MD, performed the first radical neck dissection for laryngeal and other cancers of the neck.

1907 Charles Franklin Hoover, MD, was the first to describe two physical signs, both named "Hoover's sign," that helped neurologists detect weakness in the legs and pulmonologists detect lung disease.

1910 Lakeside Hospital was the world's first hospital to perfect the manufacture of nitrous oxide gas.

1912 The nation's first school of nurse anesthesia was established at Lakeside Hospital.

1915 Henry Gerstenberger, MD; Harold Ruh, MD; and biochemist William Frohring developed an infant formula known as S.M.A. (Synthetic Milk Adapted) at Babies' Dispensary and Hospital.

1917 David Marine, MD, discovered that goiter can be prevented and cured by iodine supplementation.

1930 – 1949

1933 Claude Beck, MD, performed the first successful removal of a heart tumor.

1934 Harry Goldblatt, MD, described the role of the kidneys in hypertension (high blood pressure), laying the foundation for the discovery of renin and eventually the development of enzyme-inhibitor medications to treat chronic hypertension.

1939 Charles I. Thomas, MD, performed the first corneal transplant in Northeast Ohio.

1944 Walter Heymann, MD, began research on kidney disease in children.

1946 Louis Pillemer, PhD, developed preparations of tetanus antigen, leading to the first successful triple vaccine targeting diphtheria, pertussis (whooping cough), and tetanus (DPT), which virtually eliminated these once-fatal diseases in the United States.

1947 Claude Beck, MD, performed the first successful defibrillation of a human heart.

1947 Hymer Friedell, MD, initiated research that became the essential source of information on the long-term effects of radiation on humans.

1950 – 1969

1950 William Holden, MD, performed the first successful femoro-popliteal bypass (from the thigh to the lower leg), using a section of the patient's own vein.

1951 James Reagan, MD, pioneered cytopathology for cancer detection and introduced diagnostic terminology for reporting Pap smear results.

1952 Claude Beck, MD, helped develop cardiopulmonary resuscitation techniques and played an instrumental role in promoting their use.

1952 Use of chloramphenicol in blood disease was developed by Austin Weisberger, MD.

1953 Frank Nulsen, MD, pioneered pressure-regulated one-way valves for the treatment of hydrocephalus (water on the brain). He, along with Charles Herndon, MD, and Lester Persky, MD, also established one of the first hydrocephalus and myelodysplasia clinics for children in the country.

1953 Liver scan by radioisotopes was introduced by Hymer Friedell, MD, and Abbas Rejali, MD.

1953 Oscar Ratnoff, MD, discovered the Hageman Blood Factor. This work led to the 1975 discovery of the Fitzgerald Factor (Factor XI).

1954 Louis Pillemer, PhD, in collaboration with Irwin Lepow, PhD, and Enrique Ecker, PhD, discovered an alternative pathway for the immune response that does not involve antibodies. Drs. Ecker and Lepow also defined a chemical pathway in the body that contributes to inflammation and injury during illness.

1955 Alan Moritz, MD, known as the "Father of Forensic Pathology," worked to establish forensic pathology as a medical subspecialty and influenced the development of a professional U.S. medical examiner system, displacing lay coroners in that position.

1955 Claude Beck, MD, and Walter Pritchard, MD, performed the first successful reversal of a fatal heart attack outside of an operating room with open-heart massage.

1957 Robert Izant, MD, performed the first successful surgery on infants to connect the stomach and intestinal tract.

1957 LeRoy Matthews, MD, developed the first comprehensive treatment program for cystic fibrosis in the nation.

1958 Benjamin Spock, MD, launched his groundbreaking child-rearing study that explored breast-feeding, weaning, toilet training, and separation anxiety.

1961 Albert Potts, MD, PhD, was recognized for his studies on alcohol toxicity on the optic nerve.

1962 Joseph Foley, MD, identified a kind of tremor known as asterixis that occurs in patients with encephalopathy. He was also the first to describe a type of muscle twitching called benign fasciculations that is not associated with any muscle disease.

1965   Kenneth Ryan, MD, was the first in the world to describe how human ovaries produce estrogen from two types of specialized ovarian cells.

1966   Edward Purnell, MD, pioneered the use of B scan ultrasonography to study and diagnose eye and orbital diseases. In 1972, he developed the first hand-held ultrasound device for the eye.

1968   S.S.C. Yen, MD, developed the first radioimmunoassay techniques for the measurement of three important pregnancy hormones.

1969   Jay Ankeney, MD, performed the first successful off-pump open-heart procedure, which later became the basis for minimally invasive heart surgery.

1969   Research by Olof Pearson, MD, established the role of prolactin in breast cancer and pituitary glands.

1969   The role of cholesterol in blood vessel disease was identified by William Insull, MD.

1970s

1970   Walter Maloney, MD, developed the Maloney esophageal dilator, a surgical tool for enlarging the esophageal opening, still the most widely-used surgical instrument of its kind.

1970   The measurement of lung function using isotopes and computer drawings was developed by Scott Inkley, MD, and James MacIntyre, MD.

1971   A "glass house" was developed to reduce infection in total hip replacement surgery.

1971   Charles Herndon, MD, was one of the first surgeons in the United States to perform a hip replacement.

1971   The Angel Frame was invented by UH employee Angel Martinez for the care of newborns.

1971   John Kattwinkel, MD; Avroy Fanaroff, MD; and Marshall Klaus, MD, with David Fleming from Biomedical Engineering, developed silicone nasal prongs for the application of continuous positive airway pressure in treating respiratory distress in pre-term and near-term neonates.

1972   Robert Stern, MD, developed the heparin lock, eliminating the need for continuous hook up to an intravenous line for children needing frequent IV administration of antibiotics, which led to home IV therapy.

1972   Clyde Nash, MD; Richard Brown, PhD; and Albert Burstein, PhD, developed intraoperative spinal cord monitoring, improving the safety of complex spinal surgery.

1972   John Kennell, MD, and Marshall Klaus, MD, demonstrated the importance of maternal-infant bonding.

1972   A bypass heart surgery method using blood vessel grafts without stopping the heart was perfected by Jay Ankeney, MD.

1974   The total jaw replacement procedure was perfected by Clifford Kiehn, MD.

1974   The first practical test for antibody deficiencies in infancy was developed by Stephen Palmer, MD.

1978   Ohio's first bone marrow bank was established at UH by hematologist-oncologist Roger Herzig, MD.

1979   Jeffrey Ponsky, MD, and Michael Gauderer, MD, were co-creators of the PEG (percutaneous endoscopic gastrostomy), a low-risk surgical procedure originally developed to insert a feeding tube for children having problems swallowing. The PEG was later modified for use with adults. It is now used around the world.

1980s and 1990s

1980   Irwin Merkatz, MD, conducted the first clinical trials of ritodrine, the first FDA-approved drug to inhibit pre-term labor, at MacDonald Hospital for Women.

1980   The world's first known survivor of ricin poisoning was treated by Leigh Thompson, MD.

1980   Robert B. Daroff, MD, established the Daroff-Dell' Osso Ocular Motility Laboratory at the Louis Stokes Cleveland VA Medical Center, one of the premier neuro-ophthalmology research laboratories in the world.

1980   Martin Resnick, MD, championed the use of transrectal ultrasound-guided prostate imaging and biopsy, which became the standard of care to diagnose prostate cancer.

1980   Kingsbury Heiple, MD, pioneered improvements of artificial finger joints.

1981   Nikon Cheung, MD, and other researchers at Rainbow Babies and Childrens Hospital pioneered work treating neuroblastoma patients with antibodies, significantly advancing the field of targeted cancer immune-therapy.

1981   The first pediatric bone marrow transplant in Ohio was performed by Peter Coccia, MD.

1981   Pioneering embolization to cure high blood pressure was performed by Joseph Puma, MD; Ralph Alfidi, MD; and Ian Dresner, MD.

1982   Randall Marcus, MD, developed revolutionary improvements in the design of an interlocking nail system to repair fractures, particularly of the long bones, which improves the healing rate and reduces the risk of infection.

1982   University Hospitals was the first in the United States to house a superconducting, whole-body nuclear magnetic resonance scanner for diagnostic imaging without X-ray radiation.

1986   Arthur Zinn, MD; Douglas Kerr, MD; and Charles Hoppel, MD, published the first description and detailed characterization of a defect (in the enzyme fumarase) in the pathway required for energy metabolism known as the Krebs cycle.

1987   Jerrold Ellner, MD, and Frederick Robbins, MD, established a memorandum of understanding with Makerere University in Uganda linking Cleveland and Kampala AIDS research and care efforts. This partnership helped drive Uganda's leadership response to the emerging AIDS epidemic in Africa.

1987   Ireland Cancer Center (now known as UH Seidman Cancer Center), in collaboration with Case Western Reserve University School of Medicine, MetroHealth Medical Center, and the Louis Stokes Cleveland VA Medical Center, became the only NCI-designated Comprehensive Clinical Cancer Center in the area.

1988   Herbert Meltzer, MD, conducted the first human trials of clozapine, the only effective antipsychotic agent available today for treatment-resistant schizophrenia.

1989   Joseph Calabrese, MD, in collaboration with researchers at Case Western Reserve University, launched groundbreaking studies that showed the effectiveness of anticonvulsants and atypical antipsychotics in treating bipolar disorder.

1989   Anthony Maniglia, MD, Chairman of Otolaryngology, and Laura Cozzi, MD, established a technique for performing safe outpatient tonsillectomies and adenoidectomies, using bismuth to control bleeding.

1989   Olof Pearson, MD, and Charles Hubay, MD, pioneered the use of the drug tamoxifen for breast cancer. It is still widely used today.

1990   Anthony Maniglia, MD, was awarded the first of five patents leading to technology for developing the totally implantable cochlear implant.

1992   Henry Bohlman, MD, pioneered a new technique of anterior (frontal) decompression and fusion of the spine in the neck.

1994   Huntington Willard, MD, described Xist, the gene that is responsible for inactivation of one of two X chromosomes in females, and how it works.

1994   Susan Shurin, MD, performed the first umbilical cord transplant to treat childhood leukemia, using cord blood stem cells from the patient's newborn sister.

1995   Cliff Megerian, MD, proved the origin of inner ear tumors in Von Hippel-Lindau disease, an inherited disease that causes tumors and cysts throughout the body. In 2002, he described the first technique to remove these tumors and preserve hearing.

1995   Michael Konstan, MD; Pamela Davis, MD, PhD; and Charles Hoppel, MD, demonstrated ibuprofen's profound effect on slowing the loss of lung function in patients with cystic fibrosis.

1996   Pierluigi Gambetti, MD, developed the first classification of sporadic prion diseases, now used worldwide in diagnosing this class of dementias caused by mutation of the prion protein gene. Dr. Gambetti defined and named fatal familial insomnia and also linked the same mutation to Creutzfeldt-Jakob disease.

1998   University Hospitals became the site of one of the world's first intraoperative magnetic resonance imaging scans.

2000 – 2017

2000   Raymond Onders, MD, and colleagues developed an innovative diaphragmatic pacing system (DPS).

2001   Kumar Alagramam, PhD, identified an important gene responsible for Usher's syndrome-related deafness.

2002   Jonathan Lass, MD, and a team led by Eric Pearlman, PhD, discovered a bacteria that led to a totally new approach for using antibiotics to treat a disease of sub-Saharan Africa known as river blindness.

2002   Pamela Davis, MD, PhD, and Michael Konstan, MD, performed the first-in-human clinical trial of a non-viral gene therapy approach in patients with cystic fibrosis using DNA nanoparticles.

2002   The reporting of an ALLHAT (Antihypertensive and Lipid-Lowering Treatment to Prevent Heart Attack Trial) study by Jackson Wright, MD, showed that thiazide-type diuretics should be considered first for drug therapy in patients with hypertension.

2004   Robert J. Maciunas, MD, was the first surgeon in North America to treat Tourette syndrome with deep brain stimulation.

2004   Shawn McCandless, MD, and Suzanne Cassidy, MD, reported that chronic diseases of childhood are primarily determined by genetics.

2005   Cliff Megerian, MD, developed a minimally invasive treatment for glomus jugulare tumors—rare, non-cancerous skull bone tumors that involve the inner and middle ear.

2005   Sanford Markowitz, MD, PhD, developed a new stool DNA test for colon cancer.

2008   Mark A. Griswold, PhD, developed a parallel imaging technique for magnetic resonance imaging (MRI) that produces clearer, more accurate images in shorter time.

2008 Faruk H. Örge, MD, was the first in Ohio to use endoscopic and microsurgical techniques to drain excess fluid from the eyes in infants and young children born with glaucoma. He also was the first in Northeast Ohio to use a new class of drugs (anti-VEGF) to treat retinal disease in premature infants.

2009 The Brain Tumor & Neuro-Oncology Center, under the direction of Andrew Sloan, MD, pioneered a minimally invasive, MRI-guided laser system to treat previously inoperable brain tumors.

2010 UH became the only hospital in the country to offer three radiosurgery platforms— IMRT/IGRT TomoTherapy®, CyberKnife®, and Gamma Knife®—in the same medical complex. This triple combination offers unparalleled options for patients in need of advanced radiation techniques.

2010 Pediatric urologists Jonathan Ross, MD, and Edward Cherullo, MD, performed one of the world's first pediatric single-site nephrectomies.

2012 Jonathan Miller, MD, performed the first temporoparietoocipital disconnection in the United States. The procedure removes tiny, non-functioning sections of the brain where seizures originate, providing a cure for intractable epilepsy.

2012 Anthony Furlan, MD, demonstrated that medical therapy is equivalent to interventional therapy for treating patients with PFO (a hole between the right and left atria) and stroke. The CLOSURE study was the first comparison of its kind and led to a significant decrease in interventions performed on stroke patients.

2012 Robert Findling, MD, showed the safety and efficacy of using medications such as lithium, antidepressants, and antipsychotics to treat childhood-onset psychiatric disorders, including bipolar disorder and schizophrenia.

2013 Jonathan Lass, MD; William Reinhart, MD; and Beth Ann Benetz, MA, CRA, FOPS, participated in a National Eye Institute study demonstrating that donor age is not a significant factor in the success of corneal transplantation, significantly expanding the pool of available tissue by including older donors.

2014 Anthony Wynshaw-Boris, MD, described a new mechanism for the correction of abnormal (ring) chromosomes by converting skin cells (fibroblasts) from patients into embryonic-like induced pluripotent stem cells.

2014 Results from the Systolic Blood Pressure Intervention Trial (SPRINT) led by Jackson Wright Jr, MD, PhD, showed that maintaining a new, lower target for systolic blood pressure results in lower heart attack, stroke, and death rates.

2015 Jonathan Miller, MD, was the first in the world to demonstrate that deep brain stimulation has the potential to improve memory after traumatic brain injury.

2016 A study conducted over 30 years by Saul Genuth, MD; the late William Dahms, MD; and Rose Gubitosi-Klug, MD, PhD, demonstrated that intensive diabetes management aimed at near-normal blood glucose levels reduces an individual's risk of diabetes-related complications and mortality.

2017 Jonathan Lass, MD, discovered that corneal donor tissue can be safely stored longer than previously thought before transplantation surgery to correct eye problems in people with cornea disease. This finding significantly expands the supply of available corneas to meet the growing number of transplant patients.

2017 Anthony Furlan, MD, and Cathy Sila, MD, played leadership roles in a multi-center stroke trial, called DAWN, which proved that ischemic stroke patients recovered significantly better with a combination of mechanical thrombectomy and medical therapy compared with medical therapy alone when initiated up to 24 hours of the stroke.

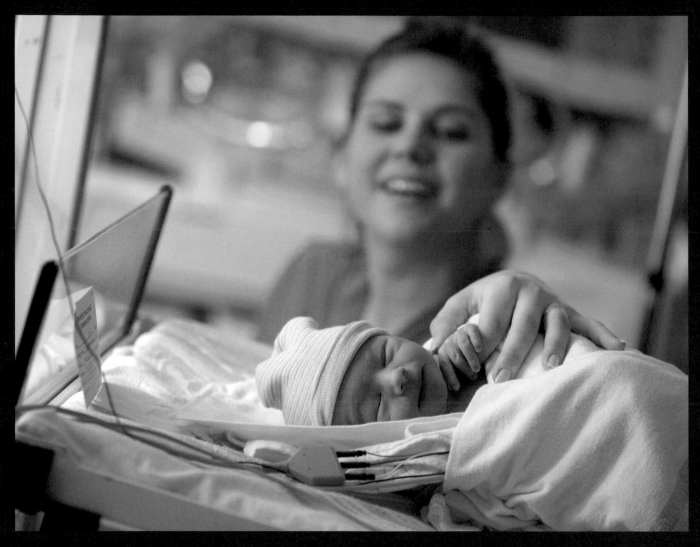

The best and most caring professionals want to work, grow, and make a difference at University Hospitals, and their compassionate quest for excellence is what defines the organization.

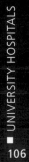

Caring

"Personalized care is a defining characteristic for us. People are people, not numbers. I had an instructor in college who said, 'Health statistics are patients with the tears wiped away.' I've never forgotten that. We need to be as efficient as possible, but we can never lose the human touch."

– Thomas F. Zenty III, CEO, University Hospitals

One day in 2012, a young patient on University Hospitals Seidman Cancer Center's sixth floor had an unexpected visitor. His name was Petie, and his presence provided a wonderful and welcome distraction. But Petie was no ordinary guest. He was a specially trained, therapeutic miniature horse, and the young woman in the bed had a lifelong passion for these animals. Her care team arranged for Petie and his owner to stop by because they wanted to cheer her up and remind her that she was still a person and not just her disease. The patient put her hand on Petie's muzzle, and everyone present saw something almost magical happen. "A weight slipped off her shoulders that afternoon, and she regained a sense of self," says Dianne Reichlin, MSN, RN, ACN, a former patient care coordinator at UH Seidman who helped bring the pony to the patient's room.

All hospitals provide medical care, and University Hospitals does it very well. This fact is confirmed by its enduring presence, 150 years of community support, and this statistic: approximately one in four people in Northeast Ohio turned to UH for diagnosis, treatment, or advice in 2016. More than 1 million patients received care from UH's expert, highly trained professionals. But they also received something more because UH prides itself on caring about individuals, not just their medical conditions. "Our nurses constantly seek ways to relate with patients on a personal level," Reichlin says, "getting to know them and their families, their likes and dislikes, things that make them comfortable and

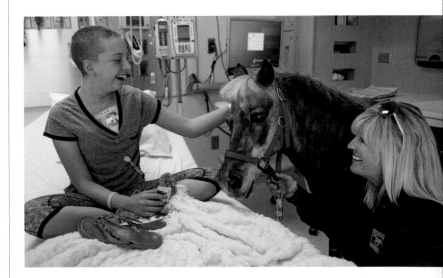

Petie's small but mighty stature brought smiles to children's faces at University Hospitals Rainbow Babies & Children's Hospital from 2011 to 2017.

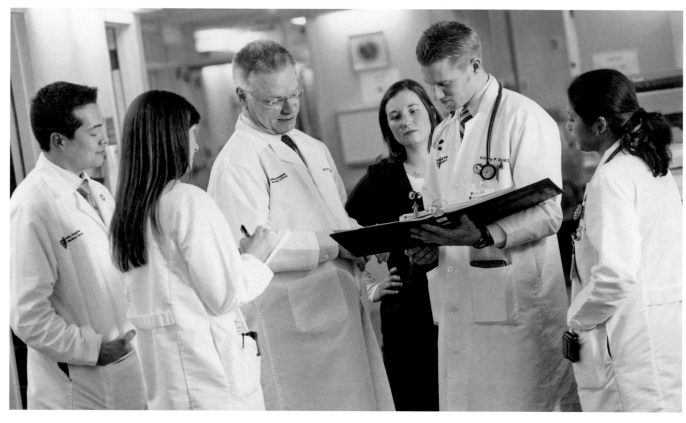

An interdisciplinary team approach during morning rounds allows staff to discuss not only medical interventions, but also the mental, emotional, and spiritual aspects of wellness and treatment.

I Remember

Rachel Vanek, CNP, a nurse practitioner, once cared for a patient with pulmonary complications who was critically ill for weeks. During his recovery, she remembers him sharing with her many untold personal stories about his life and his family. He unexpectedly died a week later. The loss hit her hard, and she attended his funeral and church reception at the family's request. "He had a very large family and many children, grandchildren, and great-grandchildren. At the reception, I was able to share with them the stories he told me. Before I knew it, I had everyone's rapt attention. It was at this moment that I realized I was not there for me, but to give them the gift of these memories."

relaxed." Caring at UI I embraces a set of ideas about how every person should be treated and an approach that goes by different names: patient-centered care, relationship-based nursing, or child life. The words are shorthand for the human side of every interaction, a way of providing care that values listening, respect, and compassion. It can be as simple as holding someone's hand, finding a few extra minutes to talk with a lonely, frightened patient, or helping a family cope with difficult news. These actions, large and small, are the difference between providing health care and truly caring for people and their health.

A Culture of Caring

Caring that goes beyond addressing people's illnesses and injuries is in the DNA of University Hospitals and its founders. Members of the Protestant Ladies Aid Society offered shelter, sympathy, and support to Civil War refugees at the Home for Friendless Strangers. A desire to help as well as heal people prompted the opening of Rainbow Cottage (1891), Maternity Home Association (1891), and the Infants' Clinic (1906). Speaking from a physician's perspective at the dedication of Lakeside Hospital in 1898, Hunter Powell, MD, told the audience, "No man should be a member of a hospital staff whose zeal for the advancement of

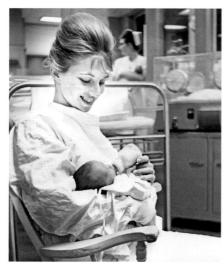
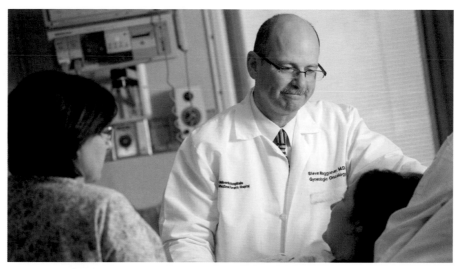
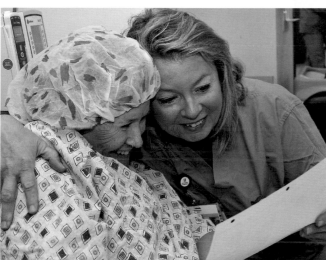
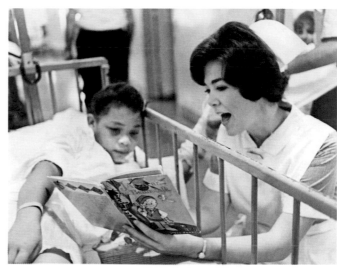
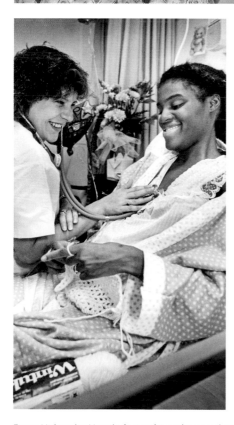
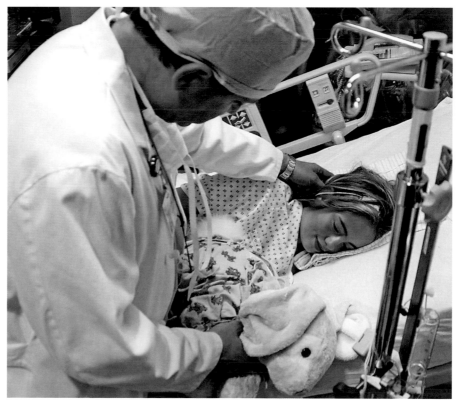

Every University Hospitals employee knows that taking care of people is more than caring about their health.

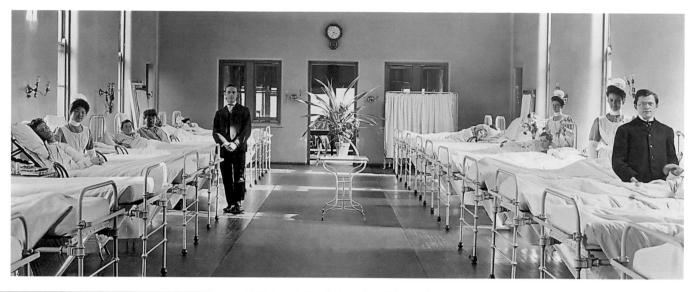

Old Lakeside Hospital ward in 1905. Patients were treated in open wards separated by age and gender.

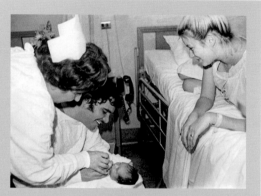

It's a Fact

In 1971, nurses at MacDonald House (now University Hospitals MacDonald Women's Hospital) launched a program to engage fathers in caring for their newborn children. A first for Cleveland, it enlisted 84 volunteer dads to come during the 6–7 p.m. feeding period for instruction on how to hold, diaper, and bottle-feed their babies. The initiative was deemed a success, and "father visits" became a regular event on Wednesday and Sunday nights.

science or the promotion of his own ambition will sacrifice the interests of his poorest patient. The waifs of humanity who seek in their weakness and distress the wards of a hospital, should find in the medical attendants men whose hearts respond to their helplessness and whose most skilled efforts will be rendered with tenderest consideration."

An article titled "The Personality of Our Hospital" appeared in the October 1949 issue of the employee newsletter *The Archway*. It reminded staff that they were the heart of the institution and that the way in which they did their jobs shaped the character of the place and determined its success or failure. "It is the quality rather than the quantity of work which makes members of the community recommend [the hospital] to their friends, or a place to which they return with confidence....Each of us, whatever our station may be, contributes to the impressions that people receive....Each of us builds some small part of ourselves into the personality which is our hospital."

Echoing that sentiment today, Terryl Homes Koeth, MS, RN, former Director of Patient and Community Programs for University Hospitals Seidman Cancer Center, says, "Everyone who works here

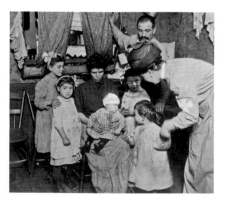

Immigrant home in Cleveland, ca. early 1900s.

contributes to the healing process. Environmental Services staff at Seidman fold towels into 'animals,' and have the option to give patients a carnation, provided by the department, on discharge day to say good-bye and good luck. Parking valets receive tours of the building so they're equipped to provide visitors with directions.

The receptionist in the lobby makes sure there's always a vase of fresh flowers on her desk. Every person, doing their job, makes this a better place and communicates that we care."

Tracy Willingham understands this. She began delivering food trays at UH in 1973 when she was 17. "I bring a lot of love and compassion to all the different positions I've held in dietary. Sometimes I can brighten a patient's day with just a few kind words. That's how we do things here, and that's how my mother raised me. She's turning 94. When she was a patient at UH, she asked me, 'You treat all the patients like you treat me?' and I told her, 'Yes, yes, I do.'"

Acts of generosity abound at UH, exponentially expanding the hospital's ability to help patients and their families beyond the walls of the hospital. Since 1999, the kindness of Albert and Norma Geller has meant that there is financial help for people who have a tough time getting to and from University Hospitals Cleveland Medical Center for radiation treatments. The couple set up an endowed transportation fund that covers the costs of van or cab service for UH Seidman patients and their families who have financial challenges.

It is the little things. That phrase shows up in countless conversations with patients and their families, and in the letters and cards of thanks they write to University Hospitals. One woman described it as "medical TLC." People express appreciation for never feeling rushed, always being greeted with a smile, and staff who demonstrate patience, put them at ease, and explain their care situation to them. *Warm, friendly, kind*—those words are also frequently used to describe doctors, nurses, and the entire spectrum of caregivers and service personnel.

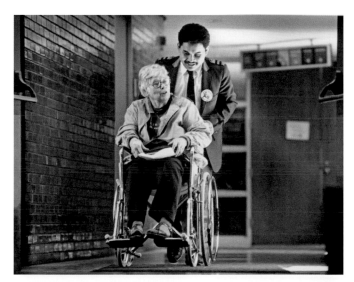

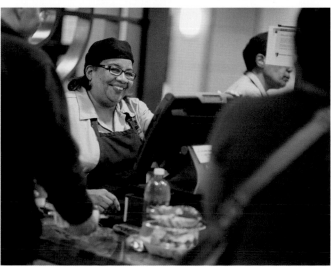

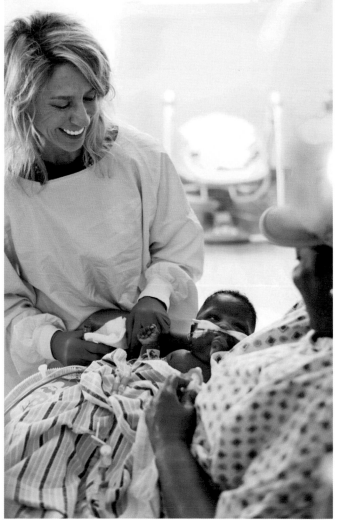

Investing in People: Employee Education

The myriad staff roles that make a hospital operational 24/7 is unfathomable. University Hospitals invests in helping their employees improve their skills, increase their opportunities, and advance their careers. "We are a learning organization," says Fred Rothstein, MD, pediatric gastroenterologist and retired President of University Hospitals Cleveland Medical Center. "We encourage people to continue their education so that they can advance at UH and take on new responsibilities."

It is a supportive culture and a commitment that changes lives. Since Jacquelyn Kirby started in the hospital's Environmental Services department more than 25 years ago, she has earned an associate's degree, a bachelor's in health care administration, a master's in health care management, and a project management certificate. She currently works as a clinical decision support analyst for the Quality Institute. "I owe all this to University Hospitals' Employee Tuition Reimbursement Program," says Kirby. "Without it, I would not have continued my education." The program dates back to 1970 and was open to all employees, providing financial aid that made it possible to obtain high school diplomas, attend college and technical schools, or take job training courses. In 1971, 100 participated. Today, the program provides support for more than 1,200 employees.

Additional career development opportunities include Bridge to Your Future, a free life skills and literacy program that builds self-confidence while improving math and reading skills. Attendees are excused from their jobs to attend sessions during work hours without sacrificing pay. The program also offers educational and career guidance. According to Thomas F. Zenty III, CEO, University Hospitals, "We make workforce development a high priority because…[w]e believe a solution to the growing shortage of health care professionals is to help [our staff] qualify for better livelihoods and pursue their career aspirations as frontline care providers."[1]

Evidence of this philosophy is the Pathways to PCA program, which allowed Fae-Dra Penna to move from the kitchen to the bedside. She received intensive training and on-the-job coaching to become a patient care assistant (PCA) at UH Cleveland Medical Center, "a place," she said, "that's full of heart." This opportunity is offered to employees in entry-level positions such as Environmental Services, Nutrition Services, and Patient Transport. Becoming a PCA was a dream come true for Penna.

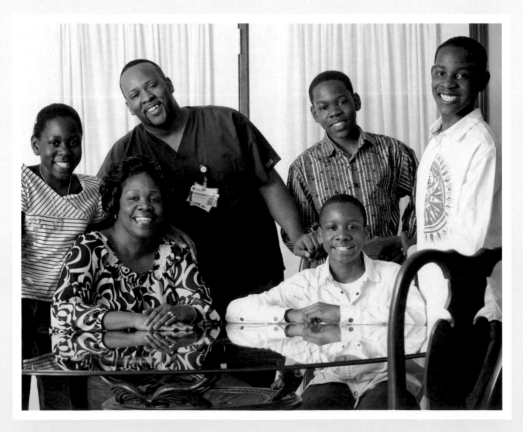

Care Coordinator Alexander Grant, RN, (back row, second from left) began his career at University Hospitals in 1994. With tuition assistance, he was able to go to school during the day to earn his nursing degree and work full time at night.

It eliminates the stress of constantly having to find someone to drive them back and forth or wait for buses when they are feeling sick. As someone who had undergone chemotherapy and been a UH volunteer, Mrs. Geller saw a need and understood the value of this assistance.

It is not always easy for patients and their families to ask questions or understand situations involving multiple specialists and complex medical issues. To make it easier for them to have their voices heard and enhance the care UH provides, the hospital established the Patient and Family Partnership Council in 1991. These volunteer groups are now active throughout the system. Chrissie Blackburn is the first Principal Advisor of Patient and Family Engagement for UH. Her job is to empower patients and their families to be informed advocates so they can play an active role in making health care decisions. Blackburn and her husband learned how important this can be the day their daughter, Lily, was born in 2007 with a rare and complex disorder that caused a variety of physical defects and deficits.

"We were living in San Diego. The doctors did not expect Lily to survive. But two weeks later, she was thriving, and we decided that we would do everything in our power to ensure that this little girl would play and eat pizza and grow up to make a difference in the world."

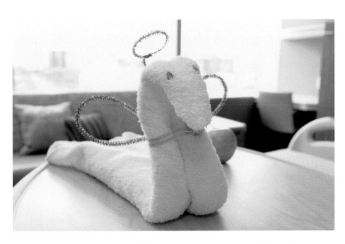

A towel "animal" is one of the many small gestures University Hospitals staff members offer to patients to brighten their day.

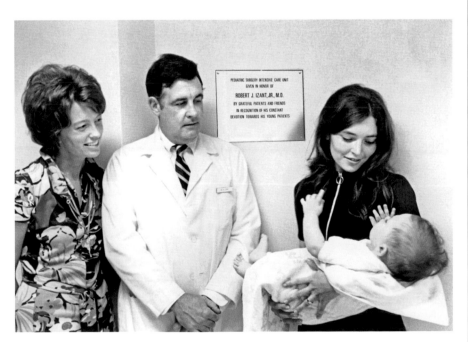

Robert Izant Jr., MD, was northern Ohio's first formally trained pediatric surgeon when he joined University Hospitals in 1958. He was known as much for his personable and comforting manner as his clinical skills. In a message, read at the dedication of his portrait in 1987, a parent of one of his patients wrote, "He glued Benjamin's split chin back together with steri-strips, a ton of concern, and a splash of humor."

I Work Here

Wanda Overton, an Environmental Services worker at University Hospitals Rainbow Babies & Children's Hospital, offers little stones and metal disks with inspirational messages printed on them from the Atrium gift shop. "I keep them in my pocket," she says, "and hand them out to cheer people up. Sometimes I give them to my co-workers. I see people having a hard time, and I can feel their pain. It's not part of my job. I do it from my heart." Shannon Edwards, Environmental Services Operations Manager, is Overton's supervisor. She explains that everyone on her team is trained to be engaged and empathetic. "We encourage staff to put themselves in other people's shoes and connect with them. Wanda does that naturally. She makes everybody feel special."

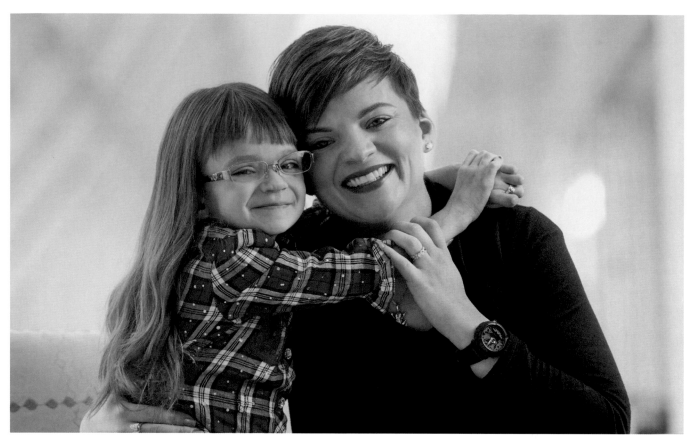

Chrissie Blackburn and her daughter, Lily, in 2014.

The couple moved home to Cleveland so Lily could be treated at UH Rainbow Babies & Children's Hospital and have the support of their family. Lily saw 17 different specialists and went through multiple surgeries. Her parents became experts in navigating the hospital system and speaking on her behalf. Lily still faces challenges, but she is flourishing.

"I wanted to give back and saw a need and way I could help," says Blackburn. In her position at UH, she addresses issues of governance, safety, quality, patient experience, and protocols to improve the quality of care that UH delivers. "I want this hospital to be the best it can be," says Blackburn. "My goal is to give patients and families a voice and use what they tell us to enhance everything that we do."

Sadly, even the best care cannot cure everyone. Karen Boyd, MBA, BSN, Director, Quality and Clinical Performance Improvement, Quality Center Services, learned this firsthand when UH physicians treated her father for advanced lung cancer. Conventional surgery was not an option for him because of his metastatic disease, but he was able to have Gamma Knife® surgery to reduce the size of the lesions in his brain. After her father's death just four months later, Boyd felt moved to write a letter to the hospital. "During his two stays in January, he was managed on Seidman 4 by a wonderful team of caregivers. It was especially important that he was able to return to the same floor both times and the same medical team." Near the end of his life, doctors supported his wish to travel to Florida for a family gathering. "It was beautiful to see how everyone at UH encouraged us to take this trip, understanding how important it was to have this time together. Dad passed away peacefully on his own terms just six days after we returned."

Caring for the Whole Person

"Bedside manner" is a familiar term that references the way physicians interact and communicate with their patients. It is about bringing courtesy, consideration, and sensitivity to every encounter; asking questions; paying attention to the answers;

and speaking in a way patients and their families can understand. Studies show that a positive doctor-patient relationship is a factor in health outcomes and can be as important as clinical skills when it comes to patient satisfaction.[2]

Edward Barksdale, Jr., MD, Surgeon-in-Chief, University Hospitals Rainbow Babies & Children's Hospital and the Robert J. Izant, Jr., MD, Chair in Pediatric Surgery, performed multiple surgeries for Sierra Bland, who had complex and serious health issues since birth. Her mother, Bethany, was impressed by his manner from their first encounter. "Sierra had already been through so much, and he was very sensitive in dealing with her anxiety. He saw us as a family and recognized how stressful the situation was for my husband and me, too."

"Being a better surgeon means being a better collaborator with patients and their families," says Dr. Barksdale.

Although Sierra passed away in 2016, during her years as a patient, she and her team of caregivers became close. Responding to one of her last requests, many of them—including off-duty nurses—gathered in her hospital room for a slumber party. Even Dr. Barksdale stopped by. The day Sierra died, 50 staff members were there with her. This is what it means to be a caring community.

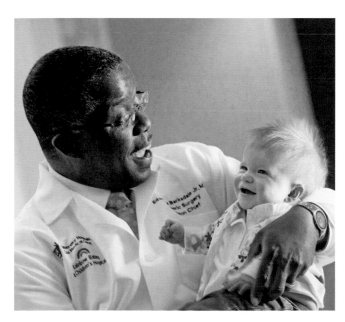

Edward Barksdale, Jr., MD, recognizes the importance of bonding with his patients.

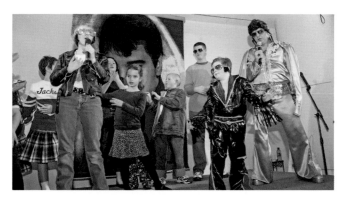

Alan Cohen, MD, aka "Alvis" and former Chief of Pediatric Neurosurgery at University Hospitals Rainbow Babies & Children's Hospital, began his 17-year career with UH in 1994. An outstanding neurosurgeon, he is perhaps best remembered for his love of Elvis Presley. Over the years, grateful patients bought him Elvis memorabilia, filling every square inch of his office. On the anniversary of Elvis' birthday, Dr. Cohen (far right) would impersonate the "King," performing a medley of Elvis songs with many of his former patients for a standing-room-only crowd of UH staff, patients, and visitors.

Catherine Koppelman, MSN, RN, who retired as Chief Nursing and Patient Experience Officer in August 2015 after eight years at University Hospitals, remembers a man in the surgical intensive care unit telling her how his nurses affected him. "He was in his mid-60s. He'd had a valve replacement and a triple bypass. 'It's the way they talk to you,' he said, 'the way they touch you, look into your eyes and approach even the most embarrassing situation so that you can keep your dignity.'" To connect like this, explains Koppelman, with empathy for what people are going through, is the goal for UH nurses. "To do that while also making sound, cognitive, science-based decisions and attending to the technical side of the work, that's the art of this profession as it is practiced here."

Tina Greig, MSN, CNP, CCRN, worked on the medical intensive care unit since 2004, became manager of the unit in 2010, and is now working as a nurse practitioner for internal medicine at University Hospitals Ahuja Medical Center. "Our patients are very sick. Nurses are kept busy, and it's easy to get caught up with the tasks that must be done. But, we go beyond that, looking at people and asking ourselves what we can do to make them a little more comfortable and a little happier. How can we help the family cope and trust us to take the best care of

In Sickness and In Health

When it comes to "matters of the heart," a doctor is not always what is needed. Sometimes a ceremony or a toast is the best medicine. Serious illness can interfere with engagements, marriage plans, and anniversary parties, but love triumphs when caregivers are willing to go the extra mile and make dreams come true.

Rev. Harry Werner, MDiv, BCC, has been providing spiritual support at University Hospitals Cleveland Medical Center since 1981 and established a volunteer program that now has 60 assistants. He remembers receiving a call requesting his immediate presence at University Hospitals MacDonald Women's Hospital. A young woman had gone into early labor. She and her partner were anxious to get married before the baby was born and wanted him to perform the ceremony immediately. "I told them I couldn't do it without a marriage license," says Rev. Werner, "and the groom tells me, 'We have one in the glove compartment' and runs out to the car to get it. The bride manages to repeat her vows in between contractions, and their child arrived after they were officially husband and wife." The couple later submitted the story about how they got married to a contest sponsored by a local radio station and won an all-expense-paid wedding.

• • •

Transport, and the company provided an ambulance at no charge with two volunteer paramedics in attendance. Members of University Hospitals medical staff also volunteered to be at the church. It took Uljanic and her team three weeks to arrange the logistics and see to every detail, which even included Nagy's barber coming to his hospital room.

"The nurses had dressed my father in his tuxedo," says Sarah Salvatore, "and he escorted me down the aisle, just as he had promised." Unable to walk or even sit in a wheelchair, Nagy was rolled on a gurney, his daughter explains, "but he held my hand and had a big smile on his face the whole time. Even though he was on oxygen, they'd put in some sort of valve so he could speak and when the pastor asked, 'Who gives away this bride?' he was able to answer, 'Her mother and I do,' and everyone cheered."

The event was covered by local and national news media. Nagy died two weeks later, after three months in the

"I am reaching out to you on behalf of one of my patients," wrote Jacky Uljanic, a nurse practitioner for the surgical intensive care unit, in an October 2013 email to her colleagues. She explained that Scott Nagy had terminal cancer and would likely die soon. "Before he does, he wishes to attend his daughter's wedding….I really want to try to make this happen for him and his family! How awesome would that be?"

There were concerns about lining up transport and medical personnel to accompany him; whether his insurance would cover any of the costs; and how to manage his medications, monitoring devices, and physical limitations. One nurse contacted a friend with a connection to Physicians Medical

University Hospitals patient Scott Nagy (center) realized his dream to escort his daughter Sarah down the aisle at her wedding—made possible by the support of his care team.

hospital. In that time, he grew close to the people caring for him as did his wife and children who had been there almost constantly. "What the people at UH did for my family and me is nothing less than amazing," his daughter says. "I am so grateful. They gave our tragedy a fairy-tale ending."

• • •

A 28-year-old woman was admitted to the Medical Intensive Care Unit on her wedding anniversary. Nurses realized that she would likely not be alive for the next one so they decided to arrange a celebration in the hospital for the couple. "Our chef Tony [Anthony Dominak, Former Executive Chef, UH Cleveland Medical Center] made them a steak dinner," says nurse practitioner Tina Greig, MSN, CNP, CCRN. "The nurses bought them a cake from a bakery in Little Italy. There was a table with a white cloth. We took her off all the machines, rescheduled her medications, got her out of the hospital gown and into a dress, and gave them time to be alone together."

• • •

On a breezy, sunny July afternoon, Maria Dobos married her high school sweetheart, Ryan Longbrake, in University Hospitals Seidman Cancer Center's Healing Garden before 25 family members, including her father, a terminally ill cancer patient.

Just two days earlier, the 25-year-old Columbus woman learned that the cancer discovered and treated in her father had surged back and spread throughout his body, leading to a grim prognosis. Doctors told the family that he may not survive until her September wedding, a grand ceremony planned at the Russian Orthodox Church where her parents were wed and she and her sister were baptized.

Seidman 6 nurses and staff mobilized to stage a wedding where 56-year-old Jeff Dobos could walk his daughter down the aisle.

No detail was left unchecked, including finalizing gown alterations, finding a minister to officiate, and decorating the art therapy room. "UH Seidman strives every day to support its patients as people first, helping them to achieve goals that cancer may make it difficult to meet," states Nurse Manager Sara Scott, BSN, RN, OCN.

Aided by a walker, Jeff slowly strolled beside his beaming eldest daughter across the sun-drenched garden. His younger daughter, Julia, the maid of honor, watched smiling, her eyes brimming with tears.

"It was perfect," said the bride. "When I was wedding planning, I cared about every little thing. But that day, when it finally happened, I had everything I needed. The staff pulled together as a team to support my dad. It was a day full of love."

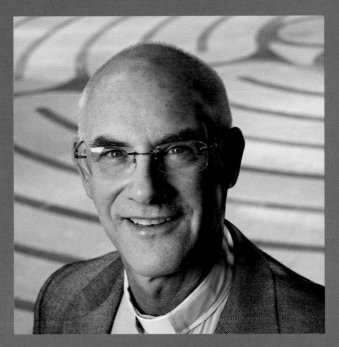

Rev. Harry Werner, MDiv, BCC.

University Hospitals' chaplain Rev. Harry Werner, MDiv, BCC, knows what it is like to be a patient. He was in his office when he had a sudden heart attack in 2012. He ended up in the cardiac catheterization laboratory with Marco Costa, MD, PhD, Director, Interventional Cardiovascular and Research Innovation Centers, reviving him. "He told me I died," recalls the chaplain. "My heart stopped beating, and I wasn't breathing. I remember hearing someone say, 'We're losing him.' But, I was calm and had a sense of peace." The team restarted his heart with a defibrillator and his breathing with chest compressions. "I came out of the experience with no more fear of dying. Sometimes, when it's appropriate I share that with patients."

I Work Here

Jacques Lynn, a former Environmental Services worker for University Hospitals who was on the job at University Hospitals Cleveland Medical Center for more than 25 years, was part of a singing group that performed around the hospital to entertain staff and patients. "We did gospel, pop, everything. Music soothes. It takes your stress away and eases your mind." Lynn is also a minister. "Nobody is a stranger with me for long. I say 'Hi' to everybody. If I see somebody upset, I stop and ask if they're OK. Sometimes they'll talk about what's happening or tell me about a loved one, and I try to offer some words of comfort. If they're believers, I'll go to the chapel and pray with them."

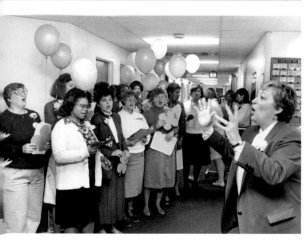

The UH Cingers were one of the many choirs, singing groups, and bands formed by University Hospitals employees over the years to entertain patients and staff.

their loved one?" Greig remembers a young man from Boston waiting for a lung transplant. "He'd been on the unit for four months and was depressed. The MICU team arranged for Trevor Crowe from the Cleveland Indians baseball team to visit him." He told the outfielder that his favorite player was Red Sox second baseman Dustin Pedroia. "The two were friends," Greig continues, "so a call was made and Pedroia overnighted a signed bat to our patient. It meant so much to him."

Marilyn Kabb, RN, was head nurse manager when a patient did not have shoes to wear home. All of the clothing he was wearing when he arrived at the hospital had to be discarded. "We kept a closet full of dated clothes for situations like this," she explained. "But this patient had very large feet. We didn't have shoes in his size and couldn't find any to purchase." However, resourceful staff and the Cleveland Cavaliers came to the rescue. "I finally had the idea to call the basketball team's front office," said Kabb. "They sent over two pairs of brand-new sneakers. We saved one in case he was readmitted."

This approach is translated into action every day throughout the system. Hearing the yearning in a cancer patient's question about the weather, a nurse takes her outside for the first time in weeks to enjoy half an hour in the sunshine. Because a nurse practitioner and a pulmonologist at University Hospitals Rainbow Babies & Children's Hospital made

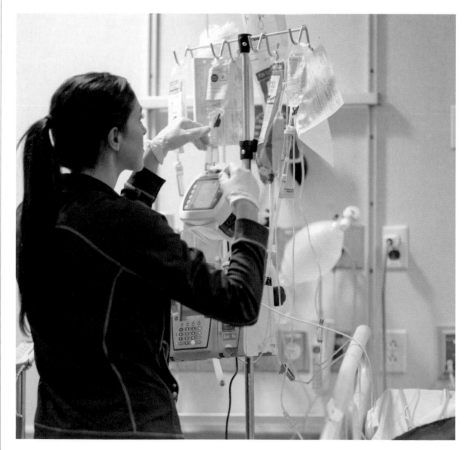

Care at University Hospitals is multidimensional, involving skilled staff and rigorous, round-the-clock monitoring and treatment.

the request, a member of the Cleveland Indians visits a young baseball fan who had been in the hospital for months awaiting a transplant. UH caregivers regularly arrange for dietary staff to send birthday cakes to patients, and they accompany patients who get a pass to attend family celebrations but are too ill to manage without assistance. But, there are happy occasions too, when parents want a baby blessed or when patients learn they are in remission or are going to get better.

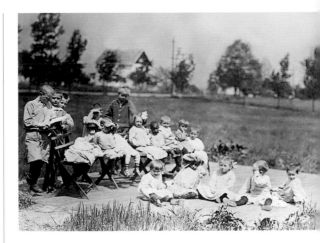

Rainbow Cottage patients at a summertime picnic, ca. early 1900s.

Caring for Kids

"Despite how sick they may be," says Patricia DePompei, MSN, RN, President of University Hospitals Rainbow Babies & Children's Hospital and University Hospitals MacDonald Women's Hospital, "children have a sense of joy. It motivates all of us to never forget about the child in the patient."

Ensuring that hospitalized children get to be children, no matter what their diagnosis, has been a priority since Rainbow Cottage welcomed its first patients during the summer of 1891. Games, toys, and books were as much a part of the furnishings as beds and chairs. A description from 1898 mentions the ideal playground provided by a "large shady lawn with spreading apple trees and thick grass," "swings and hammocks," "chickens and kittens," "picnics by the lake," and "a small sandy creek where nurses take all who are able…[to] wade and paddle to their hearts' content."[3]

Jack Horwitz, MD, a pediatric neurologist at UH Rainbow who retired in 1998, was a Rainbow resident at the South Euclid property in 1962. "We'd wheel the kids outside in carts and mobile beds and play baseball, pushing them between the bases."

It was not until the 1960s that the American Academy of Pediatrics recommended that all hospitals have playrooms, but there was one at Babies and Childrens Hospital long before that. It offered structured programs every morning and afternoon for those ages 18 months to 8 years old.

"Life in a children's ward may not be all smiles but it has its bright moments as a visitor to Babies and

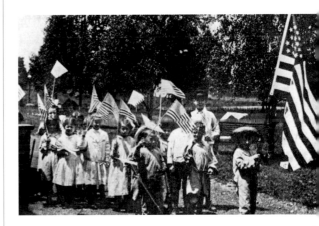

The 4th of July celebration in 1908 included donations of firecrackers, five gallons of ice cream, and a pail of candy, according to minutes from a trustees meeting.

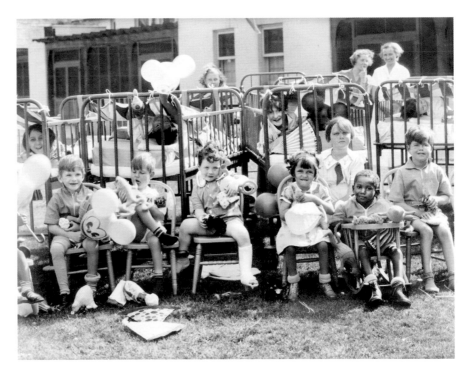

Rainbow Hospital party, 1936.

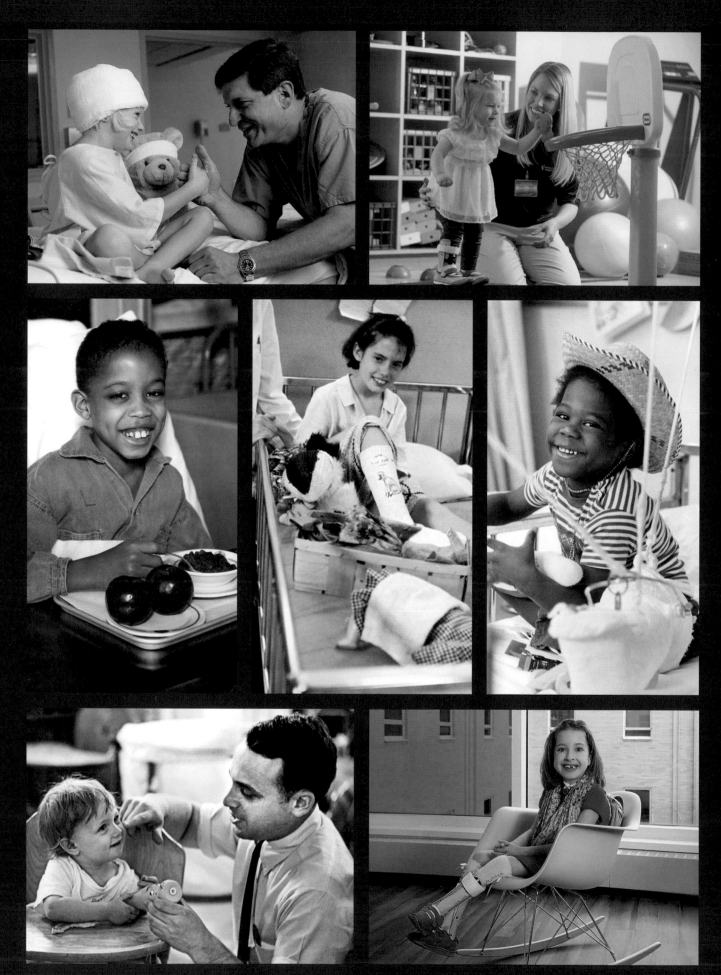

Children treated throughout the decades at University Hospitals Rainbow Babies & Children's Hospital.

Children's division of University Hospitals soon discovers....Some come in their beds, but everyone who is off isolation and able comes to the play room because there's fun to be had there between treatments, rest, and medication. For those who can't come, the diversional therapist in charge has a toy cart...[that] she takes to them. Planning the play for patients is Miss Bernice Bradley, a pretty young teacher with a soft Southern accent that brings even the most cantankerous child on her side."[4]

Providing toddlers, children, and teenagers with the best medical care also includes paying attention to their mental and emotional well-being. Social workers first joined the staff at Rainbow Hospital in 1926, and a psychologist in 1942. To ease fear and anxiety, Babies and Childrens Hospital staff began giving young surgery patients informal pre-admission tours of the hospital in 1958, and by 1961, the guided walks were scheduled weekly. Nowadays, parents of a child having surgery and staying overnight at UH Rainbow Babies & Children's can schedule a private tour to help prepare them for their procedure.

As understanding of the psychosocial needs of children grew, a more formal Child Life program took shape at Babies and Childrens starting in 1969, and it significantly changed how care was administered. In June 1970, a separate and complete emergency ward just for children, a first for the region, opened in the basement of the Wearn Building, adjacent to Lakeside Hospital, operating 24 hours a day. LeRoy Matthews, MD, then Director of Pediatrics, told a writer for *The Archway* why the facility was important. "There are frequent gruesome situations in a general emergency ward. People bleeding from wounds, a tense situation with police and domestic quarrels. All of this can be very detrimental to a child, can cause emotional problems and can harm his overall treatment." The Marcy R. Horvitz Pediatric

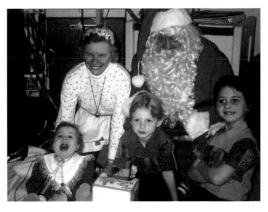

Dalia Zemaityte, MSN, RN (back row, left), dressed as one of Santa's helpers, delivered a gift to every child in the hospital on Christmas Day for 40 years. She calls it one of the joys of her life. Jeffrey Blumer, MD, former Chief of Pediatric Critical Care, outfitted in the red suit and white beard, was her companion for three decades, followed by Orry Jacobs, former Executive Vice President of UH, who played Santa for the next 10 years.

I Work Here

Celebration of Lives is presented by University Hospitals Rainbow Babies & Children's Hospital and the Center for Pediatric Palliative Care. The annual memorial gathering brings families of children who died in the past year and their University Hospitals caregivers together. The names of the children are read aloud, their pictures are displayed, and candles are lit to honor their lives.

"As a nurse, I have the opportunity to build relationships with patients and families during the most challenging and vulnerable times of their lives. Despite the acuity of the medical situation at hand, we always find reasons to shower a child with hopeful inspiration. The Celebration of Lives ceremony provides a meaningful way to recognize these precious children and their families—beyond the space of a hospital room," states Dena Mitchell, RN, CPON, assistant nurse manager, Angie Fowler Adolescent & Young Adult Cancer Institute and current Celebration of Lives chair.

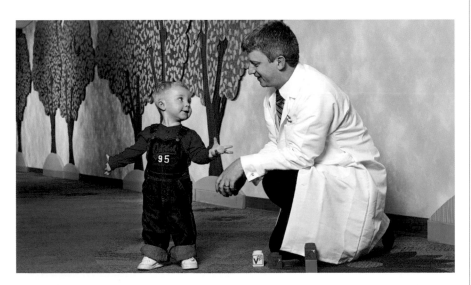

Today, hallways and rooms at University Hospitals Rainbow Babies & Children's Hospital are painted in bright colors and decorated with cartoon characters. There are multiple well-equipped activity centers and areas for adolescents to socialize.

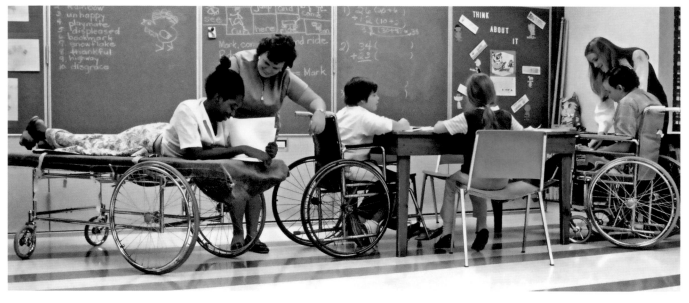

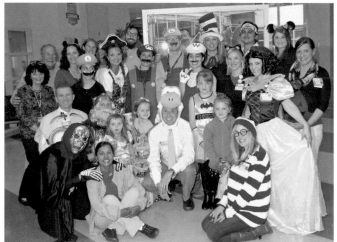

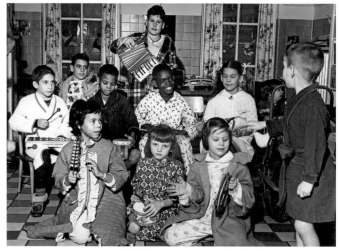

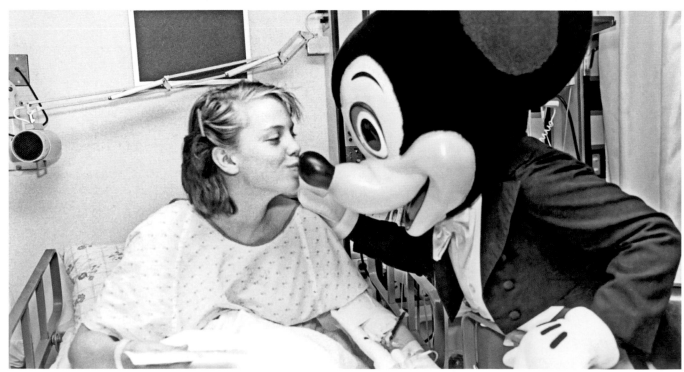

Laughter may not heal broken bones or cure disease, but it is always good medicine. At University Hospitals Rainbow Babies & Children's Hospital, every effort is made to create a homelike and cheerful atmosphere, with time and space set aside for all types of recreational and educational activities.

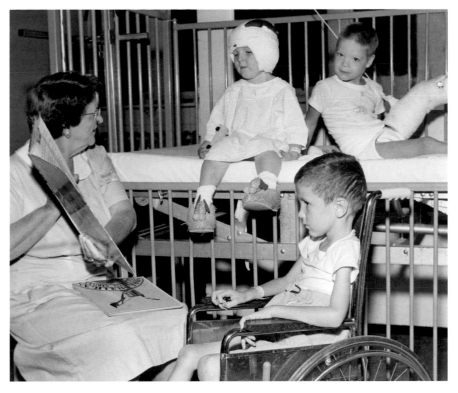

A Babies and Childrens Hospital play lady, 1960.

Emergency Center, which opened on the University Hospitals Cleveland Medical Center campus in 2011, is the latest expression of this belief. It not only isolates children from the traumas of the adult area, but also is designed with families in mind and is staffed with specially trained emergency pediatric doctors, nurses, and family liaison staff members.

Child Life services expanded after 1971 when Rainbow and Babies and Childrens became one hospital in a new, shared building. The "play ladies" entertained youngsters with stories, songs, and crayons. Today, the role has evolved to include trained art and music therapists and allied health care professionals who use research-based practices and systematized activities to help children and families cope with the stress, fear, and pain associated with illness, hospitalization, and medical procedures. The Rainbow Babies & Children's Foundation is a major supporter of Child Life services, which are not covered by insurance or billable by the hospital.

Parent participation is a key element to the work of Child Life specialists. "Rainbow Babies & Children's has led the way in making families a part of their children's care," says hospital President Patricia DePompei, MSN, RN. This reflects a larger and longstanding emphasis on the importance of family involvement that began at Babies and Childrens Hospital in the late 1950s. Prior to that, parents were typically sidelined and their presence considered a hindrance to doctors and nurses. A booklet from the 1930s details the rather restrictive visitation policies of the time: two visitors, once a week, from 2 to 3 p.m. for

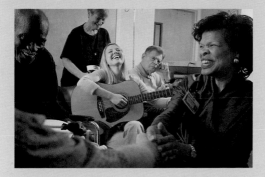

Deforia Lane, PhD, MT-BC (far right).

Pioneer

Deforia Lane, PhD, MT-BC, is recognized around the world as a pioneer in using music to address the physiological and psychological issues associated with sickness, injury, and pain. She was Associate Director, University Hospitals Seidman Cancer Center and Director of Art & Music Therapy. A cancer survivor and trained vocal performer, Lane began her work at University Hospitals after her own radiation treatment when she gave a music therapy in-service for staff to express her gratitude and to demonstrate music's benefits. She was employed by UH from 1984 until she retired in 2018, developing therapeutic approaches that include singing, composing, dancing, playing, and even learning a musical instrument, along with relaxation, guided imagery, improvisation, and musical games to help acute and chronically ill patients and their families.

Al Gore, Maureen McGovern, Wynton Marsalis, and Audrey Hepburn have accompanied Lane on rounds. In 1989, Lane invited international opera star Kathleen Battle, her college roommate, to Rainbow Babies and Childrens Hospital. The effect, according to Battle, "was magical." Comparing her career to her old friend's, Lane says, "I would never trade what I have now....This work is precious to me. I treasure the joy and hope of making a positive difference in the lives of others."

Good for Patients, People, Planet

In the past two decades, University Hospitals leaders have expanded the role of the organization to actively engage in caring for the environment. Over the last 10 years, UH has dramatically changed its approach to purchasing food, products, and services; managing waste; and constructing and operating facilities. The aim is to ensure that sustainable, earth-friendly practices are a fundamental part of business as usual.

All UH medical centers have signed a national Environmentally Preferable Purchasing Pledge. UH purchases local and sustainably sourced foods, including meat produced without routine antibiotic use; safer chemical products, including Green Seal-certified cleaning materials; and other goods and services that advance energy efficiency, as well as green construction and landscaping. Waste and recycling management programs, composting, and policies for vendors to reduce and recycle construction and demolition waste are keeping more and more materials out of landfills.

For three consecutive years beginning in 2013, UH has earned Environmental Excellence awards from Practice Greenhealth. UH was also selected by the Ohio Hospital Association's Environmental Council as the 2014 recipient of the John Chapman Award for excellence and leadership in initiating or supporting pollution prevention programs.

New construction projects at UH are required to achieve LEED (Leadership in Energy and Environmental Design) certification from the U.S. Green Building Council. The green building policies at UH focus on optimizing energy efficiency and indoor air quality, including minimizing use of chemicals of concern in construction and interior spaces. Storm water management and support for sustainable transportation are also part of UH's green building and operations practices.

"There's a universal need in this country to be more environmentally sensitive," says former Chairman of the UH board Monte Ahuja. "It makes sense economically and civically, and it is the right thing to do."

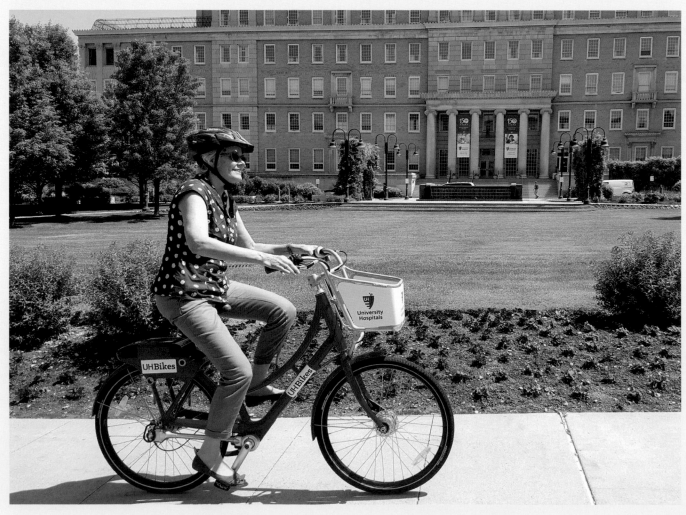

UHBikes is a bike share program in collaboration with the city of Cleveland. It encourages physical activity and environmental sustainability while also creating a new way for visitors to see and discover the city.

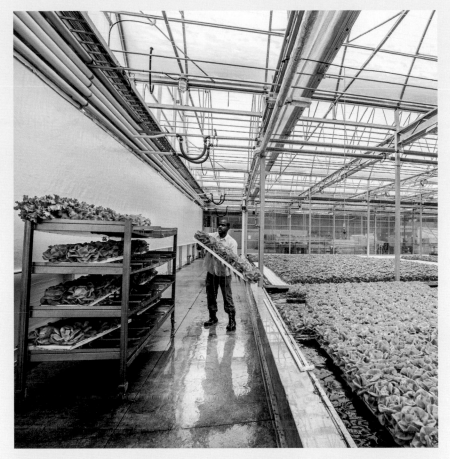

University Hospitals is a supporter and a customer of the Evergreen Cooperatives. The project is part of Cleveland's Greater University Circle Initiative, a collaboration of anchor institutions to spur redevelopment in this city neighborhood. Green City Growers, launched in December 2012, is one business in this collection of job-creating, community-building, worker-owned companies. It is a 3.25-acre hydroponic greenhouse, the largest of its kind in the country, located in the urban core. Operating year-round, it produces 3 million heads of lettuce and 300,000 pounds of herbs annually, just 4.6 miles from University Hospitals Cleveland Medical Center.

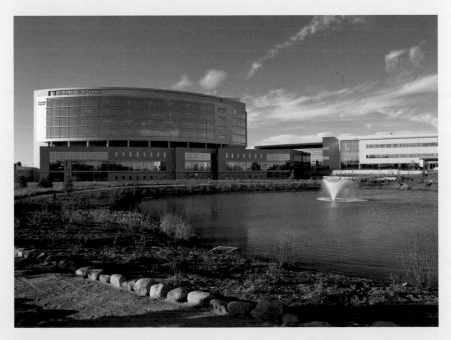

The surrounding landscape around University Hospitals Ahuja Medical Center features native plants, rainwater runoff reduction methods, and 13 acres of preserved wetlands.

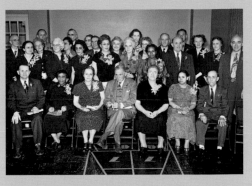

The first Quarter Century Club gala, affectionately referred to by members as the "UH family reunion," was held in 1951 in the game room at Lakeside Hospital. On the morning of the event, each woman received an orchid and each man received a red boutonnière.

I Remember

The Quarter Century Club (QCC) has been a time-honored University Hospitals tradition, recognizing people who have worked at UH for 25 years. The group had its first gathering in 1951 when 28 employees were inducted. Together, their time at the hospital totaled 808 years. The QCC currently boasts more than 2,700 active and retired members living in seven states. Arna Safar reached the 25-year mark in 2013. A former supervisor in Physicians Services, she says the Quarter Century Club is evidence of how much UH appreciates people like her. "I am not aware of another health care organization that pays such tribute and honor to its long-term employees." She also has experienced what it is like to be a UH patient. "I was sick and had surgery. It was the nursing staff and the actual caring that truly made the difference."

More Kinds of Caring

Caring as a word and an idea has multiple meanings. At University Hospitals, it extends beyond the way staff interact with patients and their families and is synonymous with a workplace culture that fosters friendships, loyalty, and supportive relationships. For 150 years, employees have banded together to assist each other on and off the job, for recreation and celebration, entertainment, and socializing. This contributes to a welcome sense of cohesion and camaraderie that is demonstrated by how long people tend to stay with the organization.

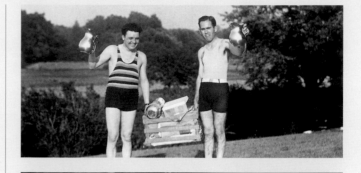

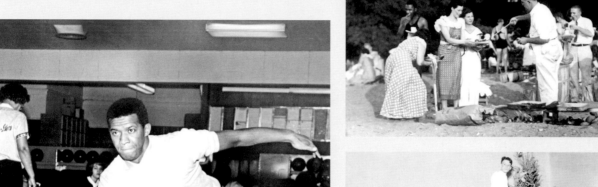

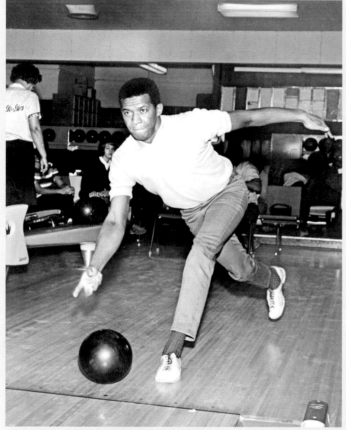

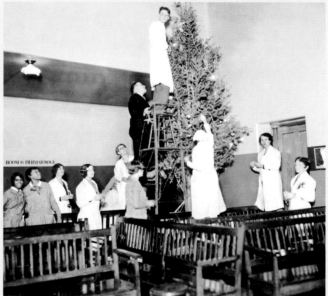

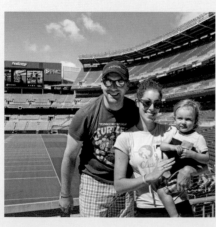

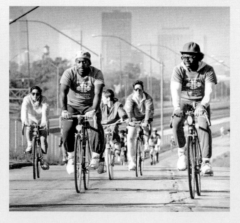

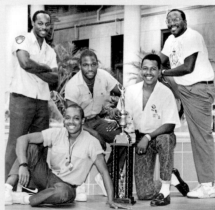

Top: Old Lakeside Hospital picnic, 1929. ***Middle (left to right):*** Bowling team, 1968; Holiday festivities,1925. ***Bottom (left to right):*** 150th anniversary employee picnic at FirstEnergy Stadium, home of the Cleveland Browns, 2016; Ireland Cancer Center Bike-a-thon, 1988; University Hospitals basketball champs, 1990.

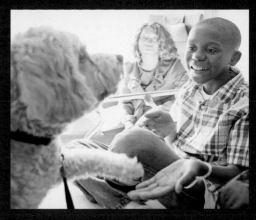

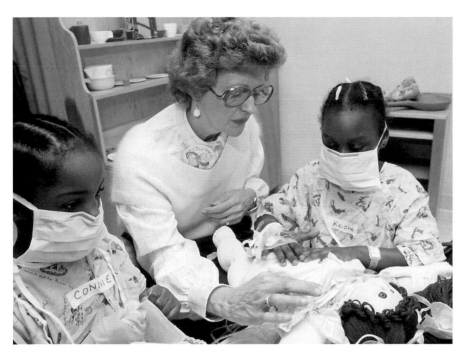

Child Life specialist Mary Barkey, MA, CCLS, ca. 1980s.

children not in isolation. "To get your child well as rapidly as possible is the aim of the Hospital….and to accomplish it, the child's welfare must be placed ahead of family considerations. Although your affections and desires may at time seem to be disregarded by hospital rules, they are really only being subordinated to the primary consideration."[5]

Pioneered at Rainbow Babies and Childrens in the late 1980s, Rainbow Comfort Measures© and Rainbow Comfort Positioning© are methods for empowering children and their parents to play active roles in their health care experiences. Child Life specialist Mary Barkey, MA, CCLS, and Barbara Stephens, MA, CRRN, a pediatric nurse, created the techniques to address the emotional and developmental needs of children receiving varying types of treatments that can often be uncomfortable, or frightening. The strategies help children and their parents manage stressful and upsetting situations, and make it easier for staff to do their jobs. "The model was well-integrated into practices at Rainbow by the early 1990s," says Lissy Zaremba, MA, Certified Child Life specialist. "They are now used worldwide. We have continued to develop and expand upon their original initiatives."

Caring is expressed in one-on-one connections. The impact is hard to measure, but the beneficial effects are easy to see. Practiced regularly, day to day, year after year, caring and the good communication it fosters between people improves clinical outcomes as well as patient and employee satisfaction. It makes the organization a better place and enhances what UH can achieve. ▼

Behind the Scenes

A bunny named Bo, donated by a veterinarian to Rainbow Babies and Childrens Hospital in 1989, was a popular resident in the playroom. Alyson Schnatz Robertson, a Child Life specialist who worked on the surgery floor, observed that the floppy-eared rabbit had a therapeutic effect on patients and staff. It prompted her to launch the Pet Pals program, which began with three dogs and their volunteer owners in 1992. Currently, more than 100 specially trained dogs are "regulars," making 160,000 visits annually to patients, families, and staff all around University Hospitals Cleveland Medical Center and at facilities system-wide. Interacting with dogs and other animals can have a positive impact on physical and psychological health, reducing feelings of stress and anxiety, lowering blood pressure and heart rate, and reducing the trauma of hospitalization by providing a pleasurable and positive experience.

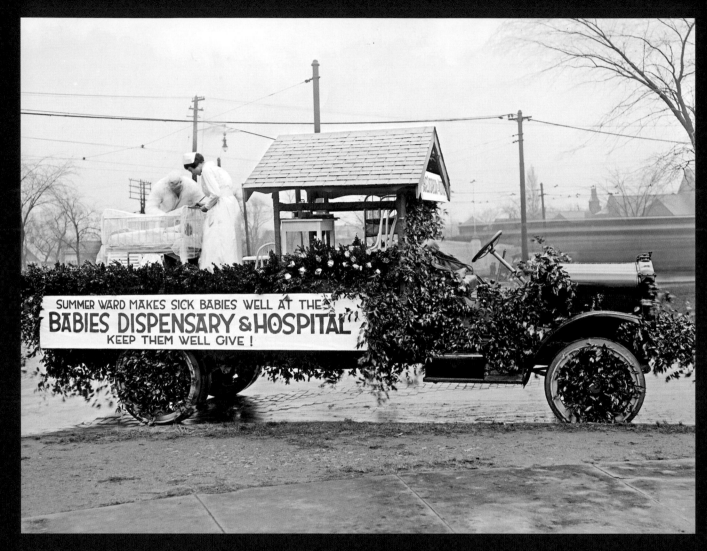

Each of the four founding hospitals began as a charitable effort, relying on donations to keep their doors open. Today, philanthropy continues to play an essential role in making University Hospitals strong. Members of the community show their support by giving generously just as they did during the 1912 fundraising campaign for Babies' Dispensary and Hospital.

Giving

"Whether you can donate a whole building or a brick, what's important is to be generous within your means. I made a donation after our son was born at Rainbow. He was premature and weighed only 2½ pounds. That was more than 40 years ago. I also became active on the board because I felt so grateful and realized University Hospitals needs time as well as treasure."

– Ann Pinkerton Ranney, Lifetime Trustee, University Hospitals

University Hospitals has always been a mission-driven charitable institution, relying upon the generosity and goodwill of the people it serves. Treating all, including those who could not afford to pay, is understood as an obligation, a principled stand that dates back to the opening of Wilson Street Hospital in 1866. But patient fees and government funds have never covered the entire cost of care. Philanthropy enabled each of the four founding institutions to fulfill their moral and social responsibilities and grow from small beginnings into the modern medical organization they have become. Survival and success were never guaranteed. Financial need was a constant challenge, the result of operating deficits, economic crisis, rising costs, and a constantly changing reimbursement landscape. There were many crossroads moments when the support of faithful friends, benefactors, and the citizens of Cleveland made the difference.

Philanthropy at UH has been synonymous with growth, renovations, expansion, and furthering medical discovery for over 150 years. In the early years, gifts often came in the form of goods to equip and operate the hospitals and clinics. Lakeside Hospital records from 1889 list donations of food, clothing, bed linens, cod liver oil, crutches, books, and a "rolling chair" from the Happy Thought Society of Miss Mittleberger's School for Girls. Businessmen often furnished loads of coal. As the hospitals professionalized over time, money was preferred so administrators could subsidize the areas of highest need, whether that was charity care, new medical equipment, the hiring of medical staff, or eventually medical research.

For every person memorialized in the name of a building, a program, or an endowed chair, there are thousands more whose names are not well-known. More than 22,000 gifts were made to UH in 2017 alone. Every contribution matters, from transformational bequests to the smallest amounts donated by ordinary citizens, according to their means. The impact of what volunteers bring is beyond any reckoning in dollars and cents. The UH story cannot be told without acknowledging all forms of giving and saluting the multiplicity of its supporters.

Most donors are inspired by UH's mission and its vision for the future of medicine and patient care. Former UH board member Bob Reitman and

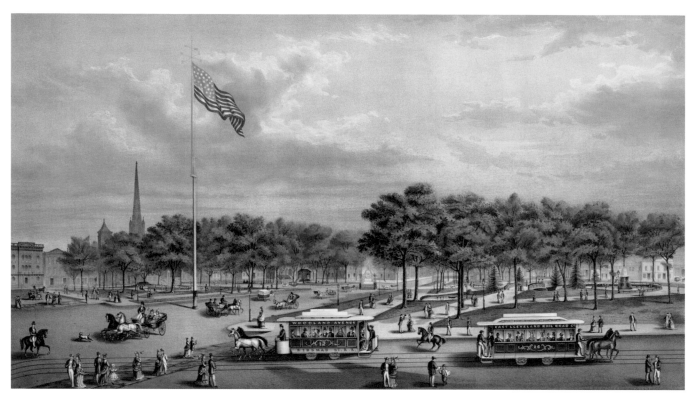

A postcard image of Cleveland's Monument Park (later known as Public Square), ca. 1873. The first fundraising event to support Wilson Street Hospital took place here in 1868.

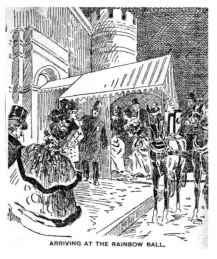

ARRIVING AT THE RAINBOW BALL.

Local newspapers often featured illustrations of the Rainbow Cottage charity ball, a much-anticipated event for Cleveland's social elite, ca. 1890s.

his wife, Sylvia, are no exception. The couple endowed the Robert S. and Sylvia K. Reitman Family Foundation Distinguished Chair in Cardiovascular Innovation in 2008, currently held by Jonathan Stamler, MD, PhD, President of Harrington Discovery Institute. Their $1.5 million contribution, jointly given to UH and Case Western Reserve University, supports clinical research to accelerate medical discoveries.

"Every gift," says Reitman, "no matter how modest, is important. Philanthropy is a way we demonstrate our humanity to our peers and to our progeny, and makes a permanent statement about who we are and what we value."

Community Support: Major Fundraising Events

Fetes, socials, bazaars, exhibitions, parties, and other forms of entertainment are time-honored methods for raising money and engaging the community. It has been a relentless and ongoing endeavor, managed mostly by women who helped to ensure the continued existence of each founding institution and the health of the unified organization they became.

Wilson Street Hospital's first fundraising event was a multi-night gala held in June 1868. A massive tent equipped with gas lighting was erected downtown on what is now Cleveland's Public Square. Crowds came for music, 50-cent plated dinners, fireworks, and refreshments. It was deemed a great success, raising more than $2,000 to cover mortgage costs and furnishings for Wilson Street.

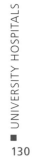

In 1875, the Calico Ball earned close to $5,000 for Wilson Street and the Bethel Relief Association, a Protestant organization that sent its homeless and sick population there for nursing care and medical treatment. The press dubbed the affair "one of the grandest social events Cleveland has ever known." Tickets cost $5, and each admitted "a gentleman and two ladies." The event drew 2,500 patrons who danced polkas, waltzes, minuets, and quadrilles until three o'clock in the morning.[1]

Events were also popular fundraisers for Rainbow Cottage. The annual Rainbow Cottage charity ball held at the Gatling Gun Armory, one of the largest banquet halls in Cleveland at the time, was another important social occasion for the city's elite families during the last decade of the 19th century. Writing in November 1895, a reporter noted that the ball was "the first big dance of the season" and provided an opportunity "to exchange greetings, renew flirtations, and display pretty new toilettes. Then, too, everyone who dances at the Rainbow ball is made twice glad by the thought that he is not only enjoying himself immensely, but is by his subscription aiding one of Cleveland's most beautiful charities."[2] Rainbow Cottage matron Louise Johnston emphasized the importance of the event in the organization's 1896 annual report. "The original plan was to take twelve children at a time and keep them two weeks only, but now we can take eighteen at a time, and we have been obliged to deviate from the rule, for in most all cases the children have come in such an enfeebled condition we have had to keep them longer; some have stayed all summer."[3]

Smaller, more intimate events were also held to cultivate philanthropic support. Potential patrons were invited to attend teas at Rainbow Cottage where they could meet the convalescent children and see firsthand the work being done there. "If the mothers of children who have enjoyed the advantages of the cottage could will it, there would be no shortage of funds to carry on and enlarge the work. Unfortunately, those in the best position to know the immense good done are the least able to give financial support."[4]

In its early years, Babies and Childrens Hospital was also fortunate to have supporters who would host events. To raise funds for the fledgling infants' clinic, philanthropists Charles A. Otis Jr. and his wife, Lucia Edwards, held a bazaar in their home in the spring of 1907. There were booths in the ballroom selling flowers, candy, Easter novelties, and toys. The latest hats from Paris were displayed in another room.

It's a Fact

Rainbow Cottage, as well as the other founding hospitals, increased its endowment through bed subscriptions, a practice common at the time of donating funds to maintain hospital beds. In 1903, the cost to endow a bed at Rainbow in perpetuity was $3,000 or $150 for a year. The fund exceeded $22,000 in 1905, allowing Rainbow to stay open year-round by 1907.

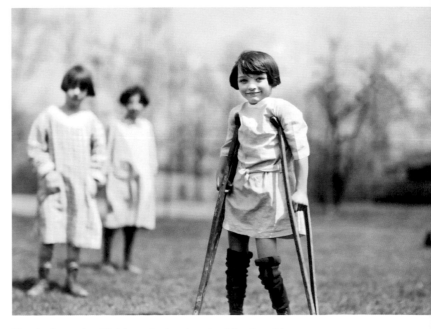

The charity work of Rainbow Cottage's early philanthropists significantly improved the health and well-being of Cleveland's youth, ca. 1920s.

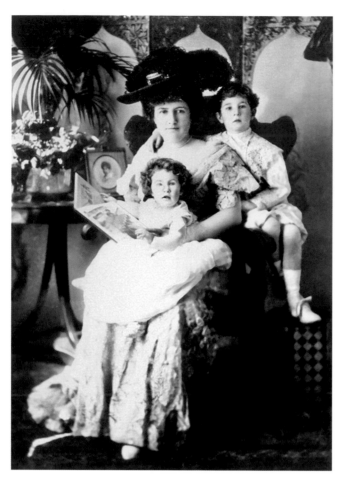

Cleveland socialite and philanthropist Lucia
Edwards Otis, ca. early 1900s.

Debutantes served tea, and their brothers played
newsboys for a day, hawking copies of *The Cleveland
News*, a newspaper owned by Mr. Otis. Admission
was 50 cents, and the event raised $2,500.[5]

The Otises settled in Cleveland in 1836 and built a
fortune in the iron and steel industry. The couple was
instrumental in the formation of Babies' Dispensary,
with Charles serving as the first President of its board
until 1914. Lucia, a member of the Rainbow Circle of
King's Daughters that founded Rainbow Cottage, also
served on the Women's Board of Babies' Dispensary.

At Maternity Hospital, social events to
encourage public support included a "harvest
gathering," the first of which was held in 1892. At
this modest affair, guests were invited to contribute
money, food, coal, and other necessities. In 1897,
the hospital's board sponsored a stage show. Actors,
musicians, and stagehands donated their time, and
the production garnered positive reviews. However,
Cleveland's infamous bad weather kept many
patrons at home. Fundraising setbacks like this were
significant because the hospital was accumulating debt amid rising
costs without an endowment. A group of singers and accompanists
came to its aid in 1899 with a free concert and later that year a show
at Association Hall with a singer and a "reader" who interpreted
works of William Shakespeare and James Whitcomb Riley. In
subsequent years, musical recitals, art exhibitions, card parties, and
trolley rides to the country and the beach were organized to benefit
the struggling hospital and its patients.[6]

When the Hotel Statler held its grand opening in downtown
Cleveland in October 1912, the Board of Lady Managers at Babies'
Dispensary transformed the occasion into a charity ball. They wisely
capitalized on the community's widespread curiosity to see what was
reputed to be the most luxurious accommodation between New York and
Chicago. The ball drew guests from as far away as Detroit, Pittsburgh,
and Buffalo. A special train brought in attendees from Detroit and picked
up more guests from towns to the west of Cleveland. Hotel owner E.M.
Statler donated the use of the hotel, 25 percent of the bar proceeds, and
all of the money raised from ticket sales. The ball, called "the largest and
most magnificent social event ever staged in Cleveland" by *The Plain
Dealer*, brought in nearly $5,000 for the Dispensary.[7]

In the first decades of the 20th century, national trends in
fundraising shifted dramatically; events were reduced in number and

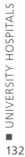

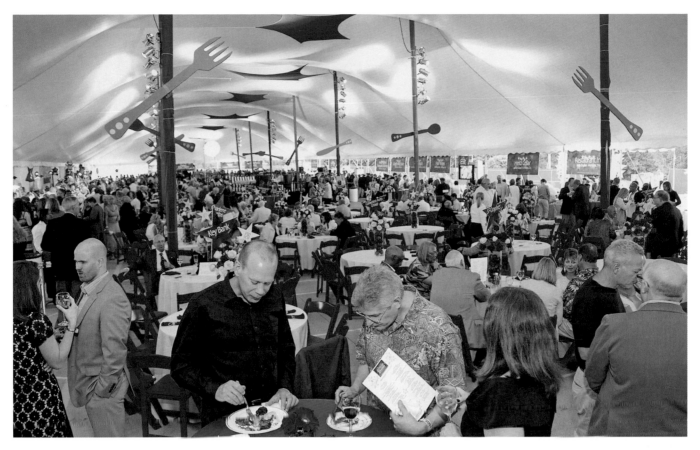

The biennial Five Star Sensation fundraiser for University Hospitals Seidman Cancer Center delivered a memorable evening of food, drink, live music, and socializing, 2013.

scale, and organized, public fundraising campaigns gained popularity. The founding hospitals followed suit, and for the next six decades, events were deemphasized. Then, in the 1980s, University Hospitals revisited the concept, melding it with some of the strategies of a professionally-run campaign to create an innovative approach to grassroots fundraising and community engagement.

Contemporary fundraising events held at UH follow the successful tradition of galas and balls of the past, but with a modern twist. In 1987, UH held the first Five Star Sensation event at the Cleveland Convention Center. It originated with committee Co-chair Lee Edwards. She contacted famed chef and restaurateur Wolfgang Puck who agreed to participate and enlist his industry friends to do the same. Eleven celebrity chefs from around the country traveled to Cleveland to prepare food for 800 people, with all of the proceeds benefiting the then-named UH Ireland Cancer Center.

While intended to be a one-time event, Five Star continued on thanks to the vision and work of Carole Carr, a personal friend of Chef Puck. The combination of Puck's star power and Carr's management skills attracted other big names in the culinary world as well as sell-out crowds. In 1995, *The Plain Dealer* observed that "[f]or one night, every other year, Cleveland is the food capital of the world."[8]

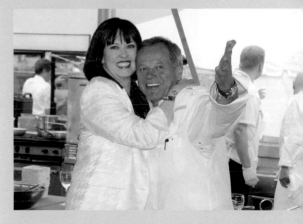

Five Star creators Carole Carr (left) and Chef Wolfgang Puck, 2009.

It's a Fact

"You know what is so extraordinary?" asked Wolfgang Puck. "That the people in Cleveland support us so well. When they do this kind of event in San Francisco, [organizers] are happy to get 500 people; here, we get three times that. At first, I was so nervous all the time to get people to come. Now it's like a homecoming."[9]

In 2015, after more than 25 years of dedicated leadership, Carr and Puck retired from Five Star, and a new era commenced. Cleveland's own star chef Michael Symon became the new culinary host of the event. Jackie Rothstein, philanthropist and wife of former University Hospitals Cleveland Medical Center President Fred Rothstein, MD, and philanthropist Jane Seidman volunteered to co-chair the event. The 2017 fundraising extravaganza featured 39 chefs and 40 vintners under two football field-sized tents. A total of nearly $20 million has been raised to benefit cancer patients since the gala's inception.

University Hospitals Rainbow Babies & Children's Hospital's largest fundraising event is a themed "Ride the Rainbow" party that has been held at an historic hotel, the county airport, museums, and the city's Public Hall. The festive biennial gathering harkens back to the Rainbow Cottage annual charity dinner dances held in the late 19th century. Ride the Rainbow has raised $8.4 million since its inaugural event in 2004. The 2014 Ride the Rainbow gala, called "Superheroes Unite," attracted 1,100 attendees and raised a record $1.4 million. It also gave one mother and son an experience they will never forget. Lisa Arnold, RN, a pediatric nursing supervisor at UH Rainbow, was the grand prizewinner of the "Superhero for a Day" raffle. After a four-course dinner, she and her teenage son, Bobby, were taken by limousine to a private, invitation-only premiere of *Captain America: The Winter Soldier*, an action movie filmed in Cleveland. Bobby knows about confronting danger firsthand. A UH Rainbow patient since birth, Bobby has a rare genetic disorder and was not expected to survive his first few years.

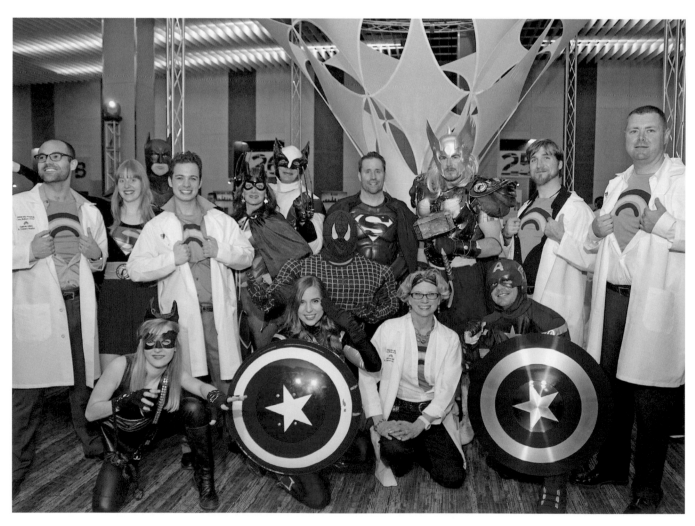

University Hospitals Rainbow Babies & Children's Hospital physicians, nurses, and other care providers embraced their inner "superhero" at the Ride the Rainbow fundraising event in 2014.

However, with the help of his doctors and a true fighting spirit, he has become a real-life superhero.

Community Support: Public Campaigns

By 1910, Cleveland was the sixth largest city in the United States. All of its health care institutions were challenged by dramatically increasing patient numbers and the need to expand. Time and again, the founding hospitals turned to the community for help in the first three decades of the 20th century, launching large-scale fundraising drives to provide the necessary capital.

In March 1907, Babies' Dispensary and Hospital held its public "Save the Babies" campaign, which raised $100,000, a portion of which was used to purchase and renovate a property on East 35th Street to serve as the dispensary's new home. Additionally, more than 500 children contributed a dollar each to pay for a nurse who went to the homes of sick babies to teach their mothers to feed and care for them. In 1910, the original wooden structure was replaced with a brick building to house milk laboratories and examination rooms.[10]

Two years later, the overwhelming need for an inpatient hospital to support the mission of Babies' Dispensary spurred another campaign. In August 1912, volunteers ranging from society matrons and downtown workers to school-age children went door-to-door for two weeks to raise $1 million on behalf of the dispensary to build and equip a full-sized inpatient children's hospital on the same site. The wealthy offered their cars and chauffeurs to transport the canvassers around the city. A call went out to enlist 5,000 girls, ages 12 and older, to help the drive. Mayor Newton D. Baker spoke to them during a rally at the Cleveland Armory to kick off the effort. To motivate the volunteers, a film about the dispensary was shown featuring scenes of a sick child and a weeping mother as well as nurses and physicians at work. The film was also screened for the public at the Alhambra Theater downtown, with uniformed nurses and little girls stationed in the lobby to accept donations. Despite a last-minute solicitation appeal that was mailed to 100 business leaders and their employees, the campaign fell short of its goal by hundreds of thousands of dollars. However, the widespread public support for the dispensary inspired Samuel Mather to begin discussions to add Babies' Dispensary to a potential new complex for Lakeside Hospital.[11]

Lack of funds caused by the outbreak of WWI delayed planning for the new hospital facilities. After the war, planning resumed, and in 1923, a city-wide fundraising campaign took place to raise money for the construction of new facilities in University Circle for what would become Babies and Childrens and Maternity hospitals. Over 400 Clevelanders, many of them prominent business people and society figures, were mobilized into eight teams to raise $2.5 million during one week in May. Every bank in Cleveland accepted contributions. Local department stores included campaign

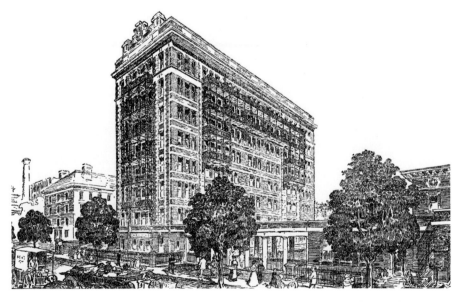

An architectural rendering of the hospital planned for Babies' Dispensary and Hospital, 1911.

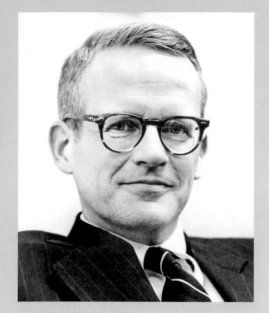

Former University Hospitals board member Allen Ford, ca. 1980.

I Remember

Allen Ford served on the University Hospitals board for three decades. His personal connection to UH, however, goes back much further; his parents assisted in the 1927 fundraising campaign for the medical center. During WWII, when he was 15 and the hospital was short-staffed, his mother, who volunteered at UH, suggested he get a summer job at the hospital. "I worked in the basement of what is now the Lakeside building in the dietetic storeroom," recalls Ford, "delivering food carts up to the floors and washing pots and pans in the main kitchen. I suspect I'm the only [board member] in the history of University Hospitals who did that. I liked getting paid, but I wasn't in it just for the money. We had rationing at that time and meat was scarce, but I got to eat hamburgers every day and when Mrs. Zack, a wonderful woman who ran the bakery, was feeling good, she would offer me a miniature pie. So, I was highly motivated."

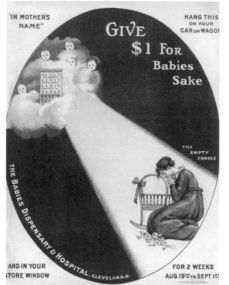

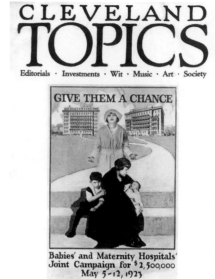

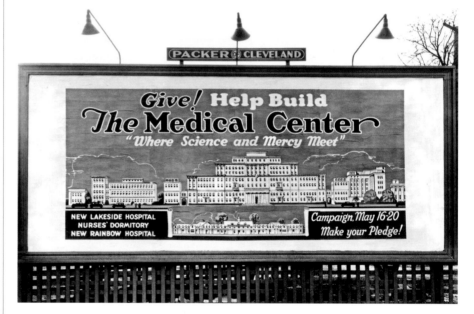

Promotional materials from the 1912, 1923, and 1927 University Hospitals' fundraising campaigns.

materials in their advertisements, and area theaters promoted the campaign on stage and on screen.

Coverage of the daily donations that shared personal stories of individual generosity made front-page news all over the city. "A mother of five children, all of whom have benefitted by medical treatment at Babies' Dispensary, and whose husband is in jail, left 30 cents for the building fund with the explanation that she wanted to do something 'for America'. Another woman…sent in $5, and another, who said she had been saving to buy a vacuum cleaner but had decided to stick to her broom awhile longer, gave $6. A man of 70 produced a quarter, two dimes and three pennies, which he said was all the money he had but gave the quarter to the building fund. A cripple painfully hobbled up to headquarters, left $2, then rested for an hour before undertaking the trip home again."[12]

As the campaign drew to a close, it had not yet reached its goal. Campaign Chairman Arthur D. Baldwin, a Cleveland attorney and civic leader, issued a last-minute appeal to every citizen in Cleveland. "It would be mighty nice if a lot of 'from-one-baby-to-another' contributions were received. There are plenty of parents of new babies who should be glad to send a dollar or more along in the names of their own children."[13] By the next day, the goal had not only been met but surpassed by more than $110,000. In addition to corporate contributions from Sherwin-Williams and the Cleveland Cliffs Iron Company, sizable gifts were received from Edward Harkness, whose family had made their fortune from Standard Oil; the Lakeside Hospital trustees; and Samuel Mather, the largest campaign donor. There were also many small donations. Thirty children in Shaker Heights marched to the home of a campaign team member and turned over their piggy banks, which contained 150 pennies.[14] The final count revealed that 6,250 donors from all walks of life had been part of this extraordinary undertaking. Two years later, the newly built Babies and Childrens and Maternity hospitals opened in University Circle and officially became part of University Hospitals.

Another ambitious and carefully orchestrated weeklong campaign was undertaken in 1927. Its objective was to raise $6 million for the construction of Lakeside Hospital in University Circle, a more modern facility for Rainbow Hospital in South Euclid, and new nursing dormitories adjacent to the new Lakeside Hospital. Promoted with the slogan "Where Science and Mercy Meet," it was the largest fundraising campaign in Cleveland's history to date. Volunteers were a veritable "who's who" of Cleveland's most prominent families, many of whose descendants have continued to be involved with supporting UH and working on the hospital's behalf up to the present day.

The drive began with a quiet phase during which Samuel Mather and campaign officials approached the wealthiest, most prominent families in Cleveland to secure commitments for their support. To attract public interest, City Manager William R. Hopkins, Chair of the citizens committee for the campaign, wrote a proclamation to encourage everyone to do his or her part. He reminded Clevelanders that this next phase in the development of UH and the academic campus would "place Cleveland in a very select group of cities at the very peak of medical progress and teaching."[15]

On May 21, 1927, *The Plain Dealer* reported on its front page that the campaign had not only met its goal but surpassed it by raising $8,034,355. It was another landmark moment in UH history. An information booklet produced by UH in 1935 emphasized the role of Cleveland's citizens in this achievement. "Never for a similar purpose

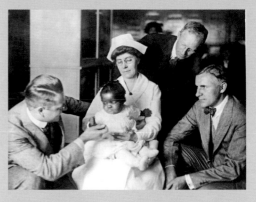

Arthur Baldwin (second from right) with patient and staff at Babies' Dispensary and Hospital, ca. 1910s.

Pioneer

Arthur Baldwin was known for devoting much of his time to charitable organizations. He was involved in the formation of the Cleveland Foundation, the Legal Aid Society, and the organization that would become United Way. He worked with Edward Cushing, MD, to establish the Babies' Dispensary and Hospital in 1907 and was its second President, a tireless advocate, a board member, and a donor.

Baldwin played an instrumental role in forming University Hospitals. "Samuel Mather put the plan together for the creation of University Hospitals," said Samuel "Jack" Horwitz, MD, former Chief of Pediatrics at University Hospitals Rainbow Babies & Children's Hospital, "but it was Arthur Baldwin who saw it through, merging the three hospitals [Babies and Childrens, Maternity, and Lakeside], and raising the money to get them all built. He was UH's first President. He led the organization through the Great Depression, helping to save it." Baldwin continued his active involvement at UH, including serving as Chairman of the board until 1940.

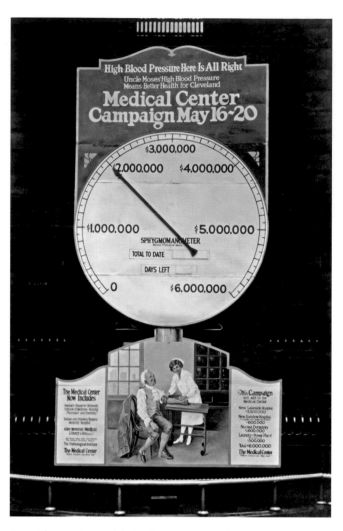

An outdoor poster used during the 1927 campaign. According to *The Plain Dealer*, "The spriest gentleman on Euclid [A]venue last night was the figure of old Mose Cleveland (figure on the left) at the corner of E[ast] 9th [S]treet. The old fellow has so much ginger, and his 'pressure' is rising so rapidly that he is expected to burst the recording instrument into smithereens by tonight."[16]

was there such a united response. Contributions poured in from people in all stations of life, and the completion of the Medical Center, as it now stands, was made possible...[It] was created not only for the community but by the community."

Thirty-five years would pass before the public was once again asked to help UH expand to meet the modern health care needs of the community. Unlike the whirlwind fundraising campaigns of the past, the 1962 "University Medical Center" drive, as it was called, was designed to be a long, slow process. Cleveland's legacy families once again enthusiastically showed their support, as did a number of new donors and Cleveland's large corporations. Even the federal government participated. As the campaign progressed, facility improvements began to take shape, changing the exterior facade of the University Circle campus. When the drive ended in the mid-1970s, a total of $55.7 million had been raised. The funds supported facility enhancements at Western Reserve University as well as at UH, including the Robert H. Bishop Building, named after Samuel Mather's son-in-law and longtime board member and hospital administrator of Lakeside and UH; the George M. Humphrey Building for ambulatory care; modernization of Lakeside; and an addition to the Leonard C. Hanna House. One of the most prominent results of the campaign was the construction of a new hospital to replace the outdated Babies and Childrens Hospital, a hospital that would now be large enough to allow Rainbow Hospital to share the space and move to University Circle, creating Rainbow Babies and Childrens Hospital.

The need for growth and expansion continued, and in 1982, UH announced the "Center of Excellence" a $42 million capital campaign to build a new Ambulatory Referral Center; a new parking garage between Cornell and Abington roads; a complete modernization of MacDonald House; and additions to Hanna Pavilion, the Robert H. Bishop Building, and Rainbow Babies and Childrens Hospital. During this campaign, UH received a $14 million grant from the state of Ohio to create the R. Livingston Ireland Cancer Center. Longtime UH board member "Liv" Ireland, who was stricken with cancer, made a personal appeal to his friend James Rhodes, the governor of Ohio, to secure the funding, and this led to naming the Ireland Cancer Center in his honor.

The next major expansion of buildings and infrastructure occurred as a result of the 1991 "Campaign for UH." A total of $61 million, surpassing the original goal of $40 million, was raised in two phases. The first phase focused on funding the Alfred and Norma Lerner Tower and the Samuel Mather Pavilion, new equipment and technology, clinical research, physician education, and the UH endowment. The second phase raised funds for capital and programmatic improvements at Rainbow Babies and Childrens, including the construction of the Leonard and Joan Horvitz Tower.

In 2006, UH unveiled Vision 2010, a far-reaching, strategic initiative that involved major facility and technology upgrades and reinvestment in the community, including University Hospitals Ahuja Medical Center in Beachwood, the Quentin & Elisabeth Alexander Level IIIc Neonatal Intensive Care Unit at University Hospitals Rainbow Babies & Children's Hospital, University Hospitals Seidman Cancer Center, and the Center for Emergency Medicine and the Marcy R. Horvitz Pediatric Emergency Center on the University Circle campus. The overall scope of the plan required the largest fundraising effort to date. To meet the financial needs of this ambitious vision for Cleveland's health care future, UH launched the *Discover the Difference* philanthropic campaign in November 2010. The response echoed the massive show of public engagement that defined earlier endeavors.

In addition to the sizable gifts that resulted in the naming of buildings and rooms as well as endowed chairs for physicians, a great deal of support came once again from grassroots events and individuals of modest means. On December 12, 2012, UH announced it achieved its campaign goal of $1 billion one year earlier than expected. As a result, hospital leadership and philanthropic supporters set their sights higher and committed to a new goal of $1.5 billion—the largest campaign in UH history and one of the largest hospital fundraising

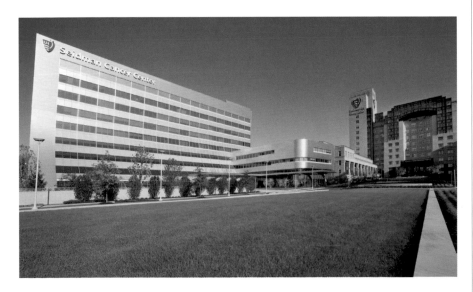

University Hospitals Seidman Cancer Center, 2011.

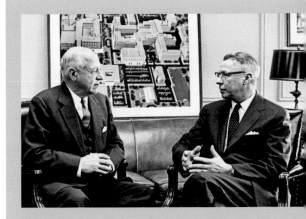

Former U.S. Secretary of the Treasury George M. Humphrey (left) with his 1962 campaign Co-chair, J.D. Wright, Chairman of the board of TRW, an automotive and aerospace component manufacturer. An architectural rendering of the proposed University Hospitals/Western Reserve University Medical School campus at University Circle is featured behind them.

Family Ties

The 1962 campaign was co-chaired by longtime University Hospitals supporter George M. Humphrey. A businessman who began his career at the M.A. Hanna Company, Humphrey served as secretary of the U.S. Treasury Department under President Dwight Eisenhower and was the President of National Steel. As a young attorney, Humphrey wrote the constitution and bylaws for the newly-organized UH. His wife Pamela participated in the 1927 campaign as a volunteer solicitor. His son Gilbert and daughter Pamela Humphrey Firman both served on the UH board, while daughter Carol Humphrey Butler served on the Rainbow Hospital board. Grandson George Humphrey II not only served on the UH board, but also chaired the 1991 Campaign for University Hospitals. Members of the Humphrey family continue to support UH today.

campaigns in the country. In 2017, UH exceeded this goal with a total of $1,511,586,803 raised, making UH one of a select few health care systems in the nation to attain such an ambitious goal. In total, campaign contributions came from more than 83,500 individual donors, 90 percent of whom were new donors, and 184,920 gifts. More than 1,200 volunteer leaders were engaged in the effort.

Visionary Benefactors: Past

There is a long tradition of charity and philanthropy among Cleveland's oldest and most prominent families. A 1925 article on the construction progress of Babies and Childrens and Maternity hospitals in University Circle noted that "[the hospitals] were made possible in large part by donations from fortunes assembled by pioneer Clevelanders."[17] Early benefactors of University Hospitals regularly appeared in the society pages of local newspapers and in the Cleveland Blue Book, a directory of the city's elite families. A strong network of kinship as well as social and business connections linked these early leaders. The same individuals served on the boards of the founding hospitals, worked there as volunteers, and supported them financially. Their children and grandchildren often carried on the family's support. These ties were critical to the formation and growth of UH and the development of the medical center campus.

Hinman B. Hurlbut, the first president of Wilson Street Hospital, was also its greatest financial benefactor. A wealthy lawyer, banker, and railroad magnate, he was an important champion and sponsor of the hospital in its crucial early years. Hurlbut provided significant

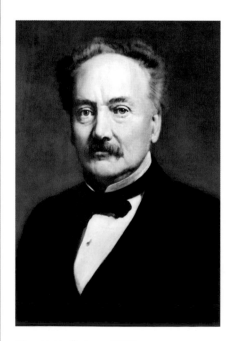

Hinman Hurlbut, ca. 1870s.

financial support, paying off the building's mortgage and covering all of the hospital's expenses for 1869 and much of 1870. After personally arranging for the lease of nearby Marine Hospital, Wilson Street's second home, he funded the building's necessary renovations and then built a new wing to house a surgical theater. He frequently wrote checks to cover monetary shortfalls at the end of each year during his presidency. When Hurlbut died in 1884, he left $200,000 to the hospital. Minutes from the board's annual report that year praise his generosity. "No one had ever shown more affection for this institution than he; no one had ever aided it so largely…When he left us and this earth it was not in forgetfulness, but he remembered this institution by a gift so munificent as to insure its stability for the future, so that, in time to come, the poor and the afflicted must rise up and bless the name of Mr. H.B. Hurlbut."[18]

When Samuel Mather became President of Lakeside Hospital, he followed Hurlbut's example of providing support for the hospital. In 1900, Samuel Mather contributed $50,000 to Lakeside's endowment, commenting, "It is a simple impossibility to carry on the work of a large modern hospital on a self-supporting basis."[19] Throughout his long tenure as Lakeside's chairman of the board, Samuel Mather's donations often assured the solvency of the hospital's finances, kept the hospital from closing, and provided opportunities for substantial growth. He came forward to cover yearly budget shortfalls and specific operating costs; made sizable donations for special projects and during fundraising campaigns; and paid for such minor but no less meaningful things as the purchase of magazines for the patients, seeds and flowers for the hospital's gardens, flower bouquets for each graduate of the nursing school, and small presents on Christmas Day for every nursing student and patient in the hospital. "Lakeside Hospital is probably Samuel Mather's chiefest hobby. If there's a deficit in the hospital finances at the end of the year, Mr. Mather is usually only too happy to write out a check that will more than make it up. This has gone on from year to year until whenever anything is broken or damaged about the place, the nurses and other employees look upon the loss as just that much out of Mr. Mather's generous pocket. If a nurse drops a saucer she will smile and remark, 'Poor Samuel!' Among many of the nurses, the remark is almost a byword when anything goes wrong."[20]

Samuel Mather and his wife, Flora Stone, were united in a philanthropic partnership. But, long before they married in 1881, Flora, born into wealth, was a philanthropist in her own right. She was inspired by pastors and teachers to lead a useful life and modeled her charitable work after that of her parents, Amasa Stone and Julia Gleason. They were members of the First Presbyterian Church ("Old Stone Church") and were among the group of parishioners that established the Home for Friendless Strangers and Wilson Street Hospital. Flora continued her family's legacy when she endowed a training school for nurses at Lakeside. Her name is associated with more than 30 organizations, all of which received bequests in her will after she died in 1909 at age 56. *The Plain Dealer* quoted one of the leaders of a charity Flora Stone Mather supported as saying, "There

It's a Fact

Samuel Mather's philanthropic influence in Cleveland ran deep and wide, and his passion for Lakeside Hospital also inspired others. A number of his partners and other executives at Pickands, Mather & Company served on the Lakeside board and also became supporters of the hospital. One of his partners, Harry Coulby, left Lakeside a gift that continues to give. Coulby, who was born in England, came to America as a young man and is said to have walked from New York to Cleveland because he did not have money for a train ticket. He amassed a fortune in the shipping business over his lifetime. He died in 1929 and left the bulk of his $3.2 million estate to the Cleveland Foundation, with half the money designated to benefit Lakeside. The Coulby endowment has generated more than $40 million for University Hospitals since it was established, and that support continues to this day.

Another bequest with a connection to Pickands, Mather & Company came from George Simmons, who worked as a groundskeeper and chauffeur to Mather's business partner, Colonel James Pickands. Simmons amassed a small fortune through smart investing in the stock market, which he learned from Colonel Pickands. In his 70s and almost blind when he died in 1959, Simmons left nearly $500,000 in his will to UH for ophthalmology research.

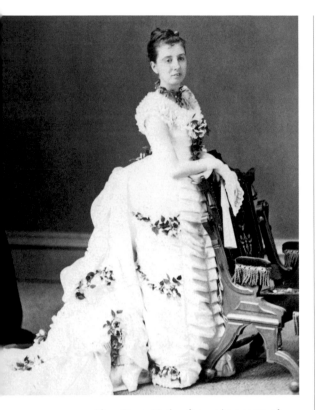

Flora Stone Mather focused on some of the most important civic and social reform issues of her era, including education for women as well as medical care and charitable support for poor women and children, ca. 1890s.

has never been such another woman in Cleveland and there never will be...There is not a philanthropic organization in the city that will not feel her loss deeply."[21] She left Lakeside an annual gift from her estate, and after her death, the new nurses' dormitory that had been built with support from Samuel Mather was renamed for Flora Stone Mather. When Lakeside relocated to University Circle and new nursing dorms were built, one continued to carry her name.

Another philanthropic family who made their mark in the growth of Lakeside was the Hannas. Brothers Leonard C. Hanna Sr. and H. Melville Hanna Sr., Cleveland industrialists who made their fortunes in coal and iron ore, joined the Lakeside board in the late 1890s and were major supporters of the hospital throughout their lives. H. Melville Hanna was key in partnering with Mather to plan the new hospital complex. When Hanna died in 1921, it was estimated that he had donated more than $1 million to Lakeside and for the proposed new Babies and Childrens Hospital in University Circle.

During the 1927 campaign, Leonard C. Hanna Jr. and his mother, Coralie, helped to underwrite the construction of a private pavilion at the new Lakeside to be named the Leonard C. Hanna House after his late father. In 1945, following the death of UH board member Howard Melville Hanna Jr., other members of the Hanna family and employees of the M.A. Hanna Company made a $1 million gift

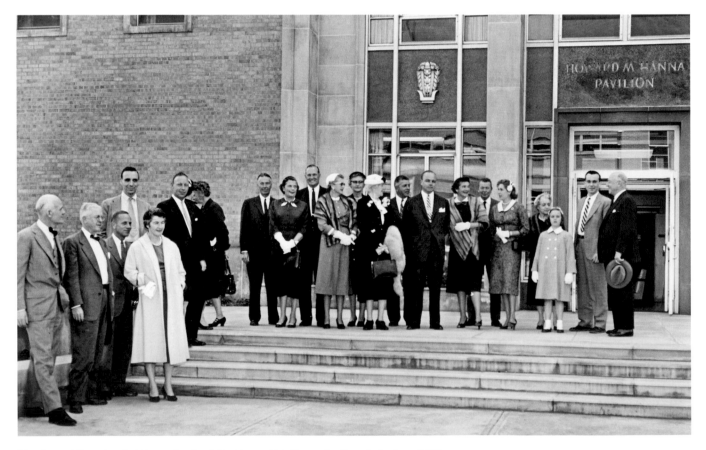

Members of the extended Hanna family at the Howard M. Hanna Pavilion dedication, 1956.

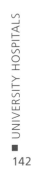

to establish a psychiatric institute at UH. When completed in 1956, the building was named the Howard M. Hanna Memorial Pavilion, often referred to as the Hanna Pavilion. Support from the Hanna family continued with a $10 million gift from the Leonard C. Hanna Jr. Fund, which has generated more than $50 million to support UH since 1957 and aided in the construction of the Joseph T. Wearn Laboratory for Medical Research adjacent to Lakeside. A later gift of more than $6 million from the fund was the largest single contribution to the 1962 University Medical Center campaign.

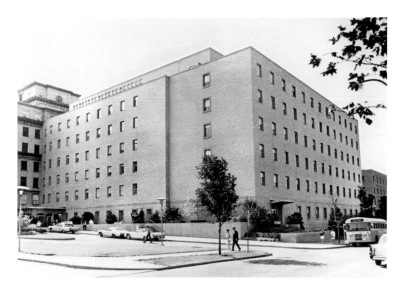

The Joseph T. Wearn Laboratory for Medical Research opened in 1962 on the University Circle campus.

The Wades were another prosperous Cleveland family whose generosity helped to expand UH facilities and infrastructure. Family patriarch Jeptha Homer Wade I made his fortune with the Western Union telegraph company, as well as railroads, banks, and industrial companies. In 1910, his grandson Jeptha Homer Wade II and his wife, Ellen Garretson Wade, who served on the Babies' Dispensary board, gave $100,000 to the Dispensary to complete and equip a new facility on East 35th Street, purchase additional property for future expansion, and pay off all of the dispensary's debts. The gift was made in honor of Anna Wade, Jeptha's mother, who devoted her charitable efforts to children's health. "It will give the association power for still greater usefulness and testifies in splendid fashion to the generosity of its donors."[22] Jeptha Homer Wade II, who also supported Lakeside, continued his financial beneficence to the dispensary by collaborating with Samuel Mather and others to quietly purchase and then donate land for a new facility in University Circle in 1915. He also donated $150,000 during the fundraising campaign of 1923. The Wade family's involvement with UH continued for several generations. The couple's daughter, Helen Wade Greene, created a trust in support of UH in 1957, and granddaughter Elizabeth Sedgwick was married to Ellery Sedgwick, longtime UH Trustee and Chairman of the UH board from 1970 to 1974.

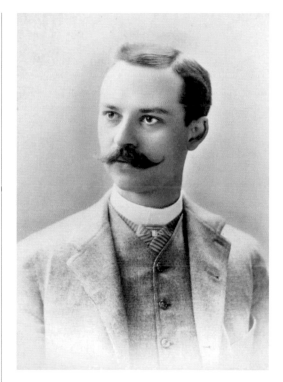

Jeptha Homer Wade II, ca. 1880s.

Transformational Benefactors: Now

Building on the strong foundation of those that came before them, several individuals and families have made pivotal gifts in the late 20th and early 21st centuries that have moved University Hospitals forward and bolstered Cleveland's reputation as one of the nation's premier health care centers.

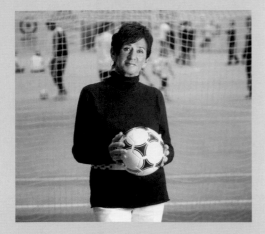

Iris S. Wolstein, 2008.

Pass It On

Bert L. Wolstein was an athlete, a sports fan, and owner of the Cleveland Force, the former professional soccer team in Cleveland. He also knew what it was like to have cancer. After he died, his wife, Iris, conceived of a fitting tribute to him. Collaborating with physicians and staff at University Hospitals Rainbow Babies & Children's Hospital, she led the way in creating Iris S. and Bert L. Wolstein's Kids Kicking Cancer, a program that makes it possible for young cancer patients and survivors to get involved in physical activities such as soccer, swimming, golf, basketball, and conditioning. In 2008, she established a $1 million endowment for the program to ensure that that these special patients could get fit and have fun just like other boys and girls. Trained coaches teach skills while health care professionals observe from the sidelines and offer safety advice along with encouragement. Reflecting on the impact of her gift, this hands-on philanthropist said,

"[W]hen I watch them at play, I know with certainty that we are creating joy for these kids."[24]

Iris S. and Bert L. Wolstein made one such gift. The research building that bears their name on the medical center campus offered a new workplace for physician-scientists from UH and Case Western Reserve University. "Bert firmly believed our gift would create an atmosphere in which to accomplish medical miracles to help the ills of humanity," said Iris. "I am certain that he would be pleased, as I am, with the diligence of the researchers in the use of this setting to stimulate solutions to the afflictions of our nation and the world beyond."[23]

A bequest of $35 million from the estates of Donald J. and Ruth Weber Goodman made in 2004 to improve cancer care and

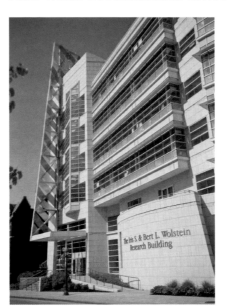

In 2003, the Iris S. & Bert L. Wolstein Research Building opened, supported by a $25 million gift from the Wolsteins.

cardiovascular disease was another defining moment. Supported by their philanthropic fund through the Cleveland Foundation, the Goodman Discovery Center at University Hospitals Seidman Cancer Center is a space specifically designed for physicians, nurses, and cancer patients involved in clinical trials where research and treatment happen side by side. At the time, very few cancer centers anywhere in the country had such a facility. Dr. Goodman, a dentist, had been treated for leukemia at UH. His granddaughter and executor,

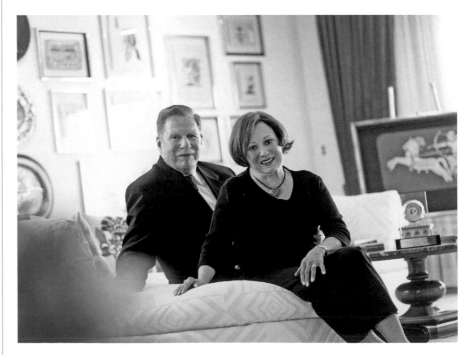

The late Donald J. and Ruth Weber Goodman, 2005.

Rainbow Babies & Children's Foundation

The Rainbow Babies & Children's Foundation, a volunteer organization of women, was formed when Rainbow Hospital and Babies and Childrens Hospital merged in 1974. Throughout its history, the charitable organization has provided funding for capital needs and facility improvements; clinical research; endowed chairs and subspecialty fellowships; the Child Life Program, which helps children and their families navigate the hospital experience; and advocacy work on behalf of children.

Circle of Friends is a community outreach endeavor that the Rainbow Foundation initiated in 2002. Individuals or groups are encouraged to band together, for a single project or event, or as an ongoing association, to help University Hospitals

Rainbow Babies & Children's Hospital. In 2015, 65 circles, generating close to $1 million annually, had been formed, raising money in a variety of creative ways, bringing volunteers into the hospital, and acting as community ambassadors.

The Rainbow Foundation's philanthropic endeavors have catapulted University Hospitals forward on several occasions. In 2006, the Rainbow Foundation gave $20.6 million to UH Rainbow, at that time, the largest single donation in the hospital's history. Five million dollars funded an "Endowed Chair Challenge" program to recruit and retain top talent in pediatric and neonatal care. The Foundation surpassed this gift in 2012 with its transformational gift of $32.5 million to the *Discover the Difference* campaign.

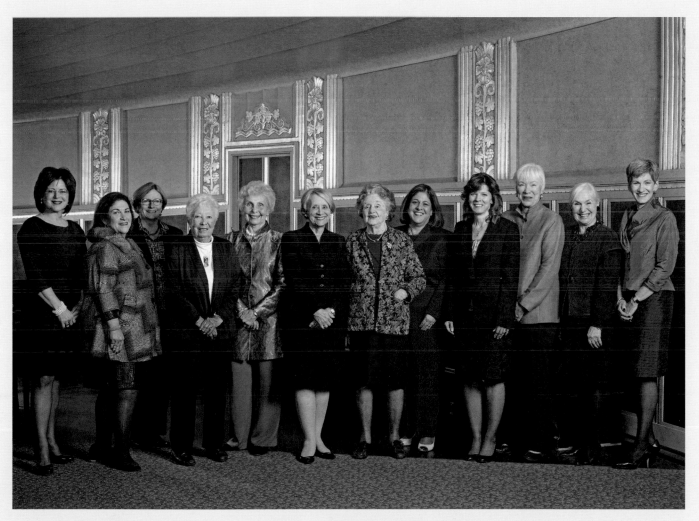

Rainbow Babies & Children's Foundation former President Margaret Marting (seventh from left) poses with five decades of Rainbow Babies & Children's Foundation presidents. Like those who preceded and followed her, Marting was moved to volunteer by compassion, her own good fortune, and a strong sense of responsibility toward others. "It broke my heart to see children who couldn't even get out of bed," she said, describing her visits to Rainbow Hospital. "My work for Rainbow took a great deal of time, but I was happy to give it because I could see that what we were doing improved things." Marting, who passed away at age 105 in 2018, continued to provide support with a bequest to the Quentin & Elisabeth Alexander Level IIIc Neonatal Intensive Care Unit at University Hospitals Rainbow Babies & Children's Hospital. From left: Dinah Kolesar, Beth Curtiss, Jane Meyer, Jane Wolf, Mary Herrick, Ann Pinkerton Ranney, Margaret Marting, Ann O'Brien, Patti DePompei, MSN, RN (President, University Hospitals Rainbow Babies & Children's Hospital and University Hospitals MacDonald Women's Hospital), Sarah Robertson, Lynne Alfred, and Julie Adler Raskind.

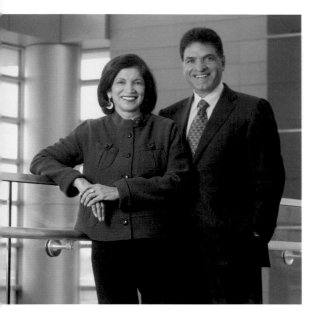

Usha and Monte Ahuja, 2011.

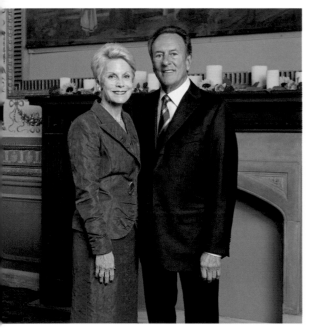

Sheldon Adelman has played a critical role in University Hospitals' modern expansion efforts through his involvement in Vision 2010 and the *Discover the Difference* campaign, as chairman of the UH Development Committee. Shelly was also the founding chair of the UH Seidman Cancer Center Leadership Council. Shelly and his wife Terry were among the first to make a significant gift to the campaign— $5 million to create the Adelman Welcome Center at University Hospitals Seidman Cancer Center. Terry, a UH volunteer during her teens, helped start the University Hospitals Neurological Institute Leadership Council, which she co-chairs today.

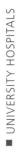

Kayleen McDowell, who sat on the Seidman Cancer Center Leadership Council at UH, said that even though they lost him to the disease, his death gave hope to others. "Through giving, my grandparents have made it possible for thousands to have a chance for a cure, and this legacy will live on for generations."[25]

As Vice Chairman and then Chairman of the UH board, Monte Ahuja has had a major impact on the direction and development of UH. His life story and his commitment to Cleveland are notable. Arriving in America with only $5 in his pocket, he built a successful automotive supply company, and his generosity and philanthropic interests in health care and education have touched the lives of thousands. Appointed to the board of Cleveland State University in 1991 by the then-Governor of Ohio, George Voinovich, Ahuja eventually served as the university's board chairman for 6 years. Additionally, the school's College of Business was named after this alumnus and benefactor. "My friend Shelly Adelman [UH board member] asked me get involved with UH," said Ahuja. "It was 2001, a time of transition for the organization. We had to modernize and concentrate on infrastructure spending. We needed to think big, think bold, and think not just about today but the future. And so we undertook projects to make the transition into the 21st century."

After joining the board, Ahuja agreed to take on the chairmanship of the strategic planning committee to develop UH's Vision 2010 initiative. Designed to redefine and improve health care in Northeast Ohio, Vision 2010 included a variety of building projects for UH, including a new free-standing hospital in Beachwood eventually named University Hospitals Ahuja Medical Center in recognition of an historic $30 million gift made by the Ahuja family in 2007.

Additionally, Ahuja served as Co-Chair of the *Discover the Difference* fundraising campaign in support of Vision 2010. A key player in the design of the medical facilities this campaign made possible, his leadership and generosity inspired others to give major donations of their own. In concert with his wife, Usha, he exemplifies civic responsibility, community stewardship, and volunteer leadership.

Ahuja's forward-thinking vision, leadership, and philanthropic contributions cement his position as one of the top visionary leaders in UH history, joining Hinman Hurlbut and Samuel Mather as far-sighted hospital chairmen who not only personally led the hospital through dramatic growth and change, but also contributed significant philanthropic support to help the hospital make those changes.

Members of the Horvitz family have been generous donors to UH for three generations. Thirteen-year-old Danielle Horvitz contributed the money she received for her bat mitzvah to furnish a playroom in

Rainbow Babies and Children's Hospital. Her grandparents, Joan and Leonard Horvitz, followed with a $7 million pledge in 1995 to build Horvitz Tower on the University Hospitals Cleveland Medical Center campus. The facility combined the latest in pediatric health care with amenities designed especially for children and their families. "If you're lucky and do well, you give back," said Leonard Horvitz. "Cleveland is where Joan and I live, and we felt we wanted to do something for our community. We hoped it would encourage other people to do the same." Danielle's parents, Marcy and Richard Horvitz, also provided $1.5 million towards medical research at UH, pediatric research at Rainbow, and in support of neurosurgeon Robert Ratcheson, MD. After Marcy died in 2003, Leonard, Richard, and Danielle gave $5 million toward the Marcy R. Horvitz Pediatric Emergency Center on the main campus to honor her memory. "She was an elementary school teacher who had a special love for children. And, we had a history with Rainbow Babies and Children's. It seemed so right," said Richard. Shortly thereafter, Leonard and Richard also funded a second pediatric emergency center bearing Marcy's name at UH Ahuja. Today, Danielle Horvitz Weiner continues the family tradition she began as a child by serving as a member of the Rainbow Babies & Children's Foundation Board of Trustees.

The personal connection between Lee and Jane Seidman and Fred Rothstein, MD, former President of UH Cleveland Medical Center, led the Seidmans to donate a $42 million gift to UH at the launch of

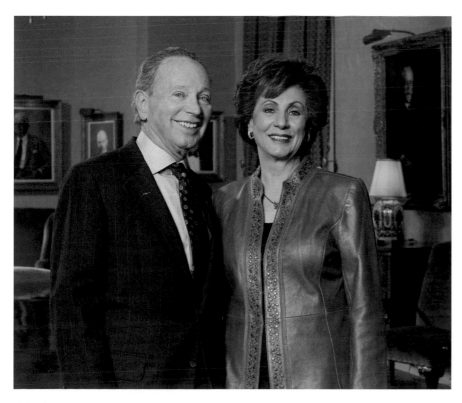

Philanthropists Lee and Jane Seidman, 2010.

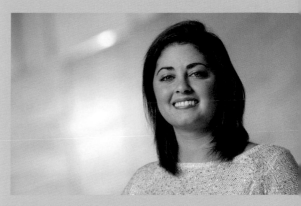

Gina Cortese, 2016.

Paying It Forward

Jane and Lee Seidman's giving inspired another family member, Gina Cortese, to also give back. While a student at Kent State University in 2012, Cortese was diagnosed with a brain tumor. Following surgery, she underwent intensive chemotherapy and radiation treatment, and in the process lost all of her hair. "When that happens, you just don't feel like yourself," she explained. "Wearing a wig was uncomfortable—they itch. I thought hats would fit my personality better, and I found some great ones." Happily there came a day when the 23-year-old no longer needed them. The decision to pass them along to others who did was the first step in organizing what would become Gina's Journey. It is a program that collects and buys new and gently used hats for male and female cancer patients of all ages that are available for free at University Hospitals. Each is dry-cleaned, put in a bag tied with a red ribbon, and given to the Pediatric and Adult Infusion centers at University Hospitals Seidman Cancer Center. Cortese receives help with the project from Jane, her mother's cousin, and Lee. "Not everyone can afford the extra expense," said Cortese. "I know this makes a difference. People pick them up when they come in for treatment, and the bins always empty quickly."

The Harrington Family: Breaking the Barriers to Discovery

During a routine stress test, Ron Harrington's UH cardiologist, Carl Orringer, MD, noticed a slight anomaly. It led to the discovery that Harrington, an apparently healthy marathon runner, had a 70 percent blockage of his arteries and required quadruple bypass surgery. In gratitude for that life-saving diagnosis and with a desire to further Dr. Orringer's work in preventive cardiology, the Harrington family was inspired to give $22.6 million in 2008 to establish University Hospitals Harrington Heart & Vascular Institute, making UH one of the nation's leading centers for cardiovascular medicine. The Harringtons' gift was one of the biggest donations to a cardiology program in the nation.

In 2012, the Harringtons made an additional transformational $50 million gift to UH, the largest single contribution in UH history. The funds were used to create the Harrington Discovery Institute at UH, a groundbreaking initiative to advance the work of gifted physician-scientists dedicated to the development of new drug therapies. Ron Harrington, who built a small local business into one of the country's largest mail-order medical supply companies, wants to create an entrepreneurial culture that attracts people with big ideas. "We are very excited about what we see as a national model that will bring new drugs to the market to help patients with heart disease, cancer, and other health conditions....We have three hopes for this awe-inspiring opportunity: We'd like to assure physician-scientists that their discoveries are carried further along to completion. Secondly, we would like to create in the Cleveland business community an investment into the health care arena. And last, but not least, we hope to save lives."

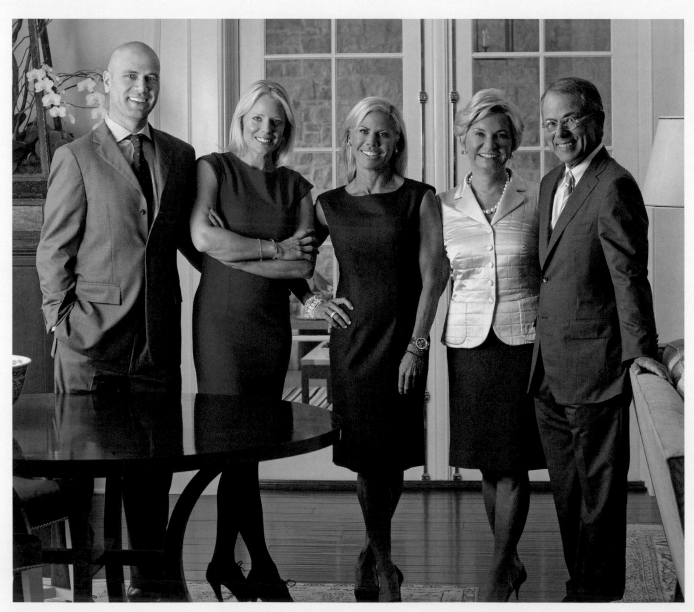

The Harrington Family (left to right): son Ron, daughter-in-law Lydia, daughter Jill, Nancy, and Ron, 2012.

the *Discover the Difference* campaign. Dr. Rothstein and his wife, Jackie, took the Seidmans out to dinner to thank them for establishing an endowed chair in 2008. "That's when he told us they were raising money to build a cancer hospital," remembers Jane. "Cancer has taken many people from us," added her husband, Lee, owner of one of the largest auto dealerships in Cleveland. "We came home, talked about it, and decided to help."

The new University Hospitals Seidman Cancer Center, which opened in 2011, was named in their honor. In addition, every cancer program across the system transitioned from the Ireland Cancer Center name to Seidman.

"It was not our first time giving, but it was our largest gift," said Jane. "We're comfortable in life. We're happy with each other and our family. We don't need a lot of fancy things…When people say, I wish I could do what you and Lee have done," says Jane, "my response is, give what you can. When you have more, give more. And remember that everybody has something to give."

Making It Personal

Gratitude is a powerful feeling, and it often prompts patients and their families to express their appreciation for medical care received by making donations to University Hospitals. Other reasons include a desire to celebrate the life of a special person, to further a medical field one is passionate about, or to meet a pressing health care need. All of these factors were motivators for Kathleen Coleman.

Her husband, Les, former Chairman and CEO of the Lubrizol Corporation, was diagnosed with stage 4 lung cancer in 2000. His oncologist, Nathan Levitan, MD, former President, University Hospitals Seidman Cancer Center, gave him the option to try an experimental clinical trial. Les, a PhD in chemistry, was eager to participate. However, after a few months of treatment, he succumbed to the disease. His participation was an investment in research, something he believed in deeply, to move cancer care forward. Kathleen, grateful that there was a way to draw something positive from the experience, decided to memorialize him with a $1.5 million endowed gift to establish the Dr. Lester E. Coleman, Jr. Chair in Cancer Research and Therapeutics in 2001. This was followed in 2007 by funds to complete the Kathleen A. and Dr. Lester E. Coleman Clinical Research Suite at UH Seidman. She also became a charter member of the Seidman Cancer Center Leadership Council, which was formed in 2005, and has been its Chair since 2008. In 2013, she invested in the *Discover the Difference* campaign with a

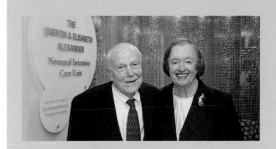

In 2006, the Elisabeth Severence Prentiss Foundation contributed $7 million for the expanded state-of-the-art NICU named The Quentin & Elisabeth Alexander Level IIIc Neonatal Intensive Care Unit in honor of Quentin and Elisabeth's (shown above) longtime board participation.

Family Ties

The late Elisabeth "Betty" Alexander's family's involvement with University Hospitals spans generations. Alexander, a Rainbow Babies & Children's Foundation Honorary Lifetime Trustee and past President, also served as Chair of the Women's Committee. Her father, John Hadden Sr., late husband, Quentin, and daughter, Pam, were all UH board members. Her mother, Marianne, served on the Women's Committee.

Alexander's great-great-grandmother, Mary Severance, and great-grandfather, Louis H. Severance, served on the Wilson Street and Lakeside Hospital boards, respectively. Alexander's great-aunt Elisabeth Severance Prentiss established the Elisabeth Severance Prentiss Foundation, which has funded UH programs in pediatric surgery, neurology, adolescent psychiatry, and joint replacement.

Benjamin Millikin, MD, Alexander's grandfather and Cleveland's first ophthalmologist, established Lakeside's Ophthalmology Department in 1893. The UH Eye Institute, created in 2008 with support from the foundation, carries on his work. Alexander's uncle, Severance Millikin, had a 40-year term on the UH board. Her brother, John A. Hadden Jr., MD, was a child psychiatrist, and his wife, Elaine, was Chair of the Women's Committee for the 1962 capital campaign.

Community Philanthrophy

Many of the community hospitals in the University Hospitals system started as charities and grew through local philanthropy. Elyria's first hospital was a gift to the community from local businessman Edgar Allen, who lost his son Homer in a terrible streetcar accident in 1907. Elyria Memorial Hospital, the forerunner of today's University Hospitals Elyria Medical Center, opened its doors in 1908 due to Allen's efforts. In 2016, another local family stepped forward to help meet Elyria's health care needs. Karen Mole and The Hampson Family Foundation gave $10.6 million to fund the Hampson Mole Community Health Project. Designed to address pressing community health needs such as obesity, heart disease, stroke, cancer, diabetes, and other serious conditions, the donation is the largest in the hospital's history, and the first transformative community hospital gift of its kind in the UH system. "Philanthropy holds great power to catalyze new healthy community approaches, and Karen Mole and The Hampson Family Foundation have set an example for the entire nation," said Thomas F. Zenty III, CEO of University Hospitals.[26]

Previously, the foundation helped establish the Hampson-Mole Breast Health Suite, which provides patients with screenings, biopsies, and other services. Foundation President Karen Hampson Mole was born at the hospital. Her late husband, Jim, and late parents, Lois and Bert, were all treated for cancer there. She views the foundation's support as a way to acknowledge what Elyria has meant to her and her family and to invest in the county where they have long lived and worked.

donation of $7.5 million for Seidman to establish the Kathy and Les Coleman Clinical Trials Center.

"These gifts to support the advancement of clinical trials honor Les' lifelong commitment to science and will have a profound impact on patients today and for generations to come," said Coleman.[27]

The fight against cancer inspired another UH supporter, Robert (Bob) Gries, to give back. A fifth-generation Clevelander whose great-great-grandfather was the first Jewish settler in Cleveland, Gries was a longtime UH board member. His grandfather Rabbi Moses Gries helped dedicate Maternity Hospital when it moved to Cedar Avenue in 1912 and, along with the other clergy at the ceremony, asked for Cleveland women to help the hospital by giving many small donations. Both his father and his father-in-law worked on the 1927 medical center campaign. Bob has lived up to the example set by his forbears. "My family has always devoted much of their resources to philanthropy, and I was brought up to believe in civic engagement. My involvement with UH began May 15, 1929, the day I was born there. My parents were treated there until they died of cancer." Bob and his sister, Ellen Cole, established the Lucile D. and Robert H. Gries Fund in Cancer Research at UH in memory of their parents in 1969. Bob was named to the UH board in 1977 and assumed a leadership role in the 1991 campaign for University Hospitals.

In 1988, Sally Gries, Bob's wife, experienced a sudden, shooting pain and mental confusion during a business meeting. She was rushed with a brain bleed to UH where her husband discussed treatment

University Hospitals' first dental clinic opened in 1911 at Babies' Dispensary and Hospital to provide treatment for poor and disadvantaged children. Over the years, the clinic ceased operations and closed its doors a number of times. In 1998, it reopened as the Irving and Jeanne Tapper Dental Center in recognition of a large donation made by former clinic Director Irving Tapper, MD, and his wife, Jeanne.

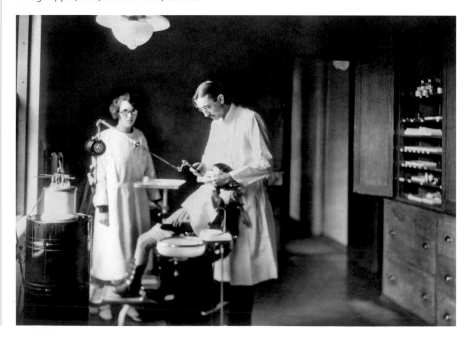

options with Robert Ratcheson, MD, then Head of Neurosurgery. "Give it to me straight, I told him," Bob recalls. "He [Dr. Ratcheson] said there are three possibilities: It will take care of itself, it won't matter what we do, or we can operate." Gries asked Dr. Ratcheson what he would choose if his own wife was the patient. "Operate," he said. Gries shared the doctor's opinion with Sally, and 27 years later her response still provokes a chuckle: "How do I know he likes his wife?"

Dr. Ratcheson performed the repair that saved Sally's life. Following a long convalescence and months of physical therapy, Sally made a full recovery. In appreciation, the couple established the Sally Gries Nursing Endowment Fund to recognize nurses who provide outstanding care for neurological patients and their families. In 2007, they made an additional contribution to the fund as well as a financial gift to University Hospitals Neurological Institute. Sally serves on the institute's Leadership Council. The couple also provided additional resources to turn a fund Bob and his sister established in their parents' names in 1968 into an endowed chair.

Personalized funds at UH not only express donors' passion and gratitude but also focus on overlooked needs. One such example is the Smiling Eyes Fund established by David and Jonny Lyons, the children of Janice Lyons, MD, Director of Breast Cancer Services at UH, and

As in the early years, philanthropy today sometimes takes the form of material as well as financial gifts. In 2016, University Hospitals Rainbow Babies & Children's Hospital patient 7-year-old Ella Tryon established the Help Me Color a Rainbow movement and collected a total of 13,132 boxes of crayons and 254 coloring books for patients at UH Rainbow. Her desire to give back stemmed from her own hospital stay for severe food allergies at UH Rainbow where crayons were in short supply due to concerns about cross-contamination from one patient to another. Her project, which has since become a non-profit foundation, has delivered more than 22,000 boxes of crayons to children's hospitals throughout the United States. This little girl with a big heart is hoping to take her project to a national level by donating 1,000 crayon boxes to every children's hospital in the country.

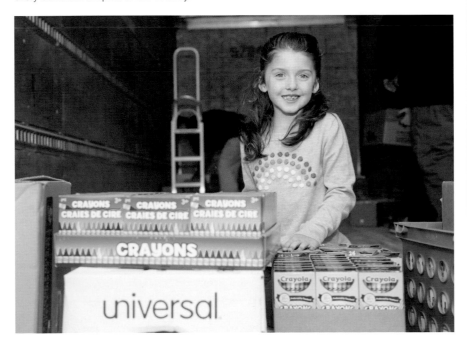

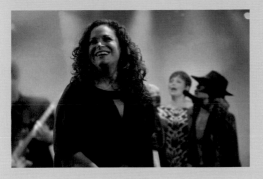

Betsy Werbel in concert, 2014.

Pass It On

Singer and actress Betsy Werbel had a desire to "take something bad and turn it into something good." She and her brother Brian grew up in Cleveland. She was interested in musical theater in high school, and he worked as a lab assistant at Case Western Reserve University School of Medicine. She moved to New York City where her theater career took her to Broadway. Brian became a scientist determined to find a cure for cancer, but died at age 29 before he was able to find one. To honor his dream, the family established a fund in his name to support summer fellows conducting oncology research at University Hospitals Seidman Cancer Center.

After Brian died, Betsy joined the national touring company of the musical *Wicked* when it made a stop in Cleveland in 2009. She and members of the cast performed a benefit show at the Hanna Theatre with proceeds earmarked for the Brian Werbel Memorial Fund. Betsy, however, was inspired to do more. She gathered a group of singers and musicians to perform in New York on the five-year anniversary of her brother's death. "It was a very special evening," said Betsy. "We got a standing ovation. But what was most gratifying to me was knowing we'd raised a lot of money for something Brian cared about passionately." In 2014, Betsy organized another successful concert in New York.

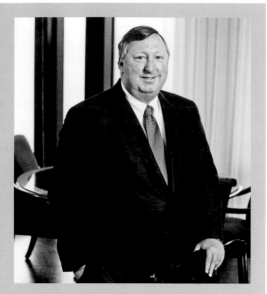

University Hospitals board member and former board chair Henry Meyer III.

Pass It On

Henry Meyer III, retired CEO of KeyCorp, joined the University Hospitals board in 1991 and became Chairman in 1999. However, his involvement with the hospital goes back much further. "My mother was on the Rainbow board for 40 years. My grandmother and my wife have chaired that board. And I was born at UH. It was the first air I breathed," says Meyer, whose maternal grandparents served as solicitors and donors for the 1927 campaign. Describing himself as a proud seventh-generation Clevelander, Meyer believes that, like him, others who serve on the board and its many committees are motivated by a love for the organization, its mission, and the important role it plays in the community. "We get involved, dig in, and are very active." Meyer's term spanned a period of great turmoil as the organization transitioned into a multi-hospital system. "We understood that decisions we were making would set the stage for what was to come."

her husband, Michael, a local chef, to provide financial support for families affected by cancer.

When a parent is diagnosed with cancer, it affects the entire family. Loss of income and treatment costs can lead to financial pressures. Suddenly, there is not enough money for necessities such as clothing or food, school fees, or presents at holiday time. Children in the family are not always able to fully understand the situation. "This fund is to help minimize the sacrifices children have to make," said Michael. "Social workers who specialize in cancer at UH screen their patients to determine those that might benefit from Smiling Eyes and submit requests. David and Jonny evaluate each application."

David started the small fund with his bar mitzvah money in 2013, and Jonny continued this legacy in 2016 when it came time for his bar mitzvah. "Our boys are learning to appreciate their own lives while creating a legacy based on taking care of others," Michael explains.

Time and Talent: Volunteers

The unpaid work of countless men and women who have given their time, energy, and expertise to University Hospitals has helped make the organization the much-admired, patient-centered place it is today. Most do their work quietly, behind the scenes, with little fanfare or public awareness. A few were well-known in their time and beyond. Some leave a lasting mark, even if their names are forgotten.

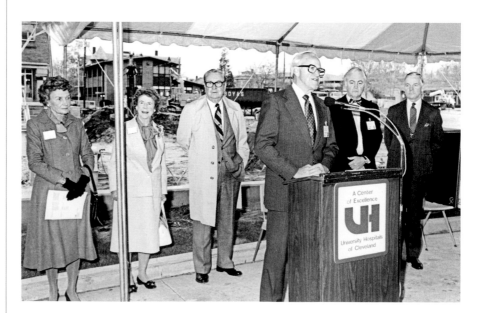

University Hospitals' Ambulatory Referral Center was renamed the Harry J. Bolwell Health Center in 1986 in recognition of Harry Bolwell's (shown at podium) achievements as UH board Chairman during the late 1970s. Bolwell established a decentralized management structure at UH, which at the time was a radical departure from how the hospital had always been organized. Designed to control costs, address changing reimbursement rates, and maintain financial stability, "his ideas were unique at the time and very controversial," says James Block, MD, UH CEO from 1986 to 1992.

The very first volunteers at Wilson Street Hospital were the board members. These committed volunteers brought their skills as successful business-people, attorneys, civic and cultural activists, leaders, and managers to the job of advising hospital administrators on financial, strategic, and operational issues as well as planning for the future. Over the years, the board members assisted in steering the organization through fiscal emergencies and changing ideas about how health care should be managed and delivered.

While social norms of the past dictated that men typically fill the ranks of an organization's board, all the founding hospitals of UH have long had a strong female board presence, culminating with Sandra Pianalto, former CEO and President of the Federal Reserve Bank of Cleveland, being named the first woman to chair the UH Board of Directors in 2015. When Wilson Street was established, women were among its first board members and were also part of a secondary board that concerned itself with daily operations and help with patient care. As time went on, their roles became more formalized, and they became known as the Board of Lady Managers. While the main hospital board focused on the finances, the Lady Managers conducted weekly hospital inspections, kept track of supplies and linens, scheduled entertainment, managed the library, and oversaw renovations and improvements to the hospital's facilities. They were in charge of fundraising events, using the proceeds to purchase clothing and other necessities for patients in financial straits, as well as to ensure each ward had a tree and each patient a present at Christmas. They collected furniture, rugs, art, and other fixtures to make the hospital rooms, as well as the nurse's dormitory, pleasant and "homelike."

As part of a corporate reorganization in 1920, the board was renamed the Ladies Advisory Committee, which later became known as the Women's Committee in 1969. A formal volunteer program began at Lakeside Hospital in 1920 with only three women, all members of the Junior League, serving as clerks in the Admitting Department. Within a few years, more than 30 volunteers worked at Lakeside. Many of them volunteered as secretaries in outpatient clinics while

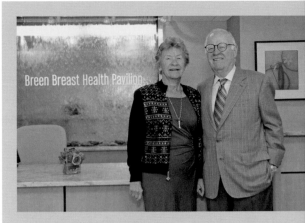

Jack Breen (right) and his wife, Mary Jane, 2011.

Giving Back

Jack Breen is a former CEO of Sherwin-Williams and a longtime UH board member and Co-Chair of the *Discover the Difference* campaign. The 80-year-old is the beneficiary of advances in health care and the expertise of those who deliver it. He has been treated at UH for prostate cancer and blood clots, received a stent for a clogged coronary artery, had knee replacement surgery, and received a kidney transplant. His wife, Mary Jane, calls him her "Miracle Man." He says, "I wore out the carpet at UH for a while, but I am living proof of what medicine can do."

Jack and Mary Jane, who was treated at UH for breast cancer, donated $5 million in 2009 to establish the Breen Breast Health Pavilion at University Hospitals Cleveland Medical Center. Early detection was critical to Mary Jane's successful outcome and remains a focus of the multidisciplinary approach that characterizes the program.

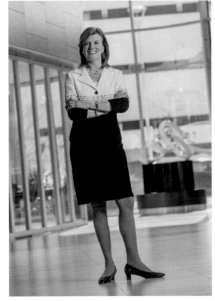

Chair of the University Hospitals Board of Directors Sandra Pianalto, 2016.

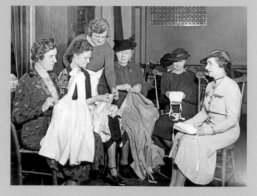

Sewing circles, comprising women volunteers, supported many of the founding hospitals' basic needs, ca. late 1920s.

It's a Fact

In the past, a number of women in Cleveland sewed many of the items used in the hospitals by staff and patients. In 1907, they mobilized an effort to outfit the new headquarters for Babies' Dispensary and Hospital. "[I]t was the debutantes…who put on their thimbles and made ready sash curtains, bedding and nurses' supplies, and since then many yards of muslin have been made into tiny garments for the frail babies cared for at the hospital."[28]

For more than eight years, female members of the Babies Aid Society met weekly to make supplies for the dispensary. At Maternity Hospital, a group of volunteers made surgical dressings in a sewing room in the basement. Outside groups gathered in private homes and churches to stitch surgical dressings as well as face masks, lab towels, blankets, diapers, and infant clothing. By the late 1930s, more than 2,000 women were engaged in this effort. Today, volunteers continue to use their needle skills to craft therapeutic heart-shaped pillows for those who have had cardiac surgery and donate their handmade quilts, blankets, hats, and booties for infants at University Hospitals Rainbow Babies & Children's Hospital.

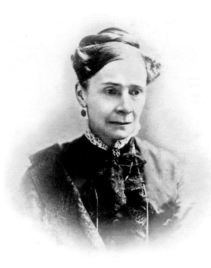
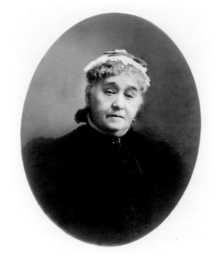

Mrs. Jane Hurlbut (left), wife of Hinman Hurlbut, and Mrs. Mary Williamson were two of many women who served on the Board of Lady Managers. Hurlbut and Williamson also served on the hospital boards of Wilson Street and Lakeside hospitals, ca. 1870s.

others ran errands, fed patients, arranged flowers, and assisted in the hospital library and dietetics department. When the new Lakeside was completed in University Circle in 1931, the Ladies Advisory Committee once again decorated and furnished the rooms.

Women were also instrumental in governing Maternity Hospital from the start and remained influential voices throughout its development. In 1899, *The Plain Dealer* reported that as a result of Maternity's move to a bigger facility, "the faithful women of the board, most of whom are mothers, and several grandmothers, are often sorely perplexed as to how to meet expenses."[29] Organizing modest but frequent fundraising events, they managed to keep the doors of Cleveland's only non-sectarian maternity hospital open and ensured that the facility was upgraded and expanded as the demand for services increased. When the hospital moved to University Circle, they continued to help by collecting revenue from a consignment shop that opened in the lobby in 1935. It offered "an attractive array of garments for infants as well as bottles of perfume, silk ruffled pillows, jams, jellies—in fact all kinds of attractive things."[30]

Women also held board positions at the Infants' Clinic and its subsequent iterations as the Babies' Dispensary and the Babies' Dispensary and Hospital. Often working alongside their husbands, they were known in their own right for their community activism and dedication to children's welfare. In addition, there was also a women's board at the Dispensary that concentrated primarily on organizing events to raise money. When the hospital's bylaws were amended in 1915 to establish a single board, the majority of its members were women. In addition, an all-female management committee oversaw daily operations at the Dispensary.

Volunteering at University Hospitals

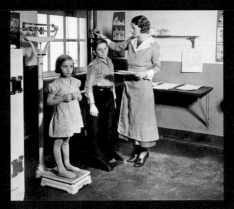
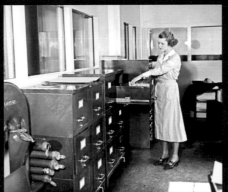
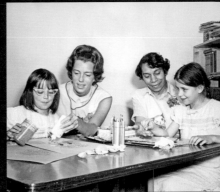

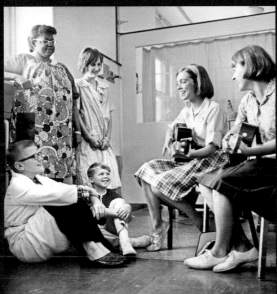
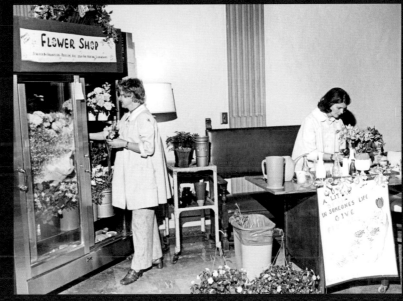

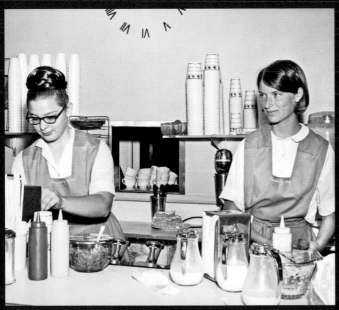
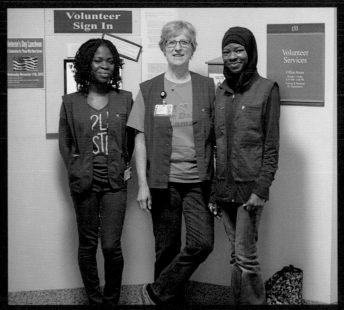

Over the years, volunteers at University Hospitals have been engaged in supporting nearly every facet of the day-to-day operations of the hospital. From left to right: (1) administering clinical care at the Pediatric Clinic at Lakeside Hospital, 1926; (2) performing clerical work, ca. 1940s; (3) participating in arts and crafts projects with pediatric patients at Rainbow Hospital, ca. 1960s; (4) entertaining patients, 1964; (5) working in the Flower Shop in the Lakeside Lobby, 1975; (6) working in the UH Coffee Shop, ca. 1960s; (7) volunteers, 2016.

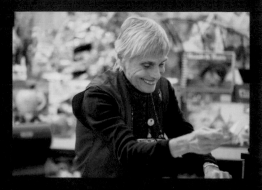

Volunteer Carolyn Oakes in the gift shop at University Hospitals, 2016.

The Spirit of Volunteerism

Carolyn Oakes has volunteered at University Hospitals since 1960. She has sold flowers in Lakeside Hospital's lobby, headed MacDonald House's women's board and was President of its auxillary, and gave tours to expectant parents. Today, "I do whatever needs to be done: sanitize rooms, restock supplies, talk to people, entertain children," said Oakes, who adds that she is only one of many. "There are a lot of people, young and old, from all walks of life who have given hours to this place, year after year. They are the unsung heroes."

Dee Kleinman has given 20,000 volunteer hours to UH. She began as a receptionist in the Rainbow Babies and Childrens Hospital in 1977, worked at the front desk at Lakeside, and has assisted patients in the Admitting Department since 1982. She also served on the Auxiliary's board. "We raised money for extras like supplying boxed lunches to chemo infusion patients at Seidman and dinners to families of patients in intensive care," she said. She was also a Rainbow Ambassador for parents when their child was admitted to the hospital. "I have a wonderful, comfortable life and have been very fortunate," said Kleinman. "I believe in giving back, and the time I spend at UH is personally fulfilling."

In 1934, UH hired an employee to oversee a formal volunteer program, and in 1936, the volunteers clocked 19,000 hours. By 1937, there were 125 volunteers, all women, working in the hospital. Volunteers staffed the front desk at Lakeside, escorted visitors, and accompanied families to the nursery to see new babies. Additionally, volunteers updated families in the waiting areas about loved ones in surgery, performed clerical work, answered telephones, did craft projects with children in the pediatric wards, and worked in the hospital library. The Volunteer Department also coordinated the volunteers at Rainbow Hospital in South Euclid and at MacDonald House, where they helped at the Pre-Natal Clinic registering patients.

Staffing levels at the hospital plunged during World War II, prompting an unprecedented need for manpower. To fill the gap, volunteers assumed much of the non-patient care duties performed by nurses. As the war progressed, staff numbers continued to drop as more men enlisted in the military or were drafted. Others found better-paying jobs in war industries. In 1942, a group of teachers and school administrators came in once a week to serve dinner trays to inpatients and help with other dietary service tasks. By 1944, the group had expanded to 44 members, giving more than 2,000 hours of service, close to 24-hours a day.

Even children got involved. A group of 40 high school girls, some from the Girl Scouts and Campfire Girls, were recruited and

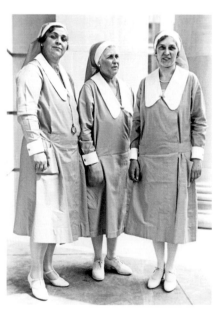

trained. By the end of 1944, they had contributed more than 1,700 volunteer hours. They were joined by Boy Scouts from five different troops who formed a "mop and broom corps" to help clean the hospital.[31] At the end of the war in late 1945, UH executives adorned the walls around their offices with murals recognizing the 1,862 volunteers who provided approximately 281,500 hours of work that freed up clinical staff to focus on providing care to patients.[32]

In 1951, members of the Women's Committee established a group to support the hospital through volunteerism as well as

Hospital volunteers in the '30s and '40s wore distinct blue outfits, which looked similar to nuns' habits. The color of their outfits allowed them to be recognized quickly without being confused with the nursing staff, earning these volunteers the title of "bluebirds."

fundraising. More than 200 women attended the first meeting, and by 1953, the size of the group had doubled. Known as the Friends of University Hospitals, the members organized and staffed a gift shop and snack bar in Lakeside and sold professional photos of newborns to their parents at MacDonald House. Later, a flower shop was added to the Friends' operations. Members could also be found performing office work and helping at patient bedsides. In 1984, the Women's Committee and the Friends joined forces, forming a new organization called the Auxiliary of University Hospitals, which still exists today.[33] The Auxiliary's efforts to raise money, as volunteers have done since the hospital's founding in 1866, continue to build bridges between the hospital and the people of Northeast Ohio. Today, there are 1,700 men and women performing many of the same services their counterparts did a century ago. More recent roles for volunteers include serving as health coaches, staffing resource centers, and participating on advisory councils and review boards. The value of these dedicated, caring individuals, past and present, goes far beyond their hours of service.

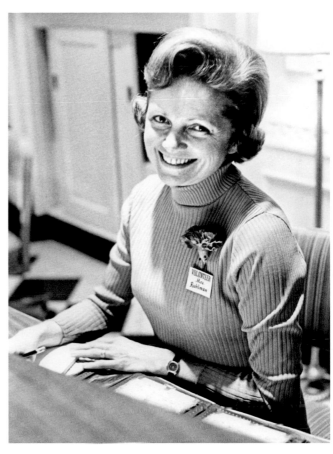

Barbara Peterson Ruhlman volunteering at University Hospitals, ca. 1970s.

"I come from a family that believes in giving back. I was born in 1932 and started volunteering at UH while a student at Laurel School," recalls Barbara Peterson Ruhlman. "Over the years, I answered phones at the front desk, served on a number of committees, and was Co-Chair of MacDonald Women's Health Leadership Council. People would be surprised how fulfilling volunteering can be."

In addition to the countless hours she has given to the hospital, Ruhlman is also a significant financial benefactor of UH, with gifts that have supported the renovation of the 11th floor of the Alfred and Norma Lerner Tower to create the Barbara Peterson Ruhlman Conference Center, an endowed chair in orthopedics, and a $6 million gift to University Hospitals MacDonald Women's Hospital in 2013 to fund capital improvements to the hospital and to create an endowment for recruiting and retaining OB/GYN physicians. In 2015, the birthing center was renamed the Barbara Peterson Ruhlman Women & Newborns Center at UH MacDonald Women's Hospital.

"I believe in UH and all the good they've done for me, for my family, and for everyone else. They really are here to care for all and serve the community. It's been a major part of my life, and the only place I'd go for my own health care. I donate because of the work they do at UH, and the way they do it, touches my heart."▼

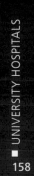

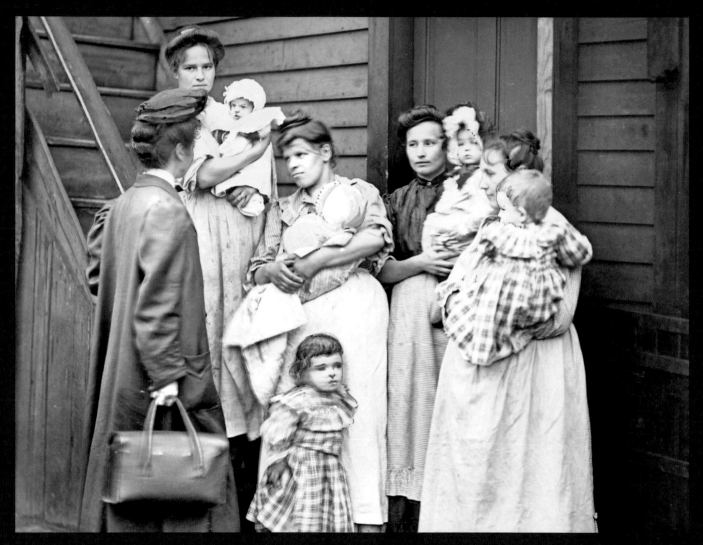

There is a history at University Hospitals of reaching into
Cleveland's neighborhoods and a precedent for extending a
welcome to those in need. In its early years, visiting nurses
from Babies' Dispensary and Hospital made house calls to the
many immigrant families living in the city, 1907.

Reach

"Our commitment to the community is in our DNA. University Hospitals has always been at the forefront of addressing pressing health care issues and has never wavered in investing its resources to serve the most vulnerable and needy."

– Heidi Gartland, Vice President, Government and Community Relations, University Hospitals

"Dr. Lowell Orbison called my high school in 1952 looking for an inner-city kid to come work in his pathology lab," remembers Edgar Jackson Jr., MD, Chief of Staff Emeritus, University Hospitals Cleveland Medical Center and former Senior Advisor to the President and CEO of University Hospitals. "He hired me, gave me books to read, and exposed me to medical students. I had wanted to be a doctor since childhood but had decided not to go to college. I thought it would be too hard. It took about a year and a half for him to convince me that I could do it."

Dr. Jackson, who is African-American, joined the staff at UH in 1973. He credits Dr. Orbison, who was white, with setting him on the path to becoming a doctor. "I have always considered him my angel. He rescued me, and it made me want to rescue kids like me."

What Dr. Orbison did was a personal effort. But it was emblematic of a philosophy that defined the four founding UH institutions and the hospital system they would become. Each was grounded in a commitment to serve the community by understanding its needs, engaging with people,

and working to improve lives. The organization's mission has been shaped by a steadily expanding understanding of who is in need, how far the sphere of influence extends, and what more can and needs to be done. "University Hospitals is a friend of all segments of Cleveland's community with respect for people regardless of race, ethnicity, or socio-economic status," says Dr. Jackson. "To do that and maintain the highest possible quality, I think, is quite an achievement."

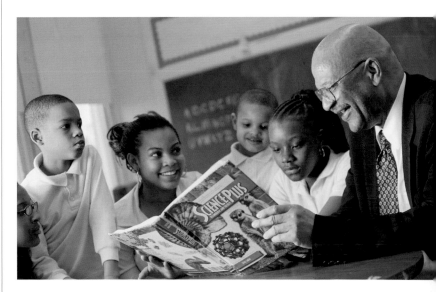

Edgar Jackson Jr., MD, reads to children in the community, 2009.

Connecting With the Community: Then

Dispensaries—the name comes from the practice of dispensing medicines—were an important part of health care in 19th and early 20th century American cities. Their historic role was to provide access to physicians and medical treatment for those who did not require hospitalization and could not afford to see a private doctor. "Is it not the call of democracy to place the new resources for health, the new powers to heal and to prevent disease, within the reach of all persons, all classes of society?...The medical and social problems which may be found in five hundred units of the human stream that rolls through the dispensary doors are as varied as life itself."[1] Physicians typically donated their time, the facilities were supported by charitable contributions, and services were provided at minimal or no charge.

Three of the four medical institutions that came together as University Hospitals operated "dispensaries." They advanced public health agendas and provided hands-on clinical training opportunities for students and specialists. Lakeside Hospital's dispensary functioned as an outpatient department and was operated jointly with the Western Reserve University School of Medicine. It had a pharmacy, a laboratory, and a waiting room that could seat 300. Admissions to Rainbow Hospital went through Lakeside and the dispensary.

The resident obstetrician of Lakeside, who was also a member of the medical school's faculty, was in charge of the hospital's Maternity Dispensary, which began operating jointly with the home delivery

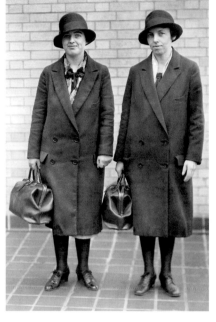

Two Maternity Hospital home nurses, ca. 1920s.

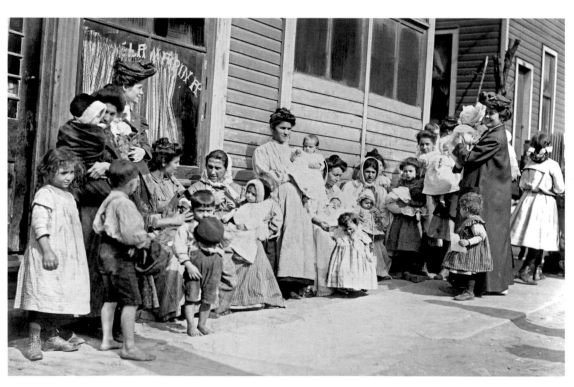

Families waiting at the Babies' Dispensary and Hospital clinic at Alta House, Little Italy, 1909. The dispensary maintained branch locations throughout Cleveland.

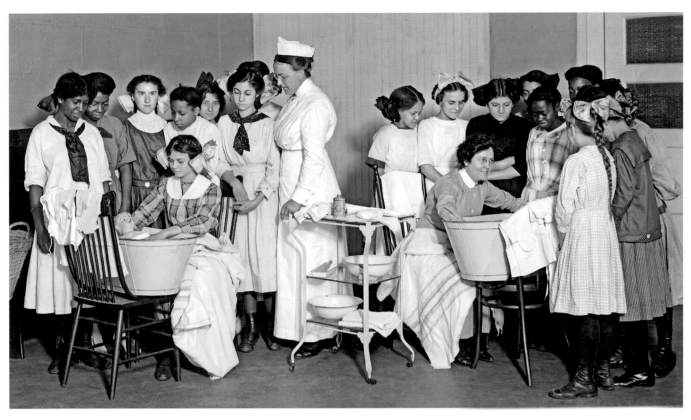

services offered by Arthur Bill, MD, and Maternity Hospital in 1909. A dispatch center was established in a rented house on East 35th Street. Maternity also had its own outpatient department that provided nursing care for mothers and newborns at home and operated prenatal clinics around the city. Physicians donated their services for charity cases. "When one considers the relief which Lakeside in one year carried to the poor in this city by 15,286 visits to their homes and [which was] obtained by these people from 45,920 visits to our Dispensary and from the many thousands of interviews with the members of our department for instruction, advice or encouragement, one cannot measure Lakeside Hospital's benevolence by the number of beds in its wards. It is something more."[2]

Babies' Dispensary and Hospital, organized in 1906 specifically to meet the needs of children three years and younger, was inspired by the most progressive medical concepts. It adopted a multifaceted approach that included preventive medicine, nutrition, and education. It was unique for the time, attracting admirers and imitators in other cities. New York pediatrician Alfred Hess, MD, speaking at Babies and Childrens Hospital's dedication in 1926, said it represented the first attempt in this country to mold an organization not only for care of sick children but also for the supervision of well babies.

Breastfeeding was encouraged, but when it was not possible or as children got older, the dispensary provided families with sterilized milk

Nurses from Babies' Dispensary and Hospital used dolls to teach public high school girls how to care for infants in 1912.

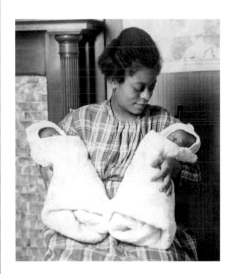

A mother, early 20th century, who received a visit from a Maternity Hospital home nurse. The babies are wearing premature jackets.

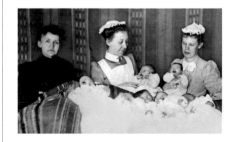

Home delivery nurses, ca. early 1900s.

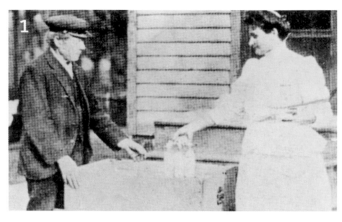

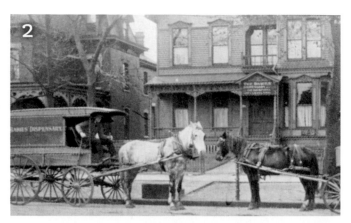

"From a hand-drawn wagon with only a few bottles of milk in 1906 to a three-quarter ton motor truck delivering 125 gallons of milk daily over a 58-mile route, is the evolution of the milk service supplied by the Babies' Dispensary and Hospital through its 63 distributing stations to babies in all parts of Cleveland and vicinity."[3]

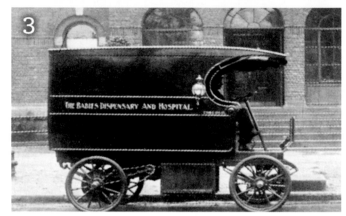

It's a Fact

Under the auspices of the Inner City Protestant Parish, an interdenominational group, 500 low-income children from Cleveland came to Babies and Childrens Hospital for physical exams—a first for many of them—in August 1965. More than 200 volunteer physicians, dentists, nurses, therapists, technicians, and clerical workers were involved. The following year, 800 children received the free exams. Those requiring further treatment were identified and referred to a doctor for additional care.

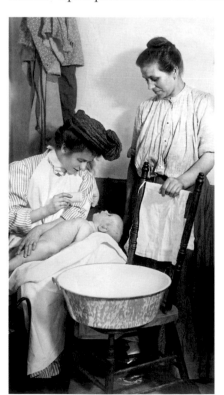

A nurse at Babies' Dispensary and Hospital instructs a mother on how to bathe her infant, 1907.

or fortified formula based on doctors' orders. The milk came from a local farm supervised by a physician and was portioned in pint and quart bottles. Upon presentation of a ticket, a family could claim the milk for free or at a nominal charge at a dispensary or at one of the many milk stations established by 1912.

In 1909, four branch clinics were established on the east and west sides of the city offering healthy baby check-ups and vaccinations. Mothers were introduced to the most up-to-date, scientific, and hygienic methods of caring for their young children. Nurses, many of whom were employees of the Visiting Nurse Association, doubled as social workers. They made home visits, showing mothers how to follow doctors' instructions, assessed living conditions, and connected families with other charitable organizations for non-medical aid.

Connecting With the Community: Now

As Lakeside, Maternity, and Babies and Childrens hospitals consolidated their missions and facilities in University Circle in the 1920s and 1930s, community outreach efforts became more concentrated there as well. This focus continued with Rainbow Hospital's move to the campus in 1971. In recent decades, there has been a renewed interest in developing programs and projects that make University Hospitals and its resources available to people both on and off the medical center campus.

Today's Medical House Calls Program, directed by William Schwab, MD, PhD, AGSF, along with Barbara Mosley, CNP, and Denise Brown, CNP, brings the home visit component back to health care for seniors who are frail, bed-bound, or disabled, or who have limited mobility or transportation challenges. Part of the UH Department of Medicine, the program aims to keep people with chronic illnesses or serious medical conditions living in their own homes and to avoid admissions to hospitals and nursing facilities. Even with the advances in technology and testing in health care today, providers equipped with a little black bag, along with training, experience, and sensitivity, can tailor care to meet the patient's goals. Following in the footsteps of providers of the past, members of the Medical House Calls team use the visits to evaluate living conditions and, when necessary, work to improve them with other services, including home health and social work.

UH supports and sponsors a wide variety of initiatives that improve quality of life, from birth through old age, and make communities healthier. Among them is Age Well, Be Well, offered through the Center for Lifelong Health, which focuses on the needs of older adults. It is free to join; provides programming throughout the UH system; and offers yoga classes, walking clubs, support groups, and social activities. Healthy eating is supported through farmer's markets and individual farm stands set up at various hospital locations. They provide a convenient source of locally grown produce for employees and area residents. UH employees can also take advantage of community-supported agriculture programs that deliver seasonal produce from area farmers to the workplace at several UH locations during the summer months. "Programs like these, as well as purchasing locally grown foods for our cafes and patient menus, are a testament to our commitment to support optimal health in the communities we serve," says Aparna Bole, MD, FAAP, Division Chief, General Academic Pediatrics and Adolescent

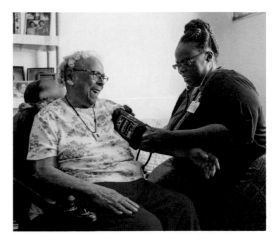

University Hospitals' Medical House Calls Program, 2016.

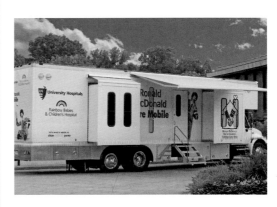

The Ronald McDonald Care Mobile® provides dental care for low-income children. The mobile dental clinic, Ohio's first, is run by the Irving and Jeanne Tapper Dental Center at University Hospitals Rainbow Babies & Children's Hospital, the area's largest primary and specialty pediatric dental practice, 2009.

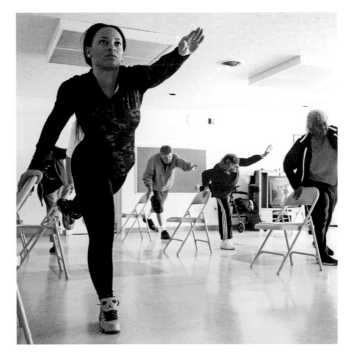

An Age Well, Be Well chair yoga class, 2016.

With support from the Rainbow Babies & Children's Foundation, Heidi Gartland, then University Hospitals Director of Child Advocacy, and UH pediatrician Lolita McDavid, MD, founded Voices for Ohio's Children in 1995. The advocacy group addresses issues and public policies that affect the physical, psychological, and social well-being of the state's youngest citizens and their families. Dr. McDavid, now Medical Director, Child Advocacy & Protection, University Hospitals Cleveland Medical Center and Gartland, who serves as UH Vice President for Government and Community Relations, also started a program called Children Who Witness Violence in collaboration with a team of physicians and researchers at University Hospitals Rainbow Babies & Children's Hospital. It offers help in the form of crisis intervention and short-term services to minimize the effects of children's exposure to witnessing violence such as murder, domestic abuse, and other forms of brutality.

Medicine, and Medical Director, Community Integration, at University Hospitals Rainbow Babies & Children's Hospital.

The UH Health Coach program is a smoking cessation initiative that integrates volunteers into primary care practices. The approach prompts patients to explore and resolve ambivalent feelings getting in the way of tobacco cessation and come up with a plan to quit that will work for them. "We know that lifestyle decisions play a huge role in well-being," says UH family medicine physician and project lead Nicholas Cohen, MD. "The idea with the Health Coach program is that instead of some authority figure telling people what they should do, which doesn't work, patients convince themselves to make different choices based on their own values and aspirations." According to Dr. Cohen, research in human psychology shows that patients are more likely to succeed under these conditions.

Parkinson's Boot Camp™, sponsored by the University Hospitals Neurological Institute Parkinson's & Movement Disorders Center, in partnership with Courageous Steps for Parkinson's and the Ohio Parkinson Foundation, Northeast Region, started in 2010 and is now an annual event. The concept, which originated in Cleveland, draws hundreds of people from around the state and the region to the free, day-long gathering. Patients participate in interactive presentations on exercise and physical activity, nutrition, and mind-body techniques for wellness as well as disease management skills. Kim Ganley, whose father died from the disease in 2016, is a member of the Neurological Institute Leadership Council and was instrumental in launching this educational outreach and support program. "It's exhilarating to watch

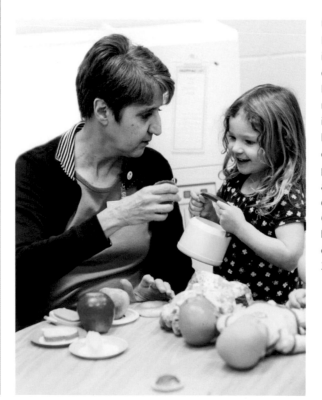

University Hospitals Parma Health Education Center is an integral part of the community focus at UH Parma Medical Center. For more than three decades, it has been a central location for EMS education, community health education programs and screenings, and a child care center for employees and the public. Gloria Gardner (left) has been a teacher at the child care center since it opened 36 years ago.

the boot camp grow and to give patients in the Parkinson's community a voice," she says. "We hope to continue to touch the lives of many."

Like the neighborhood dispensaries and milk stations that played such an important role in its past, UH continues to bring health care to where people live by growing a network of 18 hospitals, more than 50 health centers and outpatient facilities, and hundreds of physician offices throughout 15 counties in northern Ohio. In 2013, UH opened a joint venture rehabilitation hospital in Beachwood in partnership with Kindred Healthcare. The two partners then opened another rehabilitation hospital in Avon, west of Cleveland in Lorain County. UH expanded its ambulatory network into western Cuyahoga county and Lorain county in 2014, south into Akron in 2015, and even further south into Ashland county into 2016. Other expansion efforts included new health centers in North Olmsted and Broadview Heights, the latter of which offers a freestanding emergency department. Additionally, another new facility opened in North Ridgeville in 2018. "The new construction and geographic expansion exemplifies our commitment to improving access to the highest-quality care in an efficient, patient-centered environment," states Richard Hanson, President, Community Hospitals and Ambulatory Services.

Extending a Welcome

At a time when most individuals received medical care in their homes, Lakeside Hospital's board saw it as their duty "to furnish to our citizens, whose quarters are not arranged for a time of sickness, the accommodations and care which they may require" and "to provide hospitality for sick and injured strangers."[4] The annual report for 1881 noted the need to treat working men, attracted to the city by manufacturing jobs, who "are too sick to send back to the towns whence they came nor have they friends to whom to send them."

Each of the founding hospitals was grounded in a commitment to serve the poor. The city's population demographics have changed since then, but the welcome to all, regardless of ability to pay, has endured. Today, University Hospitals serves an ethnically, economically, and racially diverse community, and is actively engaged in addressing health care disparities to ensure that everyone has equal access to the best the system has to offer.

Diversity among the ranks of the medical staff, fellows, and residents, however, has been a challenge at UH that has mirrored trends in American history. In the past, the medical establishment, like the rest of American society, restricted entry into its ranks on the basis of race. UH was no exception. African-American physicians faced obstacles

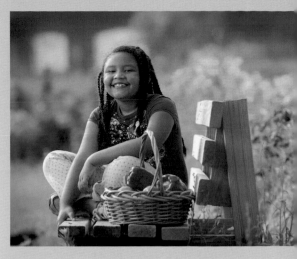

Destiny Hall, a Healthy Harvest recipient, 2014.

It's a Fact

In 2018, only 135 organizations earned a place on the Ethisphere Institute's list of the World's Most Ethical Companies®. Seven of these were health care systems, and University Hospitals was one of them. The designation recognizes extraordinary industry leaders that raise and advance the standards of ethical business practices, exemplify a culture of integrity and caring, and are committed to pairing corporate success with improving people's lives. There are many reasons that UH received this honor, the sixth time since 2012, including its workforce development program; and its outreach programs such as Healthy Harvest, which provides fresh produce and nutrition education for close to 1,000 patients yearly. The program is a joint initiative between University Hospitals Rainbow Babies & Children's and University Hospitals MacDonald Women's hospitals. Rainbow pediatric practice and UH MacDonald Women's Health Clinic patients and families receive recipes, samples to taste, and information on food assistance programs and shopping for healthy food.

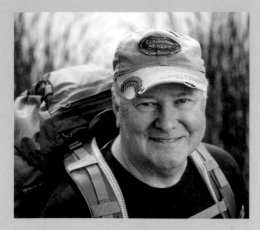

Parkinson's patient Brian Butler, RN, BSN, 2015.

Pass It On

It started with a limp. Then came tremors in his right hand. In 2012, Brian Butler, BSN, RN, was diagnosed with mild but progressive Parkinson's disease. The U.S. Army veteran is standing strong. "I do not really know what the future will hold, but one thing is for certain: I will not allow this disease to take over my active life. I have too many things I want to accomplish."

Once he learned that exercise could delay or even reverse some of the neurological damage, Butler decided to go forward with his plan to hike the Appalachian Trail, but turned this personal bucket list journey into something more. Although the University Hospitals nurse, who retired in 2015, only completed a small portion of the 2,183.3-mile route, he used the walk to increase awareness of Parkinson's and solicit pledges to support the research efforts of Benjamin Walter, MD, his neurologist at UH.

"First I survived," he wrote on his blog. "[W]e have raised over $10,000....I have started writing a book/journal of my adventure." Butler will donate any profits from the publication to Parkinson's research at UH.

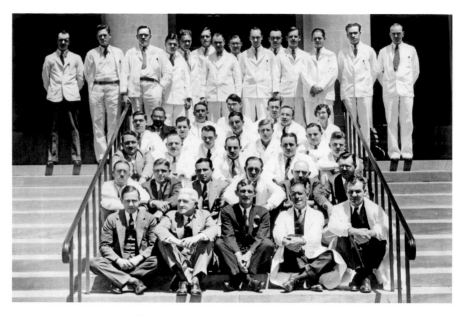

The first surgical house staff photo on the steps of the new Lakeside Building in 1931. Charles Garvin, MD, is seated (left, 5th row).

that reflected widespread and deeply rooted prejudice in the early years. But Lakeside was among the first hospitals in the city to integrate its medical staff, beginning with the appointment of urologist and surgeon Charles Garvin, MD, around 1919, followed by Leon Evans, MD, who started as Assistant Physician in Medicine in 1922, and Armen Evans, MD, a pediatrician in the outpatient department in 1925.

Society has been slow to change and minorities continued to be under-represented in the profession and the hospital. In 1990 inclusiveness became a priority. Former UH President and CEO James Block, MD, asked Edgar Jackson Jr., MD, to be Associate Chief of Staff and help him implement a diversity initiative in staff training and recruitment. "It was a choice to make this a value in our system and strive to achieve it," says Dr. Jackson.

One outcome is the David Satcher Clerkship, established in 1991 to increase diversity among the residents and fellows. It brings 10 to 15 minority medical students from around the country in their senior year to UH annually for an introduction to career opportunities in an academic medical center and in underserved urban communities.

The Edgar B. Jackson Jr., MD, Endowed Chair in Clinical Excellence and Diversity was dedicated in 2004 to recruit minority physician leaders to UH and give them an opportunity to mentor minority medical students and postgraduate trainees. It was the first permanent, endowed faculty position in an academic medical center in the United States intended to promote staff and professional diversity.

The first physician to hold the chair was Richard Grant, MD, who came to Cleveland from Howard University. He was the first African-American orthopedic surgeon to join the full-time staff of UH, and Dr. Jackson says he quickly became a role model. The current chair holder is gynecologist and obstetrician Margaret Larkins-Pettigrew, MD.

Over four years, $1.5 million was raised to fund the chair. In addition to some very large donations, many small gifts came from Cleveland's African-American community. "Most chairs are created by wealthy individuals, and we had some who made significant contributions for this one. But, many people gave $10, $15, $25," recalls Dr. Jackson. "It was incredible."

Although much remains to be done, UH has doubled its percentage of African-American physicians and increased the percentage of minority residents from 1.8 percent in 1991 to 6 to 9 percent in recent years. This rise is in part due to one noteworthy diversity initiative, the Henry L. Meyer III Faculty Minority Fellows Program, named in honor of former UH Board Chair and retired KeyCorp CEO Henry L. Meyer. These grants support young individuals who will be on the frontlines addressing health disparities and health care issues confronting the urban poor.

A Global Perspective

On December 7, 1941, the Japanese attacked Pearl Harbor and the United States entered World War II. In August 1945, Japan surrendered. In the years between those two events, the Lakeside Unit of University Hospitals cared for 45,574 people, more than any other army hospital in the Southwest Pacific.

Officially designated the Fourth General Hospital and also referred to as Base Hospital No. 4, the Lakeside Unit was reactivated on Christmas Eve 1941 in response to a request from the Surgeon General. It was the first U.S. medical unit to arrive in the Pacific Theater, just as it had been the first in France during World War I. Doctors, surgeons, and nurses, most from UH, left Cleveland in January 1942 for stateside training and arrived in Australia in March 1942. The upper floors of the Royal Melbourne Hospital were still under construction and the elevators were not functional when the Americans took over, but soon the unit's medical staff was caring for 2,000 patients in a facility designed for fewer than 700. After 23 months, 35,000 patients had been admitted.

A close and enduring association formed between the American medical personnel and their Australian counterparts. In 1944, Base Hospital No. 4 relocated closer to the frontlines, on a jungle island in New Guinea. Initially, canvas tents and pre-fabricated huts with concrete floors, open sides, and tin roofs served as "wards." The medical staff treated battle casualties, and tropical diseases such as malaria, dengue fever, scrub typhus, and jungle rot. Olga Benderoff, RN, a nurse from UH, served as Chief Nurse of the unit for the duration of the war, achieving

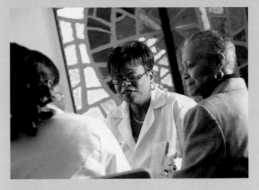

Carla Harwell, MD (center), at the University Hospitals Otis Moss Jr. Health Center.

I Work Here

Carla Harwell, MD, Medical Director of University Hospitals Otis Moss Jr. Health Center in Cleveland has been there since it opened in 1997. "I could have gone anywhere. But I'm here because of the David Satcher Clerkship I participated in as a visiting fourth-year medical student and the mentoring I received from Dr. [Edgar] Jackson." She leads a primary care facility for adults and children that serves the inner-city Fairfax neighborhood, which has been in decline since the 1970s. It is the brainchild of the former Olivet Institutional Baptist Church pastor for whom it is named. The partnership between the church and University Hospitals is unique. "We provide patient care in a culturally sensitive and spiritually supportive environment," explains Dr. Harwell. "The hospital saw a need and responded with a major investment, as part of a larger vision to revitalize this community." UH recommitted to the health center in 2017, announcing plans for a $2.5 million expansion project. New features will include a special food program, the first-of-its-kind in Northeast Ohio where patients can get groceries from the Greater Cleveland Food Bank.

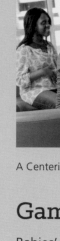

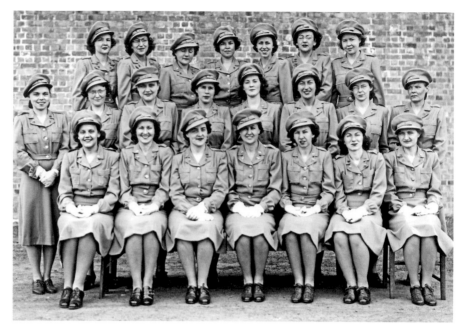

Nurses with the Lakeside Unit in World War II, 1940s. The unit, which made up the Fourth General Hospital, initially served in Melbourne, Australia, before moving closer to the front in New Guinea.

A CenteringPregnancy® support group, ca, 2010s.

Game Changer

Babies' Dispensary and Hospital greatly reduced the rate of infant mortality among Cleveland's poor. According to annual reports, the citywide death rate for infants in 1910 was 15 percent, but only 7.6 percent for dispensary patients. The next year that number decreased to 3.9 percent. Today, University Hospitals continues to search for solutions to this ongoing problem.

The CenteringPregnancy® Program aims to improve infant mortality rates in Cuyahoga County, which surpass those in many developing countries. The program focuses on at-risk mothers, between the ages of 14 and 25, providing prenatal care in a facilitated group setting with the guidance of a certified nurse midwife. "Women come to support each other, and we support them on a variety of issues ranging from nutrition and breastfeeding preparation to childbirth and family planning," explains former program director Gretchen Mettler, PhD, CNM, FACNM.

Over 1,500 low-income, expectant mothers have participated in the CenteringPregnancy® program since its inception in 2010. The program is having an impact; its participants' preterm birth rate and the low birth-weight rates are 10 percent, figures that are better than Cuyahoga County's averages.

the rank of Lieutenant Colonel. The medical staff had been transferred to the Philippines and were still aboard ship with the rest of the unit when Japan surrendered. Benderoff, who became Director of Nursing at UH, was awarded the Legion of Merit in 1946 for her service but said the credit should rightly go to all her nurses. "They did a distinguished piece of work," she said, "and Cleveland should be proud to know them."[5]

After the war, an Exchange Fellowship was established for Royal Melbourne Hospital clinical staff to conduct postgraduate

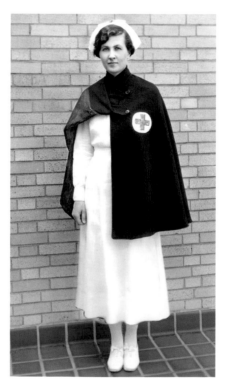

Olga Benderoff, RN, ca. late 1930s.

study at UH. The exchange eventually became reciprocal. Another outcome was an annual Thanksgiving feast, held in a Melbourne hotel, complete with roast turkey and pumpkin pie.

UH's international interactions date back to the late 19th and early 20th centuries when European immigrants made up the vast majority of patients seen at the hospitals, and American doctors went to Europe to study. "Now most patients at UH are native-born," observes John Grabowski, PhD, Historian, Case Western Reserve University, and Western Reserve Historical

Educating Future Health Care Providers

During the 1960s, University Hospitals participated in a program with Cleveland's Neighborhood Youth Corps that brought teenagers into the hospital to provide them with training and job experience. Some were high school drop-outs, and this program gave them a second chance to get their lives back on track. Many opted to remain at the hospital in full-time positions. Decades later, UH continues to find new ways to connect with students in the community.

In 2013, the hospital collaborated with the Beachwood City School District to launch a medical academy that is the first of its kind in the country. The partnership has expanded to also include students from Warrensville Heights, which is 95 percent African-American. The four-year curriculum, which includes coursework, seminars, shadowing, volunteering, and hands-on internships, offers an immersion experience that exposes young adults to the many career opportunities available in health care and gives them a competitive advantage as college applicants and job seekers.

The UH Educational Assistance Program pays the tuition for qualified trainees enrolled in programs to become allied health professionals. The forgivable loans require participants, upon graduation, to work for UH for a period of time, ensuring a pool of qualified candidates to fill positions throughout the hospital system. Teens who serve as summer youth volunteers are eligible to apply for higher education scholarships offered by the Auxiliary of University Hospitals Cleveland Medical Center.

UH also played a key role in creating the Cleveland School of Science and Medicine. It is one of nine partner institutions providing mentorship, internships, and funding. Located in the same University Circle neighborhood as UH's main campus, the college-preparatory program within a public high school serves high-achieving, low-income, and minority students interested in health care. Wilhemina Koomson, born in Jamaica to parents from Ghana, was in the first graduating class of 2010. "I discovered that I was passionate about medicine and met people willing to invest time in helping me. They gave me the courage to search for opportunities, and I found that there were great ones right across the street." Koomson worked as a volunteer in labs at Case Western Reserve University and University Hospitals Rainbow Babies & Children's Hospital during her senior year. Following high school graduation, she attended Princeton University and is currently a PhD candidate in genetics at Yale University with plans to pursue an MD degree upon completion of her postdoctoral program. "I got to do some very exciting research at Harvard Medical School at a young age," says this accomplished scholar and rising star, "and this opened doors for me."

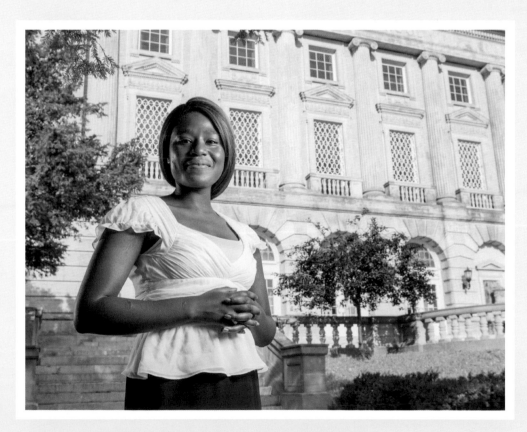

Wilhemina Koomson's participation in the Cleveland School of Science and Medicine program in high school inspired her to pursue a career in medicine.

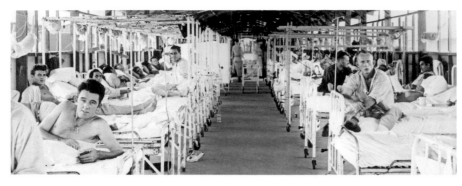

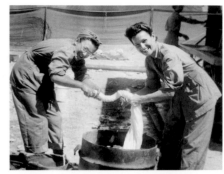

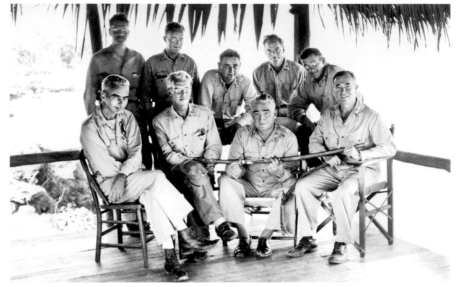

Top left: Patients in the orthopedic ward of the Fourth General Hospital in New Guinea during World War II. *Top right:* In New Guinea, personnel washed in troughs, did their own laundry by hand, and sometimes performed their duties in mud up to their knees. *Bottom:* Officers of the Fourth General Hospital in New Guinea.

Society, "and students, scientists, and physicians come to study and work here from all over the world." That reversal began, he suggests, with the passage of Medicare and Medicaid in 1965. That same year also saw the passage of a new immigration law which eliminated discriminatory nation-based quotas and encouraged people with needed skill sets to come to the U.S. "There was a shortage of nurses and physicians and pressure on the medical educational system to get more people in the pipeline. As a result, the face of UH, like hospitals around the country, began to change."

As authors, UH doctors, nurses, and administrators have an influence that extends far beyond Cleveland. One of them is Avroy Fanaroff, MD. He joined the medical staff of UH in 1975 and served as Division Chief of the Neonatal Program at UH Rainbow Babies & Children's Hospital for over 20 years. He also chaired the Department of Pediatrics from 2003 to 2008. He is an internationally acknowledged authority in neonatal and perinatal medicine. Dr. Fanaroff and Richard Martin, MD, Director, Neonatal Research Programs, UH Cleveland Medical Center, co-authored *Neonatal-Perinatal Medicine.* Now in its 11th edition,

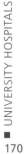

the textbook is considered the authoritative work in this area.

Dr. Fanaroff, in collaboration with his mentor, Marshall Klaus, MD, published a book *Care of the High-Risk Neonate*, which became a classic. It was translated into many languages. He recalls being at a conference when a young foreign physician approached him to

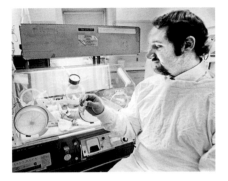

Nationally renowned neonatal expert Avroy Fanaroff, MD, ca. 1980s.

say thank you. "He told me that the book was his companion when he was alone and on call at the hospital, and [it] helped him get through a tough situation. It was very rewarding to hear that."

UH doctors have a history of taking their expertise to countries where it is desperately needed. Robert Hingson, MD, then Director of Anesthesiology, led his first medical mission to Asia and Africa in 1958. Under the auspices of an interfaith organization he founded called Brother's Brother, mission staff provided surgical, obstetric, and medical treatments in 147 hospitals. In 1962, he took a team of eight physicians and eight technicians, who were granted leaves of absence by UH administrators, to Liberia. They immunized a million people against smallpox over a two-month time period. Using jet injectors that Dr. Hingson helped to develop, they administered as many as 30,000 inoculations per day. Responding to a smallpox outbreak, 26 physicians and medical personnel, primarily from UH and Western Reserve University, went to Liberia again later that same year. They vaccinated people against that disease as well as yellow fever, poliomyelitis, and typhoid. Albert Burroughs, an anesthesia technician, remained at the request of the Liberian National Public Health Organization to train Liberian health workers in the use of the injectors.

In 1987, Frederick C. Robbins, MD, Nobel Laureate and former Dean at Case Western

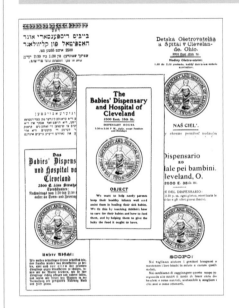

Babies' Dispensary and Hospital printed educational information on childcare in five different languages, 1908.

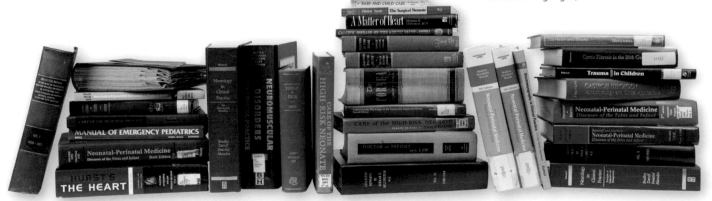

University Hospitals' ability to extend its global influence on medical education has been enhanced by the numerous UH physician-scholars, nurses, and administrators who have authored thousands of textbooks and articles throughout the decades.

University Hospitals Harrington Heart & Vascular Institute team members performed the first mitral valvuloplasty at the Mulago Hospital Catheterization Laboratory in Kampala, Uganda, 2012.

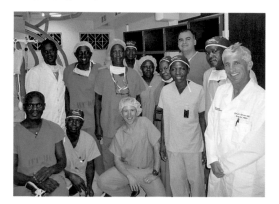

Reserve University School of Medicine, spearheaded a collaboration with Makerere University and Mulago Hospital in Uganda. "Initially, we focused on HIV, tuberculosis, and sexually transmitted infections," recalls Robert Salata, MD, UH Chair, Department of Medicine, who was a member of the original contingent that traveled to the East African nation. "Our approach was to do clinical research that would inform national guidelines for management, diagnosis, drug delivery and care, training, and technology transfer."

It was an effective strategy. Today, Ugandans living with HIV and AIDS are healthier and able to work productively. Life expectancy has increased, and the number of children born with HIV has decreased. In recent years, however, the focus has shifted. "They're starting to see the same chronic diseases we have here," says Dr. Salata. "So we're leveraging infrastructure that's already in place to address infectious diseases, cardiovascular diseases such as heart attacks, diabetes, hypertension, cancer, and strokes as well as some

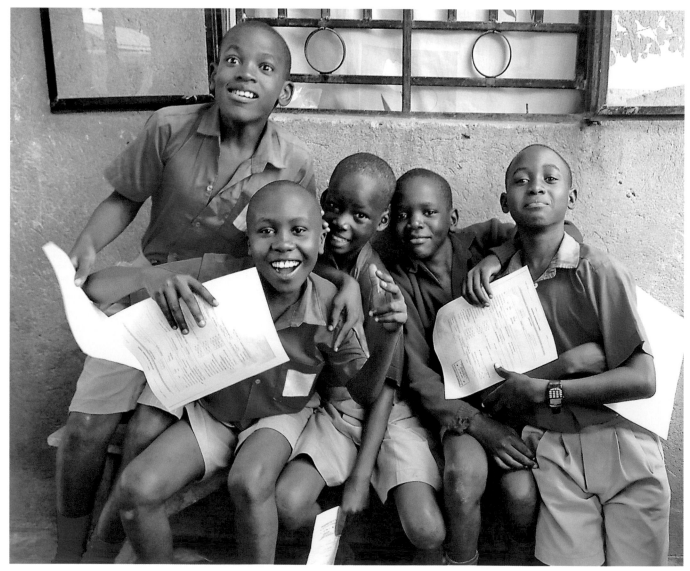

School-age boys in a village in Uganda benefit from the health care improvements made possible by University Hospitals care teams, ca. 2010s.

problems that we don't have in the United States, such as rheumatic heart disease."

Through a research collaboration with Dr. Salata, Chad Zender, MD, an otolaryngologist, partnered with UH to establish a surgical program for head and neck cancer at the Uganda Cancer Institute in the capital city of Kampala. Dr. Zender and Katrina Harrill, RN, in partnership with Ugandan health authorities, began leading surgical camps to Uganda in 2014 and continue to do so today. In addition to performing head and neck surgeries focusing on HIV-associated tumors, their teams treat patients in clinic and provide medical training to otolaryngology students and residents.

University Hospitals Harrington Heart & Vascular Institute assisted in opening Uganda's first cardiac catheterization laboratory in 2012. University Hospitals Cleveland Medical Center President and former Chief of Cardiovascular Medicine, Daniel Simon, MD, leading a team of cardiologists, including Marco Costa, MD, PhD, and Christopher Longenecker, MD, has performed more than 30 complex coronary, peripheral, and structural heart disease interventions during visits to Kampala. UH's involvement led to an epidemiology survey of cardiovascular disease and mentoring opportunities for trainees in cardiovascular medicine. Additionally, four Ugandan cardiologists have completed comprehensive, hands-on training in interventional cardiology, heart failure, cardiovascular imaging, and intensive care unit cardiovascular medicine at UH Cleveland Medical Center.

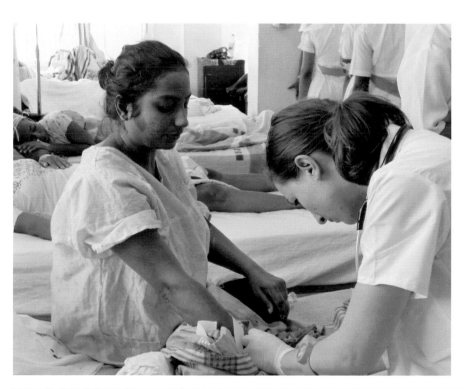

University Hospitals' health care professionals at work in Uganda, ca. 2010s.

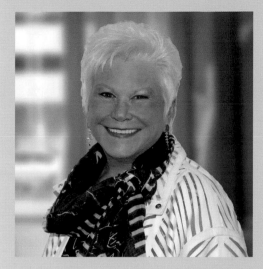

Roe Green, 2016.

It's a Fact

A Traveler's Clinic, the first of its kind in the country, was established in 1975 at University Hospitals in collaboration with the Division of Geographic Medicine at Case Western Reserve University School of Medicine. The clinic provided advice, immunizations, and prophylactic medications for people traveling abroad as well as diagnosis, treatment, and counseling for those who returned with parasites, malaria, or other conditions seldom seen in the United States.

The need for such a specialized clinic has endured and grown. The Roe Green Center for Travel Medicine is named in honor of Roe Green, whose enthusiasm for exploring the world inspired her to give $5 million in 2014 to expand and endow the program. It now operates on the University Hospitals Cleveland Medical Center campus and at the University Hospitals Chagrin Highlands and Westlake health centers. In addition to addressing the needs of international travelers, foreign visitors, and immigrants, there is a special child travelers clinic at University Hospitals Rainbow Babies & Children's Hospital.

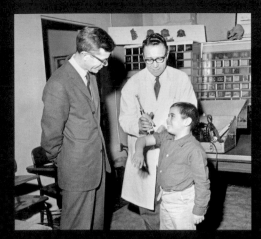

Robert Hingson, MD (center), administering a vaccine with the pistol-shaped jet injector, also known as the peace gun, ca. 1950s.

Pioneer

When Robert Hingson, MD, came to University Hospitals in 1951, he had already earned recognition for inventing a technique to deliver regional anesthesia during childbirth and improving on another that effectively prevented labor pain and reduced maternal and infant mortality. He also brought with him a prototype for an apparatus that injected liquids at high velocity. The jet injection method, known as hypospray, became an important public health tool because it was fast, efficient, and less painful and frightening than a syringe and needle. In 1956, he put it to large-scale use, inoculating Cleveland preschoolers with the Salk polio vaccine.

While at UH, Dr. Hingson, who was the first Professor of Anesthesiology at Western Reserve University School of Medicine, invented a small portable machine, nicknamed the Western Reserve "Midget," to deliver short-term gas anesthesia. It also functioned as a ventilator that could be employed by civilian first responders and military personnel for resuscitation.

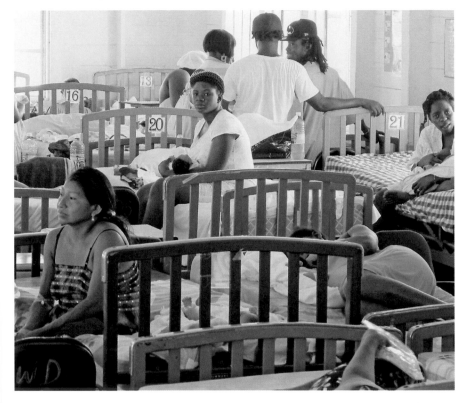

Since WONDOOR's inception in 2012, there has been a 50 percent reduction in maternal mortality in Guyana.

Other international sites where UH is involved in biomedical research and knowledge exchange include Portugal, South Africa, Kenya, Zimbabwe, Brazil, India, China, New Guinea, Australia, Mexico, and the Philippines. "Reaching out beyond our boundaries is important from a humanitarian and ethical point of view," says Dr. Salata. "Together with the School of Medicine, we have been working at global sites for well over 25 years. The hospital has consistently supported these programs and contributed to their success." Dr. Salata believes these efforts are one of UH's "jewels" and an important part of UH's story.

Another important international initiative is the WONDOOR (Women, Neonates, Diversity, Opportunities, Outreach, Research) program. It is a global health education initiative in obstetrics/ gynecology and reproductive biology sponsored by University Hospitals MacDonald Women's Hospital. Founded and led by Margaret Larkins-Pettigrew, MD, who also has a master's degree in public policy and international affairs, it is aimed at improving health care for women and their babies in low-resource countries and communities around the world and in the United States. "We are teaching humanitarianism as well as medicine," she says. There are multiple components to the program, including research, academically and clinically enriched training for resident and visiting scholars, and a postgraduate fellowship.

Current efforts focus on Georgetown Public Hospital in Guyana, which has very high mother and infant mortality rates due in large part to a shortage of specialists. The collaboration prompted Dr. Larkins-Pettigrew to ask, "How do we, who have expertise, take it somewhere else and leave that talent there? How do we do something that's sustainable?" She realized that education was the answer. As a result, WONDOOR designed and implemented Guyana's first four-year residency program in obstetrics and gynecology.

Closer to home, UH created the WONDOOR Global Health Scholars program, an educational and clinical program designed to improve the health of women for select OB/GYN residents at UH MacDonald Women's. As part of the program, which runs concurrently with the traditional OB/GYN residency requirements, former third-year resident Rachel Pope, MD, MPH, completed a rotation in Guyana. "I worked directly with Guyanese medical students. They don't get the same kind of attention we do here. There are only a few doctors to show them how to do things so they have to depend on textbooks," says Dr. Pope. "Knowing that what we're doing will help them care for women at the time of their greatest need is very special." Additionally, scholars participate in MomsFirst, a program of the Cleveland Department of Public Health that provides case management, home visits, and instruction for pregnant women and mothers until their children reach the age of 2.

People living in poverty, explains Dr. Larkins-Pettigrew, whether it is in this city or a developing country, suffer from health care disparities, especially as they relate to women, and a lack of basic health literacy. "Everyone should have access to quality health care, and we can apply what we learn abroad to what is happening right here in our own backyard." ▼

Pioneer

University Hospitals Rainbow Babies & Children's Hospital pediatrician Karen Olness, MD, was the driving force in establishing the Global Child Health Program at University Hospitals in 1987. The first pediatric residency of its kind in the country, it prepares doctors to work in under-resourced countries with the option for an overseas rotation. Dr. Olness, who directed the program for many years, also developed a unique disaster management course that trains medical professionals in the special psychological and health care needs of children and families during humanitarian emergencies. These workshops have been offered annually since 1995 in the U.S. and by the Rainbow Center for International Child Health in Pakistan, Ethiopia, Nicaragua, Panama, Syria, India, and other countries.

In 1997, doctors and nurses from the Department of Pediatrics at Khon Kaen University in northern Thailand came to Cleveland for this training. It proved invaluable in the aftermath of the tsunami that devastated their country in 2004.

Dr. Olness is also the founder and medical director of Health Frontiers, a collaborative effort with Case Western Reserve University School of Medicine, which began in 1991. The small non-government organization developed the first pediatric and internal medicine residency programs in Laos. Additionally, Dr. Olness established one of the first international adoption health service programs in the country.

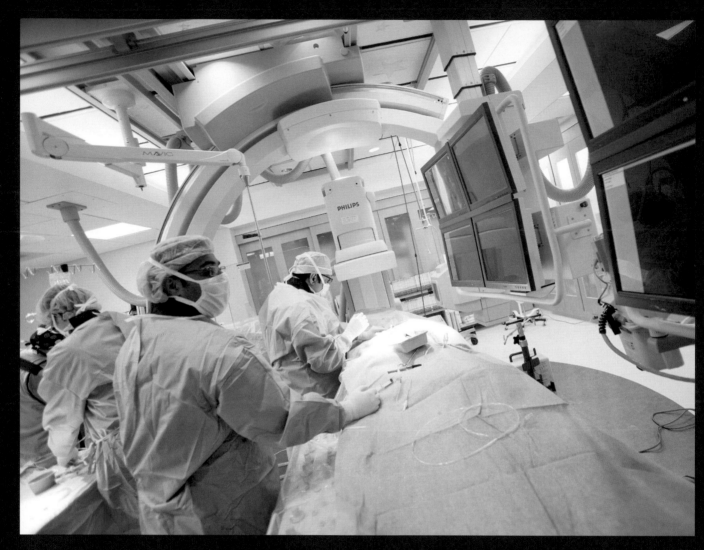

University Hospitals, like the best medical centers around the country, is constantly adapting to a changing health care landscape as it has done for the past 150 years. As UH physician-scientists push the boundaries for medical knowledge, they are giving patients hope and helping them have a better quality of life.

The Work Continues

"Innovations that cure medical conditions once thought unimaginable drive who we are and what we do at University Hospitals. This never-ending quest to advance and accelerate science requires a deeply held conviction to understand, embrace, and even stimulate change. Translating discovery into clinical breakthroughs has and will always remain central to our mission."

– Mukesh Jain, MD, Chief Scientific Officer, University Hospitals Health System and Harrington Discovery Institute, and Chief Research Officer, University Hospitals Harrington Heart & Vascular Institute

At 14, Maggie Gleason had never chatted on a cell phone, listened to music, or heard members of her family say they loved her. Born without cochleas, the small snail-shaped bones in the inner ear that make hearing possible, Maggie was totally deaf.

In 2014, Maggie was treated by a team of specialists from University Hospitals Cleveland Medical Center and University Hospitals Rainbow Babies & Children's Hospital and became the first teen in the United States to benefit from an auditory brainstem implant (ABI) for congenital deafness. This device works like an ear, translating sound waves into electrical impulses. These signals travel through the skin from a microphone-like processor to electrodes placed on the brainstem, bypassing the inner ear completely. Stimulation of nerves at the brainstem allows people like Maggie to hear sounds and distinguish pitch.

Months of healing followed the risky 10-hour surgery. Then came the day when doctors turned on the device. Maggie's father, Frank, asked, "Can you hear me?" She nodded. "I always felt I would have a lot to say to her when the moment came," Frank said, "but I was left speechless." Maggie has begun to speak and eventually, working with University Hospitals audiologists and speech therapists, her ability to verbally communicate should improve. A year after the procedure, the teen used sign language to say that her favorite sound was hearing her father call her name.

The device and the surgery to implant it were not available when Maggie was born. In the 21st

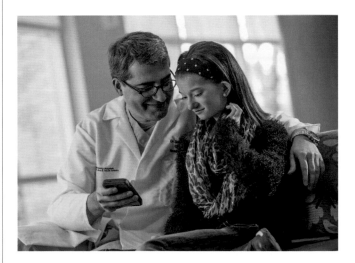

Otolaryngologists Maroun Semaan, MD (left), and Cliff Megerian, MD, in collaboration with neurosurgeon Nicholas Bambakidis, MD, and Gail Murray, MD, Director, Audiology Services, performed the auditory brainstem implant on Maggie Gleason (right), 2014.

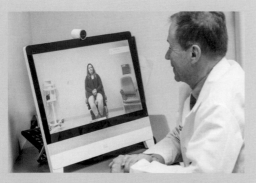

A telemedicine consultation between a patient at University Hospitals Samaritan Medical Center and the main campus at University Hospitals Cleveland Medical Center, 2017.

It's a Fact

In today's health care world, patients want seamless access to their providers and to have their health care needs addressed instantaneously. Toward this end, University Hospitals launched UH Virtual Visit in 2017, a program that allows patients to schedule appointments and meet with a primary care provider around the clock, 365 days of the year, via their smartphone, tablet, or computer. Additionally, telemonitoring is being used at UH for patients with heart disease, diabetes, and kidney transplants. A secure wireless connection is used in a patient's home for health care providers to be able to remotely check vital signs such as blood pressure, pulse, or blood glucose levels. When a deviation from the norm prompts concerns, the patient receives an alert, along with action recommendations, to correct the problem.

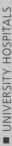

century, the advancement of medical knowledge and technology is accelerating rapidly. Standing still and maintaining the status quo is not an option. Today, medical decision-making is driven by a variety of factors, including the pressure to keep pace with evolving technology and treatments; the need to address the social, economic, and environmental factors that determine health outcomes; and a dramatic rise in consumer engagement.

"Innovation in health care is an ongoing journey for all of us," says Marco Costa, MD, PhD, President of University Hospitals Harrington Heart & Vascular Institute and UH Chief Innovation Officer. "The current state of change provides many opportunities to improve how we deliver high-quality care and the most personalized experiences to our patients."

Leading-Edge Tools and Techniques

Technology is completely changing the way diseases and injuries are diagnosed, treated, and even anticipated. Recent decades have brought advances in imaging, nuclear medicine, and robotics; tools for minimally invasive surgeries and patient monitoring; and the development of nano devices and materials. Innovations in these arenas and many others give physicians increasingly accurate and more precise information. Procedures of all kinds can be done faster, more efficiently, and with less pain, stress, and recovery time. Keeping up with the latest advancements is a hallmark of University Hospitals. Today, UH physicians are leaders in the realm of evolving technology. They are engaged in research that leads to innovation, testing, and perfecting new technological solutions to health care's most vexing problems. Most importantly, they develop recognized expertise in the application and use of this breakthrough technology at the bedside through direct patient care.

In 2010, cardiologists at University Hospitals Harrington Heart & Vascular Institute's Cardiovascular Imaging Core Laboratory were the first in the United States to perform optical coherence tomography (OCT) following FDA approval. Using light to produce high-resolution images of coronary arteries and stents in the heart, the intravascular imaging technology is so exact that it can accurately measure the diameter of arteries and the thickness of artery walls otherwise invisible or difficult to observe with older imaging techniques. This assists cardiologists in placing new stents and performing other heart procedures. OCT leads to superior outcomes and is a valuable technology for future research.

Magnetic resonance fingerprinting (MRF) takes imaging to an even more detailed level. MRF is an imaging technique based on assessing the specific tissue characteristics of a patient. Developed in collaboration with UH, Siemens Healthcare, and Case Western Reserve University School of Medicine, MRF could lead to earlier detection of many diseases, especially cancers; provide a better understanding of disease progression; and result in more personalized treatment. Pablo R. Ros, MD, Chairman, Department of Radiology, notes that MRF "has the potential to be a game-changer in disease diagnostics." When the technology is perfected, MRF scans will likely become standard procedure for annual check-ups, he adds. Current applications include using this emerging technology to determine the grade and extent of early-stage prostate cancer in an effort to optimize treatment. Other investigators are studying potential applications of MRF in the brain, breast, liver, and heart.

Technological advances also bring the ability to diagnose and treat patients in safer and more effective ways. The University Hospitals Brain Tumor & Neuro-Oncology Center designed and implemented one of the world's first intraoperative magnetic resonance imaging (MRI) operating suites, making it possible for surgeons to use MRI to track surgical progress in real time.

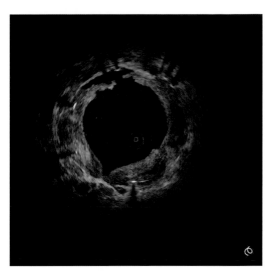

Digital optical coherence tomography (OCT) image, 2016.

UH Cleveland Medical Center surgeons were also among the first in the world to pioneer and use a minimally invasive approach known as laser interstitial thermal therapy for the removal of large glioblastoma and other types of brain tumors that have historically been challenging to access and were previously considered inoperable. The technology relies on MRI-guided lasers to destroy tumors without damaging surrounding healthy tissue. UH is one of only a few hospitals in the United States that can provide patients with this option.

High-tech devices capable of interrupting the faulty electrical signals in the areas of the brain that control movement have created an unprecedented leap forward in addressing neurologic conditions such as Parkinson's disease, multiple sclerosis,

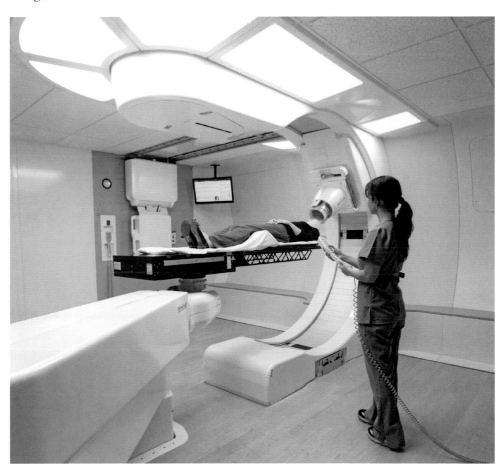

In 2016, University Hospitals opened a state-of-the-art proton therapy suite at University Hospitals Seidman Cancer Center. It is the first of its kind in Ohio and one of only six nationwide. Unlike traditional radiation, proton beam therapy is more exact, delivering a controlled and targeted form of radiation directly to cancerous growths. This results in potentially fewer side effects and minimizes the exposure of healthy tissue to radiation. It is an especially good option for children and young adults whose organs are still developing and for adults with tumors in difficult-to-reach areas such as the spine, brain, and prostate.

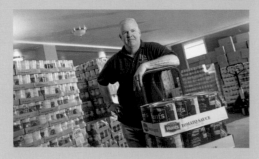

Greg Grindley after his surgery in 2016.

My Story

At age 49, Greg Grindley had suffered with Parkinson's disease for more than 10 years. A Navy veteran, he was forced to stop working, quit riding his motorcycle and scuba diving, and endured diminishing control of his limbs. His sleep was restless, and he needed a cane to walk.

There is no cure for Parkinson's, but one treatment that can help is Deep Brain Stimulation surgery (DBS). Grindley, who for years was hesitant to consider DBS fearing it would worsen his condition, elected to undergo it in 2015.

The National Geographic Channel broadcast the last two hours of the procedure around the world, performed at University Hospitals Cleveland Medical Center, live on TV. UH neurologists Camilla Kilbane, MD, and Benjamin Walter, MD, guided neurosurgeons Jonathan Miller, MD, and Jennifer Sweet, MD, to place the electrodes in the exact area of the brain where Grindley's involuntary movements originated. When the neurostimulator was activated for the first time, the tremor in Grindley's right hand disappeared. Now, he sleeps better, walks without fear of falling, and can enjoy activities he loves. During a follow-up, when doctors turned off the device, the shaking returned within 30 seconds. Reflecting on life after DBS, Grindley said, "The surgery [can't] stop the disease, but it's restored some of what I lost. It's done wonders for me."[1]

UNIVERSITY HOSPITALS

180

Tourette's syndrome, and other tremors. Instead of major, open-skull surgery, UH neurologists are among the first in the United States to treat movement disorders with a groundbreaking procedure called deep brain stimulation (DBS). It relies on a minimally invasive procedure to implant an electrical stimulator in the chest that sends signals to an electrode placed in the brain. It is hoped that applications for the technology will continue to expand and evolve in coming decades. Currently, UH researchers are testing the use of DBS to treat ailments involving neural miscommunication such as depression, bipolar disorder, and obsessive-compulsive disorder.

Access: The Right Care, Right Time, Right Place

Communication technology is having a significant impact on patient connectivity to health care, making virtual medicine a practical reality. In this new world of "telehealth," patients and physicians at University Hospitals have choices for how, where, and when they interact with each other. Instead of traveling to UH Cleveland Medical Center, patients can schedule virtual visits with UH specialists no matter where a patient lives. Interacting remotely, patients can talk with physicians about laboratory results and upcoming procedures or get a second opinion. Physicians can assess whether further diagnostic tests or face-to-face appointments are needed and discuss treatment plans. These real-time tele-consults help forge relationships between patients and providers, no matter where people live and work, and ensure an uninterrupted continuum of care. "UH provides virtual delivery of care in the emergency department, in physician offices, and at home. Our goal is to provide the power of UH at every location and for every situation to improve access to care," states Cindy Zelis, MD, Vice President, Ambulatory Services at UH.

For 19-year-old Chase Carpenter, the first person in her community to take advantage of the UH telehealth capabilities, this technology meant fewer three-hour round-trip journeys from her home in Ashland, Ohio, to Cleveland after being diagnosed with a tumor on her pituitary gland. Blurry vision accompanied by tingling and then numbness in her hands and feet sent her to the emergency room at University Hospitals Samaritan Medical Center in January 2017. Her initial MRI and the surgery were performed at UH Cleveland Medical Center, but she and her mother had pre- and post-operative tele-consults with her surgeon. "Dr. [Warren] Selman explained what he'd be doing during the operation, and we were able to ask questions. We had a second long-distance conversation afterward to talk about how I was feeling," Carpenter says. "I sat in a room that had a giant computer screen. Being able to see each other was much better than a phone call. I use Skype and FaceTime, so this was nothing new for me, but my mom really liked it, too. There was the intimacy of being together without the travel. The whole experience was easy, seamless, and comfortable."

Promoting Health and Wellness

The definition of health care has evolved dramatically since Wilson Street Hospital opened its doors to care for patients in 1868. Chronic conditions such as heart disease and diabetes have gradually replaced infectious diseases as the leading causes of mortality, and prevention is a genuine possibility. UH now strives to do more than react to the onset of illness by responding to a growing movement in medicine to keep patients out of the hospital. Services now focus on both the physical and mental well-being of patients, encouraging lifestyle habits to ward off illness before it appears and mitigate the effects when it does.

For UH, this vision to provide preventative health care reprises efforts made more than a century ago by the UH founding institutions. Home visits, neighborhood outpatient clinics, and educational initiatives to teach people how to better care for themselves and their families were hallmarks of both Babies' Dispensary and Maternity hospitals. Babies' Dispensary had branch clinics throughout Cleveland's underserved immigrant communities, providing outpatient care to the children most in need. Maternity sent nurses out to provide in-home care, not only during delivery but also afterward, as they taught new mothers how to take care of their babies. The University Hospitals Rainbow Center for Women & Children in the city's Mid Town neighborhood represents the organization's latest efforts to continue this work of caring for underserved populations where they live. Located two miles west of the UH main campus, the center will serve an area that has a large number of low-income residents, single-parent households, and one of the highest infant mortality rates in the city.

"In addition to comprehensive medical care for women and children, the new facility will address the many factors that influence the health of women, their families, and the community," says Patti DePompei, MSN, RN, President, University Hospitals Rainbow Babies & Children's and University Hospitals MacDonald Women's hospitals. Educational and support groups at the center will focus on wellness. There will be comprehensive dental and eye care programs, a group model of prenatal care for high-risk women, and programs to address basic needs such as food, transportation, and insurance benefits.

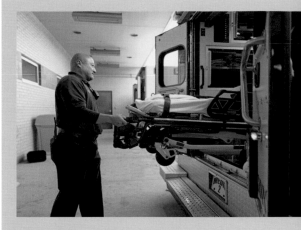

First responders at University Hospitals Parma Medical Center, 2016.

It's a Fact

First responders know the signs of a stroke, the leading cause of disability in the United States. An innovative telestroke project, piloted in the summer of 2016, is improving response times and patient outcomes. Firefighter and paramedic teams in North Royalton, Ohio, received training from the University Hospitals Emergency Medical Services Education & Disaster Preparedness Institute on how to perform a more detailed neurological assessment when dispatched to the field. Since time is critical in treating strokes, the exam is live-streamed via a computer tablet to emergency room physicians at University Hospitals Parma Medical Center. Equipped with this additional critical information about a stroke victim, ER staff can be ready to act quickly and better prepare for the patient's arrival. In 2017, two UH hospitals participated in the telestroke project, with more slated to come online.

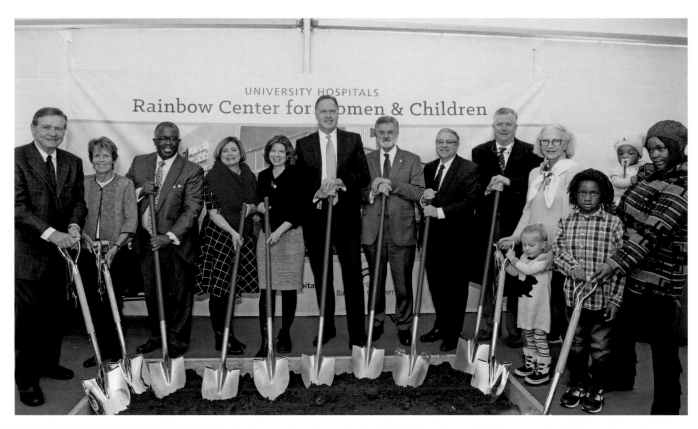

Construction began for the UH Rainbow Center for Women and Children in December 2016 (groundbreaking ceremony shown above) and opened in 2018. The center provides a new model of care that addresses the medical as well as social determinants of health, including housing, safety, education, and access to healthy food, to help build a stronger, healthier Cleveland.

Game Changer

Today, patients can shop around for doctors and hospitals and want the same conveniences they enjoy in other parts of their lives such as online scheduling, extended hours, the ability to communicate directly with providers, and access to their own medical records. They are more informed, more cost-conscious, and want instantaneous access to health care more than ever before. According to a survey conducted by the Deloitte Center for Health Solutions, more and more people are taking an active role in their own health care and increasingly see themselves and their physicians as partners making treatment decisions together.[2] Their expectations are having a transformative effect on care delivery, pushing organizations such as University Hospitals to rethink how, when, and where they connect with those they serve.

The UH Rainbow Center for Women & Children demonstrates a concern for population health, another major trend in 21st century health care. Population health addresses the health care needs of defined groups as well as individuals. The goal is to improve outcomes, reduce inequities, and provide services so that community members become healthier and avoid costly hospitalizations and procedures. Another goal of population health is to identify and manage long-term and recurring health issues in a given community. To help achieve these goals, UH is turning to "big data," a way of looking at large groups of people and trends and leveraging massive quantities of statistics to better understand factors that influence health care.

By gathering and analyzing information from millions of encounters between patients and health care providers across the UH system, experts can identify patterns of behavior and risk. UH can use this data to identify specific patient populations, track disease trends, analyze treatment plans and outcomes, and assess hospital operations. Initiatives involving data analytics provide UH with a powerful tool to deliver services more efficiently and effectively. Individual patients receive better care, and specific patient populations receive the attention they need.

Population health is also addressed at UH through accountable care organizations (ACOs), which grew nationally beginning in 2010 when Congress passed health care reform. ACOs rely on groups of doctors, hospitals, and other providers working together to deliver the most appropriate care in a coordinated manner as efficiently as possible. UH established ACOs first for its employees, and subsequently, for commercially insured patients and for Medicare beneficiaries through a Medicare Shared Savings Program. Additionally, University Hospitals Rainbow Babies & Children's Hospital established one of the first pediatric ACOs in the country, known as the UH Rainbow Care Connection, through a $12.7 million Health Care Innovation grant from the Center for Medicare & Medicaid Innovation. The ACO health care delivery model aims to support patients between doctor's appointments and to reduce unnecessary use of hospital services, including visits to the emergency room. "UH is leading the nation in this effort," states Andrew Hertz, MD, Vice President, Rainbow Primary Care Institute Medical Director, Rainbow Care Connection. The ACOs at UH have grown to be among the largest in the country and have proven successful in improving the quality of care and patient experience, while reducing overall health care costs.

Taking It to the Next Level: Better Cancer Care for Young People

According to the National Cancer Institute, cancer in adolescents and young adults (AYAs) is rare. However, it is the leading cause of death by disease in this age group, and survival rates for some cancers have lagged behind those achieved for pediatric and adult cancer patients. The Angie Fowler Adolescent & Young Adult Cancer Institute is positioned to change these outcomes. A collaboration between University Hospitals Rainbow Babies & Children's Hospital and University Hospitals Seidman Cancer Center, it opened in 2014 to address the challenge of improving outcomes for this age group. It is one of the first and few places of its kind in the United States, and the first center focused on AYA cancer within the nation's 49 Comprehensive Cancer Centers designated by the National Cancer Institute.

Teens with cancer confront issues that are particular to their age group. They often fall behind academically and miss out on important social milestones when forced to step away from their normal activities during treatment. Angie's Institute offers a holistic approach that includes state-of-the-art medical treatment and age-appropriate support for the mental and emotional needs particular to the AYA population. AYA patients receive peer counseling to help navigate the emotional and psychological aspects of their illness. Once treatment is complete,

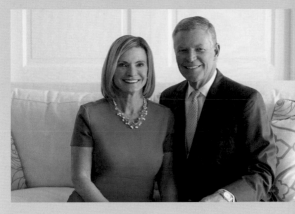

Sara and Chris Connor, 2018.

Pass It On

Chris Connor, former University Hospitals Board chair and retired CEO and chairman of the board of Sherwin-Williams, and his wife Sara gave a $1 million gift to establish University Hospitals Connor Integrative Health Network. It is a system-wide initiative launched in 2011 and based at University Hospitals Ahuja Medical Center that takes a holistic approach to healing by offering therapies and services that work in partnership with traditional medicine. The UH Connor Integrative Health Network offers evidence-based practices such as acupuncture, meditation, qigong, guided imagery, and massage. Along with art, music, and pet therapy, these practices are also used to foster relaxation and provide non-pharmaceutical ways to manage pain, stress, insomnia, and depression. Addressing the needs of the mind and the spirit as well as the body is an important component of 21st century health care, notes Chris Connor, "which emphasizes prevention and each of us taking more personal responsibility for our own heath." In 2017, the Connors further showed their support for the integrative medicine network that bears their name by donating $6.5 million to expand the program.

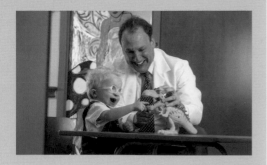

Carson Locher (left) and Richard Grossberg, MD (right), 2014.

Our Story

Carson Locher has suffered from a variety of medical problems since he was 2 months old. He was in and out of the hospital regularly and made many visits to the emergency room. In 2013, when Carson turned 2, Richard Grossberg, MD, a specialist in pediatric neurodevelopmental disabilities and his team at University Hospitals Rainbow Babies & Children's Hospital, diagnosed him with CHARGE syndrome, a condition that includes difficulties with swallowing, breathing, hearing, vision, and balance. He requires tremendous support, and so does his mother, Jessie Beals. Because he is enrolled in the Rainbow Care Connection Center for Comprehensive Care, directed by Dr. Grossberg, Carson has a dedicated team of health care professionals, including Dr. Grossberg, nurses, a dietitian, and a social worker. "He has not [been] admitted to the hospital since April 2016," says Beals. "When I call with a question, someone gets back to me within an hour or two. Dr. Grossberg is always available, even after hours. [UH] helped us get a medical bed, wheelchair stroller, and hearing aid for him."

Beals now has time and energy to be an attentive mom to her older daughter. "I believe in this approach 100 percent," she says. "It's reduced my stress level and lightened my load, and best of all, Carson is thriving."

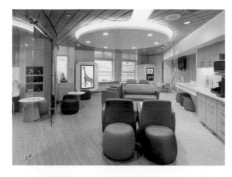
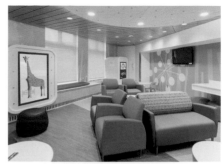
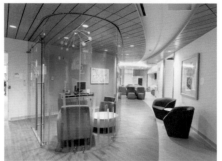
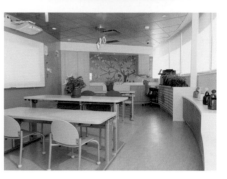

The Angie Fowler Adolescent & Young Adult Cancer Institute encompasses two dedicated floors at University Hospitals Rainbow Babies & Children's Hospital for inpatient and outpatient services. A teen lounge, bright colors, and an interactive wall contribute to a contemporary and upbeat mood. Self-contained spaces with digital access address the desire for privacy and the wish to stay in touch with the outside world.

AYA patients continue in the survivorship program that provides lifetime follow-up care to reduce the risk of recurrence or secondary malignancy and psychological help for issues that appear long after treatment is complete.

University Hospitals' adolescent cancer patients get the best of both worlds. They receive the very close attention that children need and the type of care needed by adults. AYA patients are enrolled in dozens of promising national clinical trials that offer them the opportunity to receive the latest treatments before they are available elsewhere. A partial list of studies includes trials in brain tumors, lymphoma, and soft tissue and bone tumors. Physician-scientists at Angie's Institute have led one of the largest trials for acute lymphoblastic leukemia (ALL) in the country. "Research is one of the ways in which Angie's Institute can have a major impact on the care of kids now and for generations to come," says Angie's Institute Director John Letterio, MD.

"We have enjoyed tremendous success in the treatment of childhood cancers," he continues, "but there is an important challenge that we now must address. There are health risks that a growing generation of young adult cancer survivors now face, which are either related to the therapy for their cancer or to the underlying genetic factors that placed them at risk for that first cancer. We must be dedicated to preparing our patients for happy, healthy, and productive lives after cancer."

New Frontiers in Personalized Medicine

University Hospitals physician-scientists are on the leading edge of discovery, conducting original groundbreaking research, and generating patents. They are spurring advances in their specialties by building on the research of others and working with companies to invent and improve products. Many are distinguished by their expertise in the latest, most innovative procedures. "We have a broad spectrum of new therapies that includes clinical trials," says Marcos de Lima, MD, Director of the Bone Marrow Transplant program at UH. "I would love to have the next generation see that the future is very bright....My goal is not having to treat any of these diseases in the future, meaning that everybody will be cured, and that we will find a way not only to treat, but to prevent."[3]

Exploration is especially intense in the fields of genomics, stem cells, and immunotherapy. The three are part of a broad category known as precision medicine, an evolving medical approach that replaces the one-size-fits-all mindset of the past with a perspective that considers the particularities of each individual and his or her illness. The most promising applications thus far are for cancer, but researchers have only begun to investigate the possibilities.

Genomics

Cancer used to be seen as a single, monolithic disease, and for years physicians sought treatment therapies based on this idea. However, the genomic revolution has revealed that every tumor has its own genetic composition. Profiling the exact mutation through sophisticated genetic testing is an innovative pathway to identifying the most effective response. Treatments are also tailored to each individual's distinctive genetic makeup, family medical history, and other specific risk factors. Still in the early stages of development, it is already having a dramatic impact on understanding cancer and how to fight it.

UH hematologist-oncologist Sanford Markowitz, MD, PhD, and Joseph Willis, MD, Division Chief, Pathology, and Vice Chairman, Clinical Affairs, have pinpointed 15 gene mutations in African-American men that drive higher rates of colon cancer and death in this population compared to Caucasian men. Their vision is to develop a way to specifically target cancers with these mutations so as to lead to more effective treatment of these currently highly lethal tumors.

Immunotherapy

The American Society of Clinical Oncology declared immunotherapy the 2016 advance of the year. This therapeutic modality capitalizes

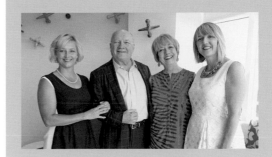

Holley, Chuck, Char, and Chann Fowler, 2014.

Pass It On

A desire to honor their child Angie, who died of cancer in 1983 at the age of 14, and create something positive out of their tragic loss prompted Chuck and Char Fowler to devote their efforts and their philanthropy to finding cures and improving survival rates for adolescents and young adults with cancer.

"This is not only a legacy to our daughter," says Chuck, "but also something that very much needed to be done."

In 2007, a gift from the Fowlers, combined with funds from Rainbow Babies & Children's Foundation, facilitated the creation of the nation's first endowed chair in the field of adolescent and young adult (AYA) cancer.

Working in concert with the medical team at University Hospitals Rainbow Babies & Children's Hospital, the Fowlers traveled the country to learn about the best AYA cancer programs and practices. "We brought those ideas home to Cleveland," says Chuck, "and combined them with what we wished had been available when Angie was sick." The result is the Angie Fowler Adolescent & Young Adult Cancer Institute, made possible by a $17 million gift in 2011 from Chuck, Char, and their daughters and sons-in-law, Chann and Ed Spellman and Holley and Rob Martens.

"We hope Angie's Institute will be a model for other AYA cancer programs across the country," Chuck says.

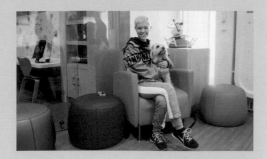

Ali Rieman, 2016.

My Story

Ali (Alison) Rieman was diagnosed with acute myeloid leukemia as a freshman in college. "I was 18, healthy, and super-active," she recounts. "Suddenly, I felt flu-like symptoms that got worse fast. I saw the doctor, had blood work done, and was admitted to Rainbow on October 6, 2015." Rieman's cancer and her treatments were aggressive. An inpatient for months, she had four rounds of chemotherapy and radiation.

"They didn't treat me like a kid. They were focused on how I was doing as a person and not just on the medical side," she recalls.

In February 2016, Ali received a half-match bone marrow transplant from her brother. Because only half of his stem cells were a match, it was necessary to suppress the other half. "This kind of expertise is one of the benefits of being treated at the Angie Fowler Adolescent & Young Adult Cancer Institute," explains Jignesh Dalal, MD, Director, Pediatric Bone Marrow Transplant.

"There were many days I didn't think I'd make it to my next birthday," says Rieman, now 21 and cancer-free. "I'm going to the gym and am back at school."

Rieman regularly visits Angie's Institute for follow-up. She also attends adolescent and young adult support group meetings. "It's great to meet other survivors. We talk about what we've been through and life after cancer."

on the power of the body's own immune system to detect and react to cancerous tumors. Finding ways to activate, boost, and direct this natural defensive response, also called biological therapy, has the potential to inhibit the growth and spread of cancer cells and to repair the damage to healthy cells caused by radiation and chemotherapy. Alex Huang, MD, PhD, pediatric oncologist with the Angie Fowler Adolescent & Young Adult Cancer Institute, is making some important discoveries in the field. "The immune system is highly sensitive and specific, and it can work better than drugs at times," Dr. Huang says.[4] "It also instills a memory of the tumor in the patient's body so the immune system will turn back on if a similar tumor ever returns again."

One trial underway at University Hospitals involves a vaccine therapy for a rare but very aggressive form of brain cancer called glioblastoma multiforme. Patients with this type of tumor have only a 25 percent chance of living two years after diagnosis, even with aggressive treatment. This approach attempts to marshal the power of the patient's own immune system to fight against tumor remnants that typically remain in the brain following surgery, radiation, and chemotherapy. Investigators plan to expand the program to study the effects of immunotherapy on other tumor types, including pancreatic, lung, colorectal, and breast cancers.

Oncology researchers at University Hospitals Seidman Cancer Center are in the vanguard of developing what could be the next generation of personalized immune therapy for melanoma, a highly fatal form of skin cancer. For example, physician-scientists are able to remove a specific type of immune cell from a melanoma patient's lymph nodes, activate them in the lab based on the genetics of the patient's tumor, and

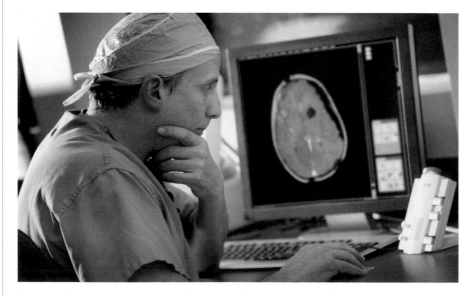

University Hospitals' neurosurgeons like Andrew Sloan, MD, are pushing new frontiers in brain cancer research, ca. 2010s.

Treatments of Tomorrow Start Today

Clinical trials test and assess the effectiveness and safety of new medical interventions and medications in human beings, and they are an essential bridge from the laboratory to the next generation of treatment. Patients who volunteer to participate in these studies have access to potentially beneficial therapies and drugs before they are widely available. This is important for seriously ill individuals who have exhausted all other options. Participating in a trial gives people hope. But not every drug proves to be effective, and in double-blind studies, only some participants actually receive the medication under investigation. "We can't promise cures," says University Hospitals neurosurgeon Andrew Sloan, MD. "No one can. But with all the research and clinical trials out there, there's always hope on the horizon."

The UH research program has grown from a dozen clinical trials available in the 1950s to over 1,200 clinical research studies offered today across the health system in more than 20 academic and clinical disciplines. University Hospitals Seidman Cancer Center, as a National Cancer Institute-designated testing site, currently has more than 500 new treatments in various stages of clinical trials.

Peter McVoy entered a UH Seidman trial for an innovative cancer treatment in late 2014. He was 62 and had been diagnosed early that year with stage 4 adrenocortical carcinoma, a very rare and aggressive cancer that is likely to be fatal. He had surgery to remove a tumor on his kidney, but scans later showed that there were lesions on his liver. He enrolled in a clinical trial and received regular infusions of a groundbreaking drug that prompted his body's immune system to attack the cancer cells. By January 2016, doctors could not detect any signs of cancer. "I was given 12 to 18 months to live," McVoy told an interviewer in 2017. "It's the third year since the trial started, which has given me two birthdays I wasn't supposed to have and another Christmas I'm going to celebrate soon and two grandsons and a granddaughter I get to share it with."[5]

transfer them back into the same patient to stimulate the immune system to attack the cancer. These doctors embody the UH mission to push the boundaries of medical discovery to provide effective treatments that improve the lives of patients.

Stem Cells

Stem cells are a versatile, powerful tool in the fight against a diverse group of diseases. They can be prompted in the lab to regenerate in many different body systems, becoming tissue- or organ-specific cells with special functions. "Stem cell therapy has great potential for treating many different diseases across specialties, offering new ways to treat HIV, different types of cancers, cystic fibrosis, rheumatoid arthritis, and inflammatory bowel disease," says Grace McComsey, MD, infectious disease specialist at University Hospitals Cleveland Medical Center, Division Chief of Pediatric Infectious Diseases and Rheumatology at University Hospitals Rainbow Babies & Children's Hospital, and Associate Chief Scientific Officer of University Hospitals Health System. Dr. McComsey also leads the Clinical Research Center of University Hospitals Cleveland Medical Center, which provides the central infrastructure for clinical trials at UH.

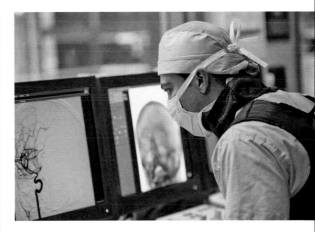

Stem cell research offers promising new treatments for stroke sufferers.

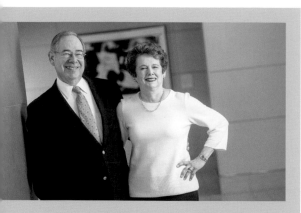

University Hospitals philanthropists Les and Linda Vinney, 2016.

Pass It On

Before she retired, Linda Vinney was a genetics counselor with a master's degree in the field. Her husband, Les, former CEO of STERIS, a medical device company, has been a longtime UH board member. Their interests came together in 2010 when the couple gave a financial gift to further genetic research at University Hospitals Seidman Cancer Center. The Linda and Les Vinney Biorepository and Genomic Facility is a place where physician-scientists can code, store, analyze, and sequence tissue samples, making it a valuable asset in the pursuit of personalized cancer treatments based on the genetic makeup of tumor types. In 2015, they established an endowed directorship in cancer genetics, which was named in their honor.

UH was a leader in early trials for treating cardiovascular disease with stem cells. Cathy Sila, MD, Program Director, Vascular Neurology at UH Cleveland Medical Center, was able to confirm that a medication derived from adult stem cells could improve outcomes for ischemic stroke patients. Early results from a small sample of people, reported in 2016, showed that one year after treatment those treated with the drug, called MultiStem®, did significantly better than others who received a placebo. Because the cells are obtained from healthy bone marrow donors rather than from the patient, they can be collected, processed in advance, and stored for future use.

The potential use of stem cells continues to expand beyond the treatment of disease to use in other fields, such as orthopedics. James Voos, MD, Chairman, Department of Orthopedics, at UH Cleveland Medical Center and Head Team Physician for the Cleveland Browns, is leading a first-time study in the use of patients' own stem cells as a therapeutic option for athletic injuries, arthritis, and other musculoskeletal issues.

The majority of stem cell research at UH has been in the field of oncology. Two trailblazers in this arena recognized for their pioneering accomplishments in bone marrow and stem cell transplantation are Hillard Lazarus, MD, Director, Novel Cell Therapy at UH, and Stanton Gerson, MD, former Director of University Hospitals Seidman Cancer Center and current head of the Case Comprehensive Cancer Center. The two physician-scientists and Case Western Reserve University biologist Arnold Caplan, PhD, are credited with the discovery and development of mesenchymal stem cells, which made UH a leader in regenerative medicine, a subset of stem cell research. These cells have the ability to support other tissues and to regenerate and replace abnormal cells. Applications in cancer and many other diseases are being developed. These cells offer the transformative possibility of permanently correcting disorders, rather than just treating them with drugs. UH operates a laboratory to isolate and grow mesenchymal stem cells for patients, using cells harvested from living donors.

"The outlook for cancer patients is improving, every year, every six months," says Dr. Gerson, who studies the interaction of stem cells, DNA, and cancer and has generated 12 patents in gene therapy and drug discovery. "We're continually learning, taking the information we have, sharing it with the world's experts, and coming up with new treatments." And sometimes, he adds, those treatments turn out to be "home runs."[6]

The Way Forward

A new model for conducting medical research has emerged in recent years. The work of discovery is no longer confined to geographical or

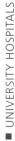

Game Changer: The Harrington Project

When it comes to moving research initiatives from the discovery stage to the marketplace, the traditional drug development system is complex and slow moving. The University Hospitals Harrington Project for Discovery & Development, established in 2012 with an unprecedented financial gift from the Harrington family, is dedicated to bridging that chasm.

Key components to this initiative include the Innovation Support Center, a non-profit pharmaceutical team that guides the process of advancing drug discovery to clinical trials, and BioMotiv, a mission-driven, for-profit accelerator. With this two-pronged approach, UH has created a bold new prototype for drug development that has attracted international attention. It has the potential to reshape the future of medicine as new, better drugs transition more rapidly and efficiently into the marketplace.

Progress thus far has been astounding. As of mid-2018, the Harrington Project has supported the launch of 20 companies and enabled five drugs to enter clinical trials, including treatments for basal cell carcinoma, Alzheimer's disease, and peripheral vascular disease. A total of five new technologies have been licensed to large pharmaceutical companies. To date, the Harrington Project has raised more than $300 million in committed funding.

"When our family got involved with this project," says Ron Harrington, "we expected the concept of discovering new drugs in order to extend life and improve people's quality of life to be well received. What we did not expect was the reception that The Harrington Project model has received in both the philanthropic and investment communities. As a result, we are far ahead of where we thought we would be at this point."

institutional boundaries. Today's modern communication technology allows physician-scientists to collaborate on a scale never seen before, making research and ideas more accessible. Free from the constraints of place, science without walls fosters a more flexible and cooperative paradigm. Physician-scientists are positioned to collect, exchange, and utilize data across the region, the state, the country, and even the world. Reflecting this shift, University Hospitals entered into a new phase in its relationship with Case Western Reserve University School of Medicine in 2016. The affiliation between the two, dating back more than 100 years, continues, but both are now free to pursue other strategic partnerships and collaborate with multiple organizations.

The Harrington Project for Discovery & Development, located at University Hospitals, is an example of the success that can be achieved when barriers to scientific collaboration are removed. It provides the mentoring, funding, and entrepreneurial expertise necessary to translate research into accessible and commercially viable drugs. "For the first time, we have an opportunity to support individual physician-scientists in truly new ways," says Jonathan Stamler, MD, President, Harrington Discovery Institute (part of The Harrington Project for Discovery & Development) and Director, Institute for Transformative Molecular Medicine at UH/CWRU. "But we can also commit to ensuring that the discoveries we think will benefit human health move forward into the marketplace."

This unique and groundbreaking opportunity is available to physician-scientists from leading institutions in this country and abroad. It is a competitive process with each year's class of Harrington Discovery Institute Scholar-Innovators selected from as many as several

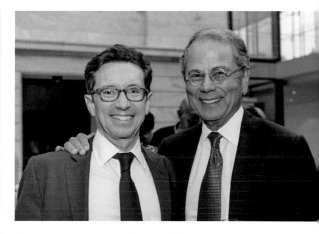

Harrington Discovery Institute President, Jonathan Stamler, MD, with the Institute's benefactor and Chairman of BioMotiv, Ron Harrington, 2016.

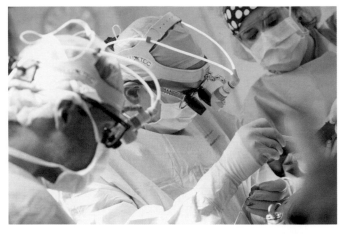

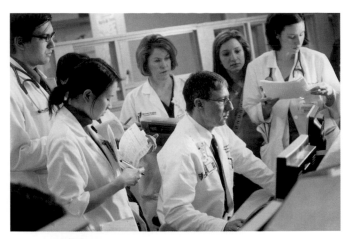

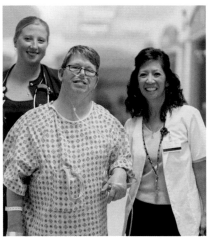

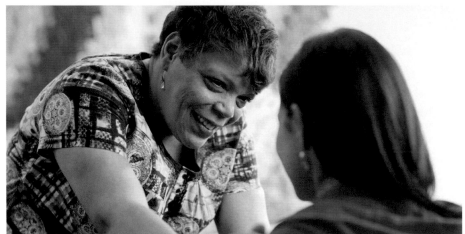

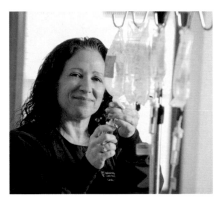

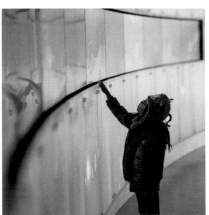

University Hospitals has survived and ultimately thrived since 1866. Only a handful of hospitals around the nation can claim similar longevity.

hundred physician-scientist applicants. Since the program began in 2012, more than 100 scholars have been selected from over 2,500 applicants representing more than 200 institutions. "This represents a commitment to our mission," explains Dr. Stamler, "by searching out the best and most promising new treatments wherever they originate."

Harrington Discovery Institute plans to leverage its expertise and resources through additional partnerships. The Oxford-Harrington Scholarship Program supports novel drug discovery research conducted at the University of Oxford. The Gund-Harrington National Initiative in Fighting Blindness represents an alliance between Harrington Discovery Institute and the Foundation Fighting Blindness, founded and headed by Cleveland-born businessman and philanthropist Gordon Gund. Efforts focus on finding treatments that could ameliorate or reverse degenerative retinal disease, a condition that took Gund's sight in 1970, when he was only 30. According to Dr. Stamler, the collaboration of an academic medical center and a disease foundation is an entirely new paradigm for drug discovery and development. Another promising collaboration involves a partnership with Takeda Pharmaceutical Company, which marks the first time Harrington Discovery Institute has joined forces with a major pharmaceutical company. Takeda's investment will aid in research and drug development in the area of rare diseases.

No one can predict the future trajectory of medical innovation. Some of today's discoveries may turn the impossible into the achievable. Studies may turn up unintended results, or even fail in their goals. As new treatments receive government approval, they may supplant those currently considered the most advanced options. It is a relentless process. What matters is that the search remains ongoing. For University Hospitals, ensuring this continuity is fundamental to its identity.

To Heal. To Teach. To Discover. This is University Hospitals' mission, distilled into three key parts. It represents a historical commitment to care for the sick and injured, to train physicians, and to foster scientific exploration, and it is more relevant today than ever. Achieving these goals decade after decade has required dedication, talent, tenacity, foresight, and funding.

The enduring viability and vitality of the organization and its ability to weather uncertainty and adapt to changing conditions hinges on its people—those who work at UH, believe in it, support it with their dollars and their time, and turn to it as a trusted partner for their health care. The social conscience that motivated the founders continues to inform today's leaders. "We see ourselves as a health care and a health caring institution," says UH Chief Executive Officer, Thomas F. Zenty III.[7]

Looking back, it is clear there are many accomplishments and successes to celebrate. A number of important developments in clinical medicine and research can be traced back to UH, an organization that is known for the compassion expressed by its caregivers and the very human, personal attention they give to each patient. Its name is synonymous with coveted opportunities for training and mentoring. The hospital has grown from treating 71 patients in its first year to helping millions, from one building and a few beds to 26,000 employees charged with serving much of Northeast Ohio's population. A seamless connection exists between primary care physicians, community hospitals, and University Hospitals Cleveland Medical Center. It is this interconnectivity that allows UH to manage health care needs from first breath to last in a coordinated way that supports wellness and offers the best options in times of illness and injury.

While there is value in celebrating the past, it is much more important to look ahead. UH remains robust and resilient, rooted in the place where it began, ready to rise to the challenge of whatever comes next.

"The important thing is not to say, 'They were great,'" insists Enid Rosenberg, member of the University Hospitals Ahuja Medical Center Board of Directors, and Chair, UH Leadership Council Chairs Committee, "but to ask 'Where are we going? Who do we want to be? How will we continue to be a resource for this community and beyond?'" ▼

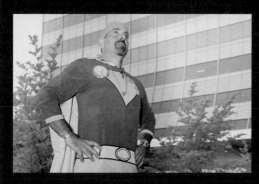

'Superman' Andy Simon, 2016.

My Story

In 2015, physicians at University Hospitals determined Andy Simon's intense headache pain was due to a stage 4 malignant glioblastoma. Following surgery to remove the tumor and radiation therapy, Simon returned to his job at a local wholesale food distributor. Because he was still able to hoist 100-pound corned beef barrels, a co-worker started calling him Superman. "Just because you're labeled with cancer," Simon says, "it doesn't have to be a negative. You can fight it. You can beat it."

But, Simon's long-term outlook was complicated. "Despite what appeared to be a clean post-operative MRI and a return to full function," said neurosurgeon Andrew Sloan, MD, "we knew we needed an aggressive approach for this type of lethal tumor." Simon was enrolled in a clinical trial designed by Dr. Sloan and based on research conducted by Stanton Gerson, MD, head of the Case Comprehensive Cancer Center. The trial uses a patient's own stem cells, which are genetically engineered to protect the body from the toxic side effects of chemotherapy, and then re-infused into the bloodstream. Simon wore a Superman costume to his final chemotherapy session in 2016. In 2018, he remains cancer-free. The results from the trial he joined have attracted national attention.

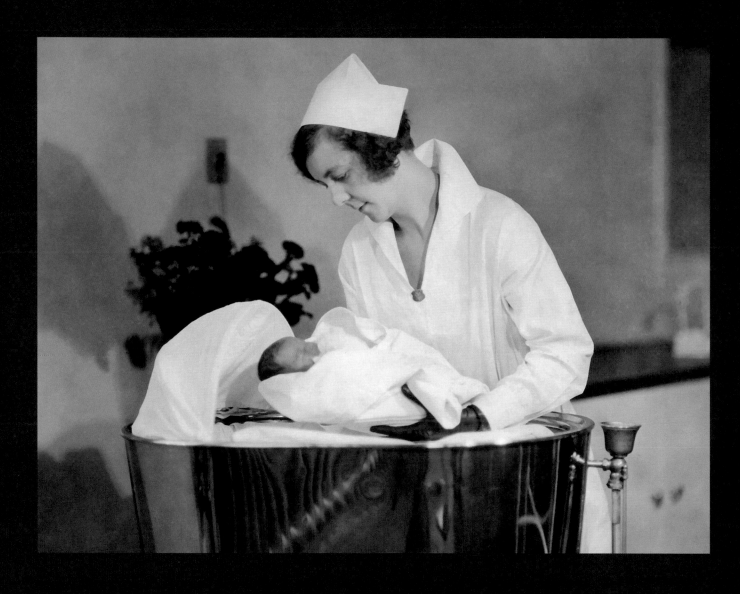

Endnotes

Chapter 1: Coming Together

1. *The Plain Dealer*, May 31, 1866.
2. *The Plain Dealer*, April 19, 1871.
3. *The Plain Dealer*, November 3, 1921.
4. Ibid.
5. Ibid.
6. *The Plain Dealer*, October 17, 1897.
7. *The Plain Dealer*, February 8, 1897.
8. *The Plain Dealer*, July 14, 1906.
9. *The Plain Dealer*, February 2, 1910.
10. "The Department of Medicine at Lakeside," *Medicine in Cleveland and Cuyahoga County*, 1977, pg. 148.

Chapter 2: Beds and Buildings

1. *The Plain Dealer*, January 24, 1898.
2. Robb, Hunter, MD. "The Opening of the New Lakeside Hospital," *The Cleveland Medical Gazette*, April, 1898.
3. *The Plain Dealer*, February 1, 1931.
4. *The Plain Dealer*, October 27, 1925.
5. *Formal Opening of the New Lakeside Hospital Building*, 1898.
6. Dittrick, Howard. "Old Lakeside," *The Bulletin of the Academy of Medicine of Cleveland*, 1953.
7. *The Plain Dealer*, January 10, 1898.
8. Pimlott, C. H. "When Old Lakeside was Young," Presentation, Annual Dinner of the Quarter Century Club of University Hospitals, Cleveland, Ohio, February 27, 1962.
9. Benderoff, Olga. Letter to The Stanley A. Ferguson Archives of University Hospitals of Cleveland, August 1993.
10. *The Plain Dealer*, October 29, 1925.
11. *The Plain Dealer*, October 27, 1925.
12. *The Official Publication of the Cleveland Hotels' Association*, February 1, 1932.
13. *The Clevelander*, March 19, 1927.
14. *The Cleveland Press*, December 4, 1928.
15. *The Plain Dealer*, February 1, 1931.
16. *The Archway*, January 1959.
17. *The Archway*, January 1958.
18. *The University Hospitals Illustrated News*, May 1936, pg. 3.
19. *The Plain Dealer*, April 4, 1956.
20. *Construction Digest*, September 11, 1969.
21. *The Cleveland Press*, June 11, 1959.
22. *Construction Digest*, September 11, 1969.
23. *The Plain Dealer*, February 13, 1994.
24. *The Plain Dealer*, February 1, 1931.

25. *The Plain Dealer*, April 6, 1997.

26. Tuten, Tera. "The 20 Most Beautiful Hospitals in the U.S. 2012 ..." Soliant Health. August 22, 2012. http://blog.soliant.com/most-beautiful-hospitals/2012/.

27. Landro, Laura. "More Hospitals are Using the Healing Powers of Public Art; Hospitals are Giving Artwork a Higher Priority." *The Wall Street Journal*, August 18, 2014.

Chapter 3: Purpose and Promise

1. *The Plain Dealer*, July 1, 1900.

2. *The Plain Dealer*, December 22, 1971.

3. *The Plain Dealer*, February 18, 1901.

4. *The Plain Dealer*, May 25, 1902.

5. Gerstner, Patsy. "Smallpox: A City on the Edge of Disaster," online exhibit, Dittrick Medical History Center, http://artsci.case.edu/dittrick/online-exhibits/smallpox/.

6. Influenza Encyclopedia, University of Michigan Center for the History of Medicine, http://www.influenzaarchive.org/cities/city-cleveland.html.

7. Lakeside Hospital, 1918 Annual Report.

8. Schonberg, Cicely. "Deadly Diphtheria: The Children's Plague," Dittrick Museum Blog, https://dittrickmuseumblog.com/2014/04/29/deadly-diphtheria-the-childrens-plague/.

9. *The Plain Dealer*, November 4, 1921.

10. Unattributed recollection obtained through an anonymous survey of University Hospitals physicians.

11. *The Plain Dealer*, October 5, 2010.

12. *The Plain Dealer*, June 13, 1976.

13. The Diabetes Control and Complications Trial/Epidemiology of Diabetes Interventions and Complications Study at 30 Years: Summary and Future Directions," *Diabetes Care*, January 2014.

14. *The Plain Dealer*, July 1, 1900.

15. Dittrick, Howard. "Old Lakeside," *The Bulletin of the Academy of Medicine of Cleveland*, 1953.

16. *The Archway*, March 1950.

17. *The Plain Dealer*, June 11, 1905.

Chapter 4: Breakthroughs

1. Sherwin, Henry. "What Fifty Years Have Wrought — 1866–1916." Sherwin-Williams Co., Cleveland, 1916.

2. Kennedy, James Harrison. "A Century of Medicine," *A History of the City of Cleveland*. (The Imperial Press, Cleveland, Ohio, 1897), pgs. 236–237.

3. Friedewald, Sarah M.; Rafferty, Elizabeth A., et al. "Breast Cancer Screening Using Tomosynthesis in Combination with Digital Mammography. *Journal of the American Medical Association (JAMA)*, June 25, 2014.

4. Mazany, Terry and Perry, David C. "A Mandate to Innovate," *Here for Good: Community Foundations and the Challenges of the 21st Century*. (Routledge), 2014.

5. Thatcher, Virginia S. *History of Anesthesia with Emphasis on the Nurse Specialist*, American Association of Nurse Anesthetists, 1953.

6. Ibid., pg. 76.

7. Kimball, O. P. "History of the Prevention of Endemic Goitre," *Bulletin of the World Health Organization*, (1953), pgs. 241–248.

8. Gerstenberger, H.J.; Ruh, O.; et al. "Studies in the Adaptation of an Artificial Food to Human Milk: A Report of Three Years' Clinical Experience with the Feeding of S.M.A. (Synthetic Milk Adapted)," *American Journal of Diseases of Children*, Vol. 17, 1919.

9. *The Plain Dealer*, January 29, 1922.

10. *Cleveland News*, August 1954.

11. *The Cleveland Press*, February 18, 1935.

12. *The Plain Dealer*, December 11, 1947.

13. *The Archway*, November 1977.

14. Leathers, Shirlee. *The First 100 Years: A Centennial History of University Hospitals of Cleveland*. (Cleveland: University Hospitals of Cleveland, 1965), pg. 32.

15. *The Archway*, July 1965.

16. *The Plain Dealer*, February 17, 1961.

17. *The Hematologist*, a publication of the American Society of Hematology, January–February 2008, Volume 5, Issue 1.

18. Trefzger, Leo and Siedel, Frank. "1286 – The Ohio Story: "Anita Gilger's Quest," *The Ohio Story* Radio Scripts, http://www.ogsarchive.org/items/show/878.

19. *The Archway*, May 1972.

20. Benjamin Rose Institute on Aging. "Mythbuster: Dr. Joseph Foley," http://www.benrose.org/mythbusters/mb-foley.cfm.

21. *Milwaukee Journal*, April 8, 1980.

22. University Hospitals Public Relations Department. Fundraising brochure, 1984.

23. *The Chicago Tribune*, September 5, 1990.

24. Wallis, Claudia and Willwerth, James. "Awakenings: Schizophrenia: A New Drug Brings Patients Back to Life," *Time Magazine*, July 6, 1992.

25. Department of Institutional Relations and Development, University Hospitals. "Transforming Patient Care and Driving Discovery through Endowment," fundraising brochure, 2014.

26. American Cancer Society. "Top 5 Reasons People Don't Get Screened for Colorectal Cancer," http://pressroom.cancer.org/Top5reasonscolorectalcancer.

27. CWRU Medicine. "Katie Couric Tours Case Western Research Lab Run by Dr. Sandy Markowitz to Study Colon Cancer." *YouTube* video, duration 1:51. Posted May 2010. https://www.youtube.com/watch?v=oQ7uw2twod4.

Chapter 5: Caring

1. University Hospitals, 2012 Annual Report.

2. *The Wall Street Journal*, August 18, 2014.

3. *The Plain Dealer*, July 24, 1898.

4. *The Cleveland Press*, January 1, 1947.

5. "Instructions to Parents of Patients in the General Wards," University Hospitals, 1930. The Stanley A. Ferguson Archives of University Hospitals of Cleveland.

Chapter 6: Giving

1. *The Plain Dealer*, January 7, 1875.

2. *The Plain Dealer*, November 7, 1895.

3. *The Plain Dealer*, December 2, 1896.

4. *The Plain Dealer*, November 29, 1896.

5. *The Plain Dealer*, March 22, 1907.

6. *The Plain Dealer*, February 1, 1899; September 2, 1899; and March 5, 1905.

7. *The Plain Dealer*, October 12, 13, 16, and 19, 1912.

8. *The Plain Dealer*, July 2, 1995.

9. *The Plain Dealer*, June 23, 1999.

10. Horwitz, Samuel J., et al. *For the Children: 120 Years of Rainbow Babies and Children's Hospital*. Cleveland: University Hospitals, 2007.

11. *The Plain Dealer*, August 14, 1912–September 1, 1912.

12. *The Plain Dealer*, May 13, 1923.

13. *The Plain Dealer*, May 14, 1923.

14. *The Plain Dealer*, May 15, 1923.

15. *The Plain Dealer*, April 10, 1927.

16. *The Plain Dealer*, May 20, 1927.

17. *The Plain Dealer*, October 25, 1925.

18. Cleveland City Hospital, 1884 Annual Report.

19. *The Plain Dealer*, March 17, 1900.

20. *The Plain Dealer*, October 31, 1908.

21. *The Plain Dealer*, January 20, 1909.

22. *The Plain Dealer*, December 16, 1910.

23. University Hospitals *Legacy Magazine*, Fall 2007.

24. University Hospitals *Legacy Magazine*, Winter 2008.

25. University Hospitals, 2009 Annual Report.

26. *The Morning Journal*, January 4, 2016.

27. University Hospitals *Legacy Magazine*, Summer 2013.

28. *The Plain Dealer*, February 23, 1908.

29. *The Plain Dealer*, April 2, 1899.

30. *The Plain Dealer*, May 2, 1935.

31. *The Plain Dealer*, May 6, 1944.

32. *The Plain Dealer*, September 4, 1945.

33. *The Plain Dealer*, May 28, 1951; and *The Archway*, January–February 1953.

Chapter 7: Reach

1. Warner, Andrew, MD, and Davis, Michael, MD. *Dispensaries, Their Management and Development: A Book for Administrators,*

Public Health Workers and All Interested in Better Medical Service for the People. New York: MacMillan, 1918.

2. Social Service Department of Lakeside Hospital, First Report, 1911.

3. *The Plain Dealer*, October 29, 1913.

4. Lakeside Hospital, 1877 Annual Report.

5. *The Plain Dealer*, March 4, 1946.

Chapter 8: The Work Continues

1. Chang, Geoffrey. "Dancing with my wife again: Greg Grindley on life one year after Brain Surgery Live." Parkinsonslife.eu/dancing-with-my-wife-again-greg-grindley-on-life-one-year-after-brain-surgery-live/.

2. Deloitte Center for Health Solutions 2015 Survey of US Health Care Consumers.

3. University Hospitals. "Dr. Marcos de Lima." *YouTube* video, duration 1:18. Posted December 18, 2015. https://www.youtube.com/watch?v+75mLC-QXeQ.

4. University Hospitals. "Immunotherapy Working Group Ready to Take Its "Moonshot" Against Cancer." January 2017. https://www.uhdoctor.org/news/immunotherapy-working-group-ready-to-take-its-moonshot-against-cancer.

5. WVIZ Ideastream, "Defeating Cancer: Precision Medicine and Personalized Care." Cleveland, OH: WVIZ-PBS TV, March 30, 2017.

6. Ibid.

7. Zenty, Thomas III and Onie, Rebecca. "Advancing Health Where We Live, Work and Play," video, duration 7:54. Posted by Health Evolution, September 21, 2017. https://www.healthevolution.com/interviews/advancing-health-where-we-live-work-and-play.

Photograph Credits

The sources from which photographs used in the book were obtained are listed here, with grateful acknowledgment.

Photographers

Studio Associates, Inc./Ed Nano
Alfred Associates
Keith Berr
Dudley Brumbach, *The Plain Dealer*
Century Photography/Janet Century
Chase, Washington
Perry Cragg, *Cleveland News*
Billy Delfs
Albert Fenn, *Life Magazine*
Joe Glick
Anthony Gray
Julie Hahn
Hanson Photographic
Hastings-Willinger and Associates
Russell Lee
Ralph Marshall
Roger Mastroianni
Mevion Medical Systems
Daniel Milner

Nick Murphy
Bill Pappas Photography, Inc.
Marty Pytel
Karl J. Rauschkolb, *The Plain Dealer*
Frank Reed, *Cleveland Press*
Donn Rothenberg
Score Photography
Herman Seid, *Cleveland Press*
Parade Studios, Inc.
Gary Yasaki

Archival Resources

Cleveland Public Library/Photograph Collection
Michael Schwartz Library, Cleveland State University
Dittrick Medical History Center, Case Western
    Reserve University
Library of Congress
The Stanley A. Ferguson Archives at
    University Hospitals
University Hospitals Marketing and Communications
University Hospitals Institutional Relations
    and Development
The Western Reserve Historical Society,
    Cleveland, Ohio

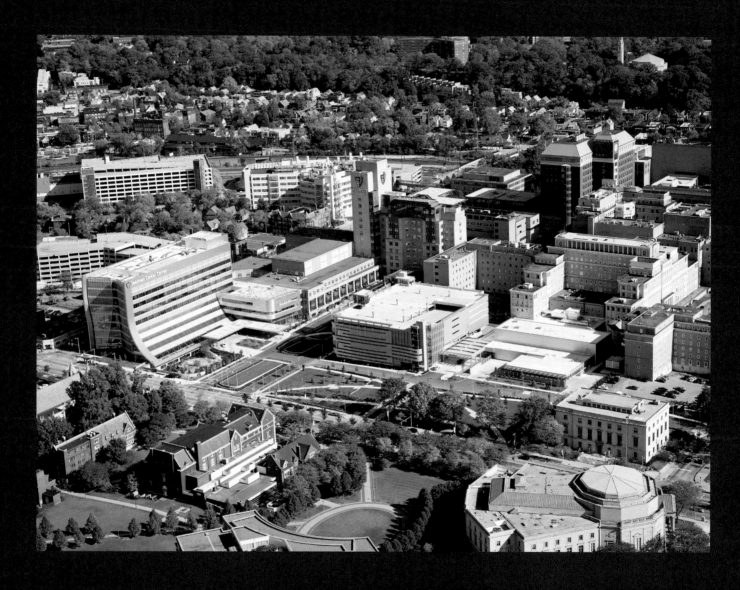

Index

A

Academy of Nutrition and Dietetics, 22
Acute Care for the Elderly (ACE), 93–94
Adelman, Sheldon, *146*
Adelman, Terry, *146*
Adult Sickle Cell Disease Center, 3
Age Well, Be Well, *163*
Agre, Peter, 101
Ahuja Medical Center
    (*see University Hospitals Ahuja
    Medical Center*)
Ahuja, Monte, 42, 124, *146*
Ahuja, Usha, *146*
Alagramam, Kumar, 104
Alexander, Elisabeth, *149*
Alexander, Quentin, *149*
Alfidi, Ralph, 103
Alfred and Norma Lerner Tower, *39,
    40,* 44, 139, 157
Alfred, Lynne, *145*
Allen, Dudley Peter, 23, 62, 73, *74,* 94
Allen, Edgar, 150
Alta House, *160*
Ambulance Americaine, 77
American Association of Nurse
    Anesthetists, 78
Angie Fowler Adolescent & Young
    Adult Cancer Institute, *29,* 121,
    183, *184,* 185–186
Ankeney, Jay, 103

Atomic Energy Medical Research
    Project, 83
Atrium, 38–39, 113
Audiology & Cochlear Implant
    Center, 60
Avon Health Center (*see University
    Hospitals Avon Health Center*)

B

Babies and Childrens Hospital, xii,
    10, *12,* 14–16, 18–19, 21, *25,*
    26–28, 30, 33, *36,* 37–38, 44, *50,*
    54, *62–63,* 75, 76, 79, 83, 85, 87,
    88–89, 119, 121, *123,* 131, 138,
    142, 145, 161–163, 171
Babies' Dispensary and Hospital, xii,
    10–12, 13, 15, 27, 31, 44, 51, 68,
    78, 102, *128,* 135, 137, *150,* 154,
    158, 160, 161, *162,* 168, *171*
Baker, Newton D., 135
Baldwin, Arthur, 31, *137*
Bambakidis, Nicholas, 177
Barkey, Mary, *127*
Barksdale, Edward, Jr., *115*
Base Hospital No. 4, *77,* 167
Battle, Kathleen, 123
Beals, Jessie, 184
Beck, Claude, *33,* 80, *81,* 82, *83,*
    99, 102

Bedford Medical Center
    (see *University Hospitals
    Bedford Medical Center*)
Benderoff, Olga, 25, 167, *168*
Benetz, Beth Ann, 87, 105
Benjamin Rose Institute on Aging,
    93, 94
Bill, Arthur, *8,* 10, 161
BioMotiv, 189
Bishop, Bessie, 140
Bishop Building (*see Robert H.
    Bishop Building*)
Bishop, Hudson, 140
Bishop, Robert, 34
Blackburn, Chrissie, 113, *114*
Blackburn, Lily, 113, *114*
Black, Lester, 33
Bland, Bethany, 115
Bland, Sierra, 115
Block, James, 39, 152, 166
Blossom, Dudley, 54
Blumer, Jeffrey, *121*
Board of Lady Managers, 132, 153
Bohlman, Henry, 95, 104
Bole, Aparna, 163
Bolton, Frances Payne, *67*
Bolwell, Harry J., *152*
Bond, Douglas, 74
Boyd, Karen, 114

Bradley, Bernice, 121
Brain Health & Memory Center, 94
Brain Tumor & Neuro-Oncology
    Center, 105, 179
Breen Breast Health Pavilion, 153
Breen, Jack, *153*
Breen, Mary Jane, *153*
Brian Werbel Memorial Fund, 151
Brown, Denise, 163
Brown Memorial Hospital
    (*see University Hospitals
    Conneaut Medical Center*)
Brown, Richard, 103
Buell, Mary, 45
Burroughs, Albert, 171
Burstein, Albert, 103
Butler, Brian, *166*
Butler, Carol Humphrey, 139

C

Calabrese, Joseph, 104
Calico Ball, 131
Canfield, Martha A., 8
Caplan, Arnold, 188
Cardiopulmonary resuscitation
    (CPR), 82
Carpenter, Chase, 180
Carr, Carole, *133*, 134
Carter, John, 30
Case Comprehensive Cancer Center,
    43, 188, 191
Case Western Reserve University
    School of Medicine, 35, 65,
    73–74, 91, 92, 99, 104, 151,
    171–172, 173–175, 179, 189
Case Western Reserve University
    (*see also Western Reserve
    University*), 2, 43–44, 51, 97,
    104, 130, 144, 168–169, 188
Cassese, Anthony, 85
Cassidy, Suzanne, 104
Celebration of Lives, 121
Center for Assessment and Care of the
    Elderly, 93
Center for Bone & Joint
    Reconstruction, 57
Center for Emergency Medicine, 31,
    41, 44, 139
Center for Lifelong Health, 163
Center for Pediatric Palliative Care, 121
Centering Pregnancy, *168*
Central Friendly Inn, *10*, 11, 44

Chagrin Highlands Health Center
    (*see University Hospitals Chagrin
    Highlands Health Center*)
Chapman, Frank, 32, 40
Cherullo, Edward, 105
Cheung, Nikon, 103
Child Life Program, 121, 145
Children Who Witness Violence, 164
Circle of Friends, 145
Clarke, Graham W., 77
Clark, J.L., 17
Clark, Mary, 17
Cleveland Browns, *56*, 126, 188
Cleveland City Hospital Association,
    xii, 4, 6, 15, 44, 140
Cleveland City Hospital (*see Cleveland
    City Hospital Association*)
Cleveland Clinic, 43
Cleveland Eye Bank, 87
Cleveland Foundation, 19, 76, 137,
    141, 144
Cleveland Homeopathic Hospital
    College, 9
Cleveland Medical Center
    (*see University Hospitals
    Cleveland Medical Center*)
Cleveland Visiting Nurses
    Association, 67
Coccia, Peter, 103
Cohen, Alan, *115*
Cohen, Nicholas, 164
Cole, Ellen, 150
Coleman, Kathleen, 149
Coleman, Les, 149
Conneaut Medical Center
    (*see University Hospitals
    Conneaut Medical Center*)
Connor, Chris, *183*
Connor Integrative Health Network
    (*see University Hospitals Connor
    Integrative Health Network*)
Connor, Sara, *183*
Corlett, William, 102
Cortese, Gina, *147*
Costa, Marco, 99, 117, 173, 178
Coulby, Harry, 141
Cozzi, Laura, 104
Crane, Erin, *47*
Crile, George, 43, 76–77, 102
Crowe, Trevor, 118
Curtiss, Beth, *145*
Cushing, Edward Fitch, *10*, 13, 137

Cutler, Elliot, *33*
Cystic Fibrosis Center, 84–85

D

Dahms' Clinical Research Unit, 74
Dahms, William, *55*, 74, 105
Dalal, Jignesh, 186
Darkow, Daniel, 97
Darling, Lettie, 14
Daroff, Robert, 93, 103
David Satcher Clerkship, 166–167
Davis, Pamela, 85, 104
de Lima, Marcos, 185
DePompei, Patricia, 47, 119, 123,
    145, 181
Digestive Health Institute (*see
    University Hospitals Digestive
    Health Institute*)
Discover the Difference campaign,
    139, 145–146, 149, 153
Dittrick, Howard, 23, 61
Dobos, Jeff, 117
Doershuk, Carl, 64, 84, *85*
Dominak, Anthony, 117
Dresner, Ian, 103

E

Ear, Nose & Throat Institute
    (*see University Hospitals Ear,
    Nose & Throat Institute*)
Eckardt, Robert, 19
Edwards, Lee, 133
Edwards, Lucia, 131
Edwards, Shannon, 113
Elisabeth Severance Prentiss
    Foundation, 36, 149
Ellner, Jerrold, 104
Elyria Medical Center (*see University
    Hospitals Elyria Medical Center*)
EMS Education & Disaster
    Preparedness Institute
    (*see University Hospitals
    EMS Education & Disaster
    Preparedness Institute*)
Evans, Armen, 166
Evans, Leon, 166
Evergreen Cooperatives, 125
Eversight Ohio, 87
Eye Institute (*see University Hospitals
    Eye Institute*)

F

Falleti, Chrissy, 84–85
Fanaroff, Avroy, *36*, 38, 73, 89–90,
 91, 103, 170, *171*
Fanaroff, Jonathan, *91*
Fanaroff, Kristy, 91
Feren, Maury, 92
Fertility Center (*see University
 Hospitals Fertility Center*)
Findling, Robert, 105
Firman, Pamela Humphrey, 139
First Presbyterian Church (*see Old
 Stone Church*), xi, *4*, 141
Five Star Sensation, *133*
Fleming, David, 103
Flemming, John, 21
Flexner, Abraham, 21, *62*
Flexner Report, 62, 67
Foley, Joseph, *93*, 102
Ford, Allen, 24, *136*
Forsythe, Paula, 89
Fourth General Hospital, *167, 168, 170*
Fowler, Chann, *185*
Fowler, Char, 28, *185*
Fowler, Chuck, 28, *185*
Fowler, Holley, *185*
Frances Payne Bolton School of
 Nursing, 69
Frank, Gerold, 34
Friedell, Hymer, *83*, 102
Friends of University Hospitals, 157
Frohring, William, 78, 102
Furlan, Anthony, 105

G

Gambetti, Pierluigi, 104
Ganley, Kim, 164
Garbett, Jean, *56*
Gardner, Gloria, *164*
Garfield, Abram, 30
Gartland, Heidi, 159, 164
Garvin, Charles, *166*
Geauga Medical Center
 (*see University Hospitals
 Geauga Medical Center*)
Geller, Albert, 111
Geller, Norma, 111
Geneva Medical Center
 (*see University Hospitals
 Geneva Medical Center*)
Genuth, Saul, 55, 105
George M. Humphrey Building, 138

Gerson, Stanton, 188, 191
Gerstenberger, Henry, 13, 27, 78, *79*,
 102
Gilger, Anita, 87
Gilman, Alfred, 101
Gleason, Frank, 177
Gleason, Julia, 141
Gleason, Maggie, *177*
Global Child Health Program, 175
Goldberg, Victor, 94
Goldblatt, Harry, 80, 102
Goldfarb, James, 58, 59
Goodman Discovery Center, 144
Goodman, Donald J., *144*
Goodman, Ruth Weber, *144*
Gorenshek, Nancy, 41
Grabowski, John, 168
Grant, Alexander, *112*
Grant, Richard, 166
Graves, Lulu, 22
Greater Circle Living program, 19
Greater University Circle Initiative,
 18–19, *125*
Green City Growers, 125
Greene, Helen Wade, 143
Green, Roe, *173*
Greig, Tina, 115, 117–118
Gries, Robert, 150–151
Gries, Sally, 150–151
Grindley, Greg, *180*
Griswold, Mark A., 104
Grossberg, Richard, *184*
Gubitosi-Klug, Rose, 55, 105
Gund, Gordon, 190
Gund-Harrington National Initiative in
 Fighting Blindness, 190

H

Haaga, John, *46*
Hadden, Elaine, 149
Hadden, Jr., John A., 149
Hadden, Sr., John, 149
Hall, Destiny, *165*
Hampson Family Foundation, 150
Hampson-Mole Breast Health Suite, 150
Hampson Mole Community Health
 Project, 150
Ham, Thomas Hale, 63
Hanna, H. Melville, 142
Hanna House (*see Leonard C.
 Hanna House*)
Hanna, Jr., Howard Melville, 142

Hanna, Jr., Leonard C., 31, 142
Hanna, Leonard C., 142
Hanna Pavilion (*see Howard M.
 Hanna Memorial Pavilion*)
Hanson, Richard, 165
Harkness, Edith, 7
Harkness, Edward, 137
Harkness, William, 7
Harrill, Katrina, 173
Harrington Discovery Institute, 130,
 148, 177, 189–190
Harrington Heart & Vascular
 Institute (*see University
 Hospitals Harrington Heart &
 Vascular Institute*)
Harrington, Jill, *148*
Harrington, Lydia, *148*
Harrington, Nancy, *148*
Harrington Project for Discovery &
 Development, 189
Harrington, Ronald G., *148*, 189
Harrington, Ronald M., *148*
Harry J. Bolwell Health Center, 39,
 44, *152*
Harvey, Kate Hanna, 31
Harwell, Carla, *167*
Healthy Harvest program, 165
Heiple, Kingsbury, *94*, 104
Hellerstein, Elizabeth, 92
Hellerstein, Herman, 91, *92*
Henry L. Meyer III Faculty Minority
 Fellows Program, 167
Herndon, Charles, 36, *55*, 102–103
Herrick, Mary, *145*
Hertz, Andrew, 183
Herzig, Roger, 103
Hess, Alfred, 161
Heyard, Richard, 82
Heymann, Walter, 102
Hingson, Robert, 171, *174*
Hodgins, Agatha, 76–77, 78
Holden, William, 102
Home for Friendless Strangers, 4,
 108, 141
Hoover, Charles Franklin, 102
Hopkins, William R., 3, 137
Hoppel, Charles, 104
Horvitz, Danielle, 146–147
Horvitz, Joan, 147
Horvitz, Leonard, 147
Horvitz, Marcy, 147
Horvitz, Richard, 147

Horvitz Tower (*see Leonard and Joan Horvitz Tower*)

Horwitz, Samuel "Jack", 119, 137

Howard M. Hanna Memorial Pavilion, *35*, 36, 44, 138, *142*, 143

Huang, Alex, 186

Hubay, Charles, 49, 104

Hubbard, Gabriela, *58*

Hulme, Mary Ann, 78

Humphrey Building (*see George M. Humphrey Building*)

Humphrey, George M., *139*

Humphrey, Gilbert, 139

Humphrey, II, George M., 13, 139

Humphrey, Pamela, 139

Hurlbut, Hinman, 61, *140*, 141, 146

Hurlbut, Jane, *154*

Huron Road Hospital, 8, *9*, 140

I

Ilcin, Chris, 58, *59*

Ilcin, Julie, 58, *59*

Infants' Clinic, 10, 15, 44, 108, 131, 154

Inkley, Scott, *35*, 39, 65, 103

Innovation Support Center, 189

Institute for Transformative Molecular Medicine, 189

Insull, William, 103

Ireland Cancer Center (*see R. Livingston Ireland Cancer Center*)

Ireland, Jr., Robert Livingston, 13, 138

Iris S. and Bert L. Wolstein's Kids Kicking Cancer, 144

Iris S. & Bert L. Wolstein Research Building, *144*

Irving and Jeanne Tapper Dental Center, *150*, 163

Izant, Jr., Robert, 102, *113*

J

Jackson, Frank G., 19

Jackson, Jr., Edgar, *159*, 166–167

Jacobs, Orry, *121*

Jain, Mukesh, 177

Johns Hopkins Hospital, 8, 13, 22, 24, 62, 67

Johnson, Lorand, 87

Johnston, Louise, 131

John T. Carey Special Immunology Unit, 51

Joseph M. Foley ElderHealth Center, 93

Joseph T. Wearn Laboratory for Medical Research, 44, 74, 121, *143*

Junod, Jr., Henri Pell, 13

K

Kabb, Marilyn, 118

Kalydeco, 86

Kathleen A. and Dr. Lester E. Coleman Clinical Research Suite, 149

Kathy and Les Coleman Clinical Trials Center, 150

Kattwinkel, John, 89, 103

Kennell, John, *88*, 103

Kerr, Douglas, 104

Kiehn, Clifford, 103

Kilbane, Camilla, 180

Kimball, Oliver, 78

King's Daughters, 7, 132

Kirby, Jacquelyn, 112

Klaus, Marshall, *88*, 103, 171

Kleinman, Dee, 156

Kline, Stuart, 28

Kline, Theresia, 28

Knowles, James Seward, 40

Koeth, Terryl Homes, 45, 110

Kolesar, Dinah, *145*

Konstan, Michael, 85–86, 104

Koomson, Wilhemina, *169*

Koppelman, Catherine, 71, 115

Kubu, Mary Lou, 70

L

Ladies Advisory Committee, 153–154

Lakeside Hospital, 4, 6–8, 10, *12*, 13–15, 21–25, 27–28, 30–35, 39–40, 43–44, 48, *49*, 50, 52, *53*, 55, 61, 62, 63, 66–68, 70, 73–78, 80, 82, 102, 108, 110, 121, *125*, *126*, 129, 135, 137, 140–141, 149, 153, *154*, *155*, *156*, 160–161, 165

Lakeside Hospital Training School for Nurses, 67, 70

Lakeside School of Anesthesia, 76

Lakeside Unit, *77*, *167*, *168*

Lamb, Delphine, 49

Landau, Bernard, 54

Lane, Deforia, *123*

Larkins-Pettigrew, Margaret, 167, 174–175

Lass, Jonathan, 87, 104–105

Lazarus, Hillard, 188

Lederman, Michael, 51

Lee, Mary Blossom, 54

Lekan, Ryan, *57*, *60*

Lenkoski, L. Douglas, 35

Leonard and Joan Horvitz Tower, 28, 36, *40*, 44–45, 139, 147

Leonard C. Hanna House, 31, 33, 39, 41, 44, 69, 138, 142

Leonard C. Hanna Jr. Fund, 143

Lepow, Irwin, 102

Lerner Tower (*see Alfred and Norma Lerner Tower*)

Letterio, John, 58, 184

Levitan, Nathan, 43, 149

Liebman, Jerome, 64

Liu, James, 58

Locher, Carson, *184*

Lockhart, Robert, 51

Longbrake, Ryan, 117

Longenecker, Christopher, 173

Lough, Marvin, 85

Louis Stokes Cleveland VA Medical Center, 95, 97, 103–104

Lowman, Isabel Wetmore, 10, 31

Lowman, John, 10

Lüders, Hans, 59

Lynn, Jacques, 118

Lyons, David, 151–152

Lyons, Janice, 151

Lyons, Jonny, 151–152

Lyons, Michael, 152

M

MacDonald, Calvina, 27

MacDonald House, 15, 27, *68*, 78, *88*, 110, 138, 156–157

MacDonald Hospital (*see University Hospitals MacDonald Women's Hospital*)

MacDonald Women's Health Clinic, 165

MacIntyre, James, 103

Maciunas, Robert J., 59, 104

Makley, John, 56

Maloney, Walter, 103

Maniglia, Anthony, 104

Mannix, John, 34

Marcus, Randall, 94–95, 103

Marcy R. Horvitz Pediatric Emergency Center, *41*, 44, 139, 147

Marine, David, 78, 102

Marine Hospital (see U.S. Marine Hospital)

Markley, John, 32–33

Markowitz, Sanford, 98–99, 104, 185

Martens, Holley, 185

Martens, Rob, 185

Martinez, Angel, 103

Marting, Margaret, 145

Martin, Richard, 170

Mary and Al Schneider Healing Garden, 28, 29

Maternity Home Association, 8, 15, 108

Maternity Home, 8, 15, 44

Maternity Hospital, 8, 9, 14–15, 18, 20, 21, 26, 27–28, 30, 44, 132, 140, 150, 154, 159–161

Mather, Flora Stone, 31, 34, 141, 142

Mather Pavilion (see Samuel Mather Pavilion)

Mather, Samuel, xii, 6–7, 13, 14, 16, 22, 24, 26, 30, 31, 34, 61, 62, 135, 137–138, 141–143, 146

Matthews, LeRoy, 83, 84–85, 102, 121

McCandless, Shawn, 104

McComsey, Grace, 51, 187

McDavid, Lolita, 164

McDowell, Kayleen, 146

McGinty, John, 60

McGuigan, Paul, 55

McVoy, Peter, 187

Medical House Calls Program, 163

Megerian, Cliff, 57, 60, 104, 177

Meltzer, Herbert, 96, 104

Merkatz, Irwin, 103

MetroHealth System, 6, 94, 104

Mettler, Gretchen, 168

Meyer, III, Henry L., 152, 167

Meyer, Jane, 145

Milk Fund Association, 10

Miller, Jonathan, 59, 105, 180

Miller, Max, 52

Millikin, Benjamin, 149

Millikin, Severance, 149

Mitchell, Dena, 121

Mole, Jim, 150

Mole, Karen Hampson, 150

Moritz, Alan, 82, 102

Morley, John, 61

Moskowitz, Roland, 95

Mosley, Barbara, 163

Murad, Ferid, 101

Murray, Gail, 177

N

Nagy, Scott, 116

Nash, Clyde, 103

Neurological Institute (see University Hospitals Neurological Institute)

Neurological Institute Parkinson's & Movement Disorders Center, 164

Nochomovitz, Michael, 97

Novak Villa, 7, 44

Nulsen, Frank, 102

O

Oakes, Carolyn, 156

O'Brien, Ann, 145

Ohio Bone & Joint Institute, 17

Old Stone Church (see First Presbyterian Church)

Olivet Institutional Baptist Church, 167

Olness, Karen, 175

Onders, Raymond, 97–98, 104

Orbison, Lowell, 159

Örge, Faruk H., 105

Orkambi, 86

Orringer, Carl, 148

Otis, Jr., Charles A., 131

Otis, Lucia Edwards, 131–132

Otis Moss Jr. Health Center (see University Hospitals Otis Moss Jr. Health Center)

Overton, Wanda, 113

Owens, Ned, 95

Oxford-Harrington Scholarship Program, 190

P

Palmer, Stephen, 103

Parkinson's Boot Camp, 164

Park, Soon, 101

Parma Medical Center (see University Hospitals Parma Medical Center)

Pathways to PCA, 112

Patient and Family Advisory Council, 45

Patient and Family Partnership Council, 113

Payne, Oliver Hazard, 140

Pearce, Roy, 76

Pearson, Olof, 103, 104

Peltz, Cathy, 56–57

Penna, Fae-Dra, 112

Persky, Lester, 49, 102

Petie the Pony, 107

Pet Pals, 127

Phelps, Charlene, 69

Philips Healthcare, 43

Pianalto, Sandra, 153

Pickands, James, 141

Pillemer, Louis, 102

Pimlott, Charles, 24

Plecha, Donna, 74

Ponsky, Jeffrey, 103

Ponsky, Lee, 47

Pope, Rachel, 175

Portage Medical Center (see University Hospitals Portage Medical Center)

Potts, Albert, 102

Powell, Colin, 39

Powell, Hunter, 108

Prentiss, Elisabeth Severance, 149

Pritchard, Walter, 69, 102

Puck, Wolfgang, 133, 134

Puma, Joseph, 103

Pung, Kali, 97

Purnell, Edward, 103

Q

Quality Institute, 112

Quarter Century Club, 125

Quentin & Elisabeth Alexander Level IIIc Neonatal Intensive Care Unit, 41, 90, 139, 145, 149

R

Rainbow Babies & Children's Foundation, 123, 145, 147, 149, 164, 185

Rainbow Babies and Childrens Hospital (see University Hospitals Rainbow Babies & Children's Hospital)

Rainbow Babies & Children's Hospital (see University Hospitals Rainbow Babies & Children's Hospital)

Rainbow Care Connection Center for Comprehensive Care, 183–184

Rainbow Center for International Child Health, 175

Rainbow Center for Women &
    Children (*see University
    Hospitals Rainbow Center for
    Women & Children*)
Rainbow Circle of King's Daughters,
    7, 132
Rainbow Cottage, xii, 7, 13, 15,
    18, 44, 96, 108, *119, 130,*
    131–132, 134
Rainbow Flex surgical bed, *91*
Rainbow Hospital for Crippled and
    Convalescent Children, 7, 8, *12,*
    14–16, 26, *28,* 30, 36–37, 44,
    87, *119,* 121, 137–139, 145, *155,*
    156, 160, 163
Rainbow Primary Care Institute, 183
Rand, III, James, 81
Rankin, Jr., Alfred, 43
Ranney, Ann Pinkerton, 43, 129, *145*
Ransom, Albert, 82
Raskind, Julie Adler, *145*
Ratcheson, Robert, 147, 151
Ratnoff, Oscar, 51, *84,* 102
Reagan, James, 102
Reeve, Christopher, *97*
Reichlin, Dianne, 107
Reinhart, William, 87, 105
Reitman, Bob, 129–130
Reitman, Sylvia, 130
Resnick, Martin, 103
Rhodes, James, 138
Ricci, Kenn, 86
Richard, Ronald, 76
Richards, Letha, 3
Richmond Medical Center
    (*see University Hospitals
    Richmond Medical Center*)
Ride the Rainbow, *134*
Rieman, Ali, *186*
Risman, Bob, 42
Risman, Eleanore, 42
Risman, Kathy, 42
R. Livingston Ireland Cancer Center
    (*see also University Hospitals
    Seidman Cancer Center*), 104,
    126, 133, 138, 149
Robb, Hunter, 21, 61, 67
Robb, Isabel Hampton, 31, *67,* 70
Robbins, Frederick C., 101, 104,
    171–172
Robert H. Bishop Building, *38, 39,*
    44, 138

Robertson, Sarah, *145*
Robinson Memorial Hospital
    (*see University Hospitals Portage
    Medical Center*)
Roe Green Center for Travel
    Medicine, 173
Ronald McDonald Care Mobile, *163*
Rosenberg, Elizabeth, 36
Rosenberg, Enid, 191
Ross, Jonathan, 105
Rothstein, Fred, 64, 80, 112, 134,
    147, 149
Rothstein, Jackie, 134, 149
Royal Melbourne Hospital, 167–168
Ruh, Harold, 78, 102
Ruhlman, Barbara Peterson, *157*
Ryan, Kenneth, 103

S

Safar, Arna, 125
Salata, Robert, 172–174
Sally Gries Nursing Endowment
    Fund, 151
Salvatore, Sarah, 116
Samaritan Medical Center
    (*see University Hospitals
    Samaritan Medical Center*)
Samuel Mather Pavilion, *39, 40,* 41,
    44, 139
Sanders, Thomas, 19
Schlotfeldt, Rozella, 69
Schneider, Albert, 28
Schneider, Mary, 28
Schulak, James, 43, *52*
Schwab, William, 163
Score, Herb, *49*
Scott, Cartez, 3
Scott, Sara, 117
Seaman, David, 52
Sedgwick, Elizabeth, 143
Sedgwick, Ellery, 143
Seidman Cancer Center
    (*see University Hospitals
    Seidman Cancer Center*)
Seidman Cancer Center Leadership
    Council, 146, 149
Seidman, Jane, 43, 134, *147,* 149
Seidman, Lee, 43, *147,* 149
Selman, Warren, *98,* 99, 180
Semaan, Maroun, *177*
Severance, Louis H., 149
Severance, Mary, 149

Sherwin, Henry, 73
Sherwin-Williams, 73, 137, 153, 183
Shumaker, Jr., Harris, 82
Shurin, Susan, 104
Siegel, Christopher, 52
Siemens Healthcare, 179
Sila, Cathy, 105, 188
Simmons, George, 141
Simon, Andy, *191*
Simon, Daniel, *99,* 100–101, 173
Sisters of Charity of St. Augustine, 17
Sloan, Andrew, 101, 105, *186,* 187, 191
S.M.A. (Synthetic Milk Adapted),
    79, 102
Southwest General Health Center, 18
Spellman, Ed, 185
Spock, Benjamin, 88, 102
Stamler, Jonathan, 130, *189,* 190
Standley, Steven, 19, 33, 71
Stephens, Barbara, 127
STERIS, 188
Stern, Robert, 84–85, 103
St. John Medical Center
    (*see University Hospitals
    St. John Medical Center*)
Stone, Amasa, 141
Surgical Theater, 98–99
Sweet, Jennifer, 180
Symon, Michael, 134

T

Takeda Pharmaceutical Company, 190
Tapper, Irving, 150
Tapper, Jeanne, 150
Thomas, Charles I., 87, 102
Thompson, George, *96*
Thompson, Leigh, 103
Transplant Institute (*see University
    Hospitals Transplant Institute*)
Tryon, Ella, *151*
Turley, Bob, *49*
Two hundred fifty-sixth Combat
    Support Hospital, 170

U

UHBikes, *124*
UH Cingers, *118*
University Circle, xii, 2, 3, 9, 10, *12,*
    13–16, 18–19, 21, *24,* 26–28, 30,
    33, 36, 39, 44, 87, 93, *125,* 135,
    137–140, 142–143, 154, 163,
    169, 171

University Group Diabetes Program, 52

University Hospitals, xi–xiii, xv–xvi, 3–4, *11*, 13–19, *20*, 22–24, 30–35, 38, 40, 42–45, 47, 49, 51, 52–53, 55, *56*, 57–59, 61, *63*, *64*, 65, 67, 69–71, *72*, 73, *74*, 75, 77–78, 80, 82–83, 86–88, 90–94, 96–101, 103–104, *106*, 107–108, *109*, 111–113, 115–117, *118*, 121, 123–126, *128*, 129, 133, 136–137, 139–141, 143, 145, *146*, 147, 149–150, 152, *153*, 155–157, *158*, 159–160, 162, 164–170, *171*, *172*, 173–175, *176*, 177–180, 182–191

University Hospitals Ahuja Medical Center, 18, 41, *42*, 44, *45*, 64, *68*, 115, *125*, 139, 146–147, 183, 191

University Hospitals Avon Health Center, 57

University Hospitals Bedford Medical Center, 17, *64*, 94

University Hospitals Chagrin Highlands Health Center, 173

University Hospitals Cleveland Medical Center, 2, 3, 15–16, *18*, 23, 28, 32, *33*, *38*, 42–43, 49, 51, 64–65, 80, 86, 93, 95, 98, 100–101, 111–112, 116–118, 123, *125*, 127, 134, 147, 152, 159, 159, 164, 169–170, 173, 177, *178*, 179–180, 187–188, 191

University Hospitals Conneaut Medical Center, 17

University Hospitals Connor Integrative Health Network, 183

University Hospitals Digestive Health Institute, 42

University Hospitals Ear, Nose & Throat Institute, 60

University Hospitals Elyria Medical Center, 17, *56*, 64, 150

University Hospitals EMS Education & Disaster Preparedness Institute, 64, 181

University Hospitals Eye Institute, 87, 149

University Hospitals Fertility Center, 42, 58

University Hospitals Geauga Medical Center, 17, 64

University Hospitals Geneva Medical Center, 17

University Hospitals Harrington Heart & Vascular Institute, 17, 42, 65, 99–100, 148, 172–173, 177–178

University Hospitals MacDonald Women's Hospital, 15, 27, 47, 78, 103, 110, 116, 119, 140, 145, 157, 165, 174–175, 181

University Hospitals Neurological Institute, 42, 94, 146, 151, 164

University Hospitals Otis Moss Jr. Health Center, 167

University Hospitals Parma Medical Center, 17, *64*, *94*, *164*, *181*

University Hospitals Portage Medical Center, 17

University Hospitals Rainbow Babies & Children's Hospital, 3, 15–16, 28, 36–38, 40–41, 44–45, 47, 49, 55, *56*, 58, 60, 64, 73–74, 84–85, 89–91, 96, 98, 103, *107*, 113, 114–115, 118–119, *120*, *121*, *122*, 123, 127, 134, 137, 138–139, 144–145, 147, 149, 151, 154, 156, *163*, 164–165, 169–170, 173, 175, 177, 181, 183–185, 187

University Hospitals Rainbow Center for Women & Children, 181–182

University Hospitals Richmond Medical Center, 17, 36, 94

University Hospitals St. John Medical Center, 17

University Hospitals Samaritan Medical Center, 17, *64*, *178*, 180

University Hospitals Seidman Cancer Center, 17, 28, *29*, 41, 44, *45*, 58, *74*, 104, 107, 110, 117, 123, *133*, 139, 144, 146–147, 149, 151, *179*, 183, 186–187, 188

University Hospitals Transplant Institute, 52

University Hospitals Urology Institute, 42

University Hospitals Westlake Health Center, 173

University Suburban Health Center, 16, 44

Urology Institute (*see University Hospitals Urology Institute*)

U.S. Marine Hospital, *5*, 6, 15, 22, 44, 61, 140

V

Vanek, Rachel, 108

Vincent, Harry, 49, 52

Vinney, Les, *188*

Vinney, Linda, *188*

Vinson, Robert, 14

Vision 2010, 19, 31, 33, 41–43, 139, 146

Voices for Ohio's Children, 164

Voos, James, *56*, 188

W

Wade, Anna, 13, 143

Wade, Ellen Garretson, 143

Wade, II, Jeptha Homer, 13, *143*

Wade, I, Jeptha Homer, 143

Waldo, Albert, *65*

Wales, Florence, 14

Walsh, Michele, 91

Walter, Benjamin, 166, 180

Walters, Farah, *18*

Waxon, Gayle, *59*

Wearn Building (*see Joseph T. Wearn Laboratory for Medical Research*)

Wearn, Joseph Treloar, 62, 63

Weiner, Danielle Horvitz, 147

Werbel, Betsy, *151*

Werbel, Brian, 151

Werner, Harry, 116, *117*

Western Reserve University (*see also Case Western Reserve University*), 6–7, 10, 12, 13–14, 19, 21, 26, 30, 35, 61–63, 67, 69, 74, 80–81, 83, 87, 138–140, 160, 171

Westlake Health Center (*see University Hospitals Westlake Health Center*)

Wiesenberger, Trudy, 45

Wiggers, Carl, 81

Willard, Huntington, 104

Williamson, James Delong, 14

Williamson, Mary, *154*

Willingham, Tracy, 111

Willis, Joseph, 185

Wilson Street Hospital, *4–5*, 15, 44, 47, 48, 61, 67, 73, 129, *130*, 140–141, 149, 153, 154, 181

Wolf, Jane, *145*

Wolstein, Bert L., 144

Wolstein, Iris S., *144*

WONDOOR, *174*, 175

World War I, *50*, 77, 135, 167

World War II, xii, 24, 35, 38, 80, 82, 136, 156, 167, *168*, *170*

Wright, Jackson, *80*, 104–105

Wright, J.D., *139*

Wyckoff, Chauncey, 13–14

Wynshaw-Boris, Anthony, 105

Y

Yen, S.S.C., 103

Z

Zaremba, Lissy, 127

Zelis, Cindy, 180

Zemaityte, Dalia, *89*, *121*

Zender, Chad, 173

Zenty, III, Thomas F., xv, *xvi*, 18–19, 96, 107, 112, 150, 191

Zinn, Arthur, 104